Illustrated Anatomy OF THE Head AND Neck

5th EDITION

Illustrated Anatomy OF THE Head AND Neck

MARGARET J. FEHRENBACH, RDH, MS
Oral Biologist and Dental Hygienist
Adjunct Instructor, Bachelor of Applied Science Degree
Dental Hygiene Program
Seattle Central College
Educational Consultant and Dental Science Writer
Seattle, Washington

SUSAN W. HERRING, PhD
Professor of Orthodontics and Oral Health Sciences
School of Dentistry
Adjunct Professor of Biological Structure
School of Medicine
Adjunct Professor of Biology
College of Arts and Sciences
University of Washington
Seattle, Washington

ELSEVIER

ELSEVIER

3251 Riverport Lane
St. Louis, Missouri 63043

ILLUSTRATED ANATOMY OF THE HEAD AND NECK, ISBN: 978-0-323-39634-9
FIFTH EDITION

Notices

Knowledge and best practice in this field are constantly changing. As new research and experience broaden our understanding, changes in research methods, professional practices, or medical treatment may become necessary.

Practitioners and researchers must always rely on their own experience and knowledge in evaluating and using any information, methods, compounds, or experiments described herein. In using such information or methods they should be mindful of their own safety and the safety of others, including parties for whom they have a professional responsibility.

With respect to any drug or pharmaceutical products identified, readers are advised to check the most current information provided (i) on procedures featured or (ii) by the manufacturer of each product to be administered, to verify the recommended dose or formula, the method and duration of administration, and contraindications. It is the responsibility of practitioners, relying on their own experience and knowledge of their patients, to make diagnoses, to determine dosages and the best treatment for each individual patient, and to take all appropriate safety precautions.

To the fullest extent of the law, neither the Publisher nor the authors, contributors, or editors, assume any liability for any injury and/or damage to persons or property as a matter of products liability, negligence or otherwise, or from any use or operation of any methods, products, instructions, or ideas contained in the material herein.

Previous editions copyrighted 2012, 2007, 2002, 1996 by Saunders, an imprint of Elsevier Inc.

Library of Congress Cataloging-in-Publication Data

Names: Fehrenbach, Margaret J., author. | Herring, Susan W., author.
Title: Illustrated anatomy of the head and neck / Margaret J. Fehrenbach, Susan W. Herring.
Description: 5th edition. | St. Louis, Missouri : Elsevier [2017] | Includes bibliographical references and index.
Identifiers: LCCN 2015038498 | ISBN 9780323396349 (pbk. : alk. paper)
Subjects: MESH: Head—anatomy & histology. | Head—anatomy & histology—Programmed Instruction. | Neck—anatomy & histology—Programmed Instruction. | Neck—anatomy & histology.
Classification: LCC QM535 | NLM WE 705 | DDC 611/.91–dc23
LC record available at http://lccn.loc.gov/2015038498

Content Strategist: Kristin Wilhelm
Senior Content Development Specialist: Rebecca Leenhouts
Publishing Services Manager: Patricia Tannian
Senior Project Manager: Carrie Stetz
Design Direction: Ashley Miner

Printed in Canada

Last digit is the print number: 9 8 7 6 5 4

Working together
to grow libraries in
developing countries

www.elsevier.com • www.bookaid.org

PREFACE

OVERVIEW OF NEW EDITION

To meet the needs of today's dental professional, the fifth edition of *Illustrated Anatomy of the Head and Neck* offers more than basic information on head and neck anatomy. Clinical considerations are noted throughout the textbook. Special emphasis is given in the chapter on the temporomandibular joint on the joint's complex anatomy and its associated disorders. Also included are chapters on the anatomic basis of local anesthesia for pain control and the spread of infection related to the head and neck.

FEATURES IN THIS EDITION

To facilitate the learning process, chapters are divided into the various anatomic systems, ending in the considerations for the anatomic basis for local anesthesia and the regional study of fasciae and spaces as well as the spread of infection.

Each chapter begins with learning objectives and a list of key terms with pronunciation guides from the 32nd edition of *Dorland's Medical Dictionary*. The pronunciation of each anatomic structure is also included within each chapter when introduced. The anatomic terms follow those outlined in the internationally approved official body of anatomic nomenclature; older terms are included in many cases for completeness.

Each chapter features two different types of highlighted terms. The terms appearing in bold and red are key terms and appear in the key terms list at the beginning of the chapter. The terms that appear in bold and black are anatomic terms that are important to the material being discussed in the chapter and are therefore emphasized. Both types of highlighted terms can be found in the Glossary.

All chapter topics discussed in depth have been chosen for their relevance to the needs of the dental professional and to build on former topics. Within each chapter are cross-references to other figures or chapters so the reader can review or investigate interrelated subjects. The content of this edition incorporates additional input from students and educators as well as the latest information from scientific studies and experts.

High-quality, full-color original illustrations and photographs are included throughout the text to reinforce a three-dimensional understanding of anatomy. We are excited to have added new osteology figures as provided for by Neil S. Norton, PhD, Professor of Oral Biology, School of Dentistry, Creighton University. He is the editor of the outstanding atlas, *Netter's Dental Anatomy*. Other in-depth figures have also been added or expanded within this new edition to improve overall anatomic understanding.

Tables and boxes summarizing important information appear throughout the text. Flow charts have been included to help with coordination of structures. Identification exercises and updated review questions are included for each chapter; both are great tools for self-study as well as study group discussion.

At the end of the book are two appendices. Appendix A is an updated bibliography that references published works relevant to head and neck anatomy. Appendix B provides a review of the procedures for performing extraoral and intraoral examinations. Following Appendix B are a Glossary containing both key terms and anatomic terms that uses short, easy-to-remember definitions and a detailed index to quickly look up topics.

This textbook is coordinated with *Illustrated Dental Embryology, Histology, and Anatomy* by Margaret J. Fehrenbach and Tracy Popowics and can be considered a companion textbook to complete the curriculum in oral biology. Many of the figures in this text also appear as hand-drawn outlines in the *Dental Anatomy Coloring Book*, edited by Margaret J. Fehrenbach.

NOTABLE IN THIS EDITION

The important anatomy-related key chapters on the temporomandibular joint, local anesthesia anatomy, and spread of infection have been significantly revised to allow for the latest updated evidence-based information. **Thirty-six full-color flashcards** are located in the back of the text. The cards are perforated for easy removal from the text and are an excellent study tool for students who want to test their knowledge of head and neck anatomy.

The **Evolve website** continues to be an important component, as it was in the last edition, and has been expanded. This site provides a variety of resources for both instructors and students. Included for instructors are an image collection, answer keys, and a test bank. For students, we have included discussion questions for each chapter and practice quizzes.

In addition, we have continued to have the resource of **TEACH** online, an exciting coordinated effort for instructors, which includes a Lesson Plan Manual for all topics covered in the textbook. It features updated online PowerPoint slides with notes that can be individualized for custom presentations. There are also other related materials for both students and instructors. Elsevier sales representatives will be able to help demonstrate the latest in this exciting digital format; student dental professionals can check with their instructors.

As authors, we have tried to make the text easy to understand and interesting to read. We hope that it challenges the reader to incorporate the information presented into clinical situations.

Margaret J. Fehrenbach, RDH, MS
Susan W. Herring, PhD

ACKNOWLEDGMENTS

Our families and friends need to be thanked for their understanding of our devotion to the Work. Finally, we would like to thank Editors Kristin Wilhelm, Rebecca Leenhouts, and Carrie Stetz as well as the staff of Elsevier for making this latest edition possible.

Margaret J. Fehrenbach, RDH, MS
Susan W. Herring, PhD

CONTENTS

CHAPTER 1

Introduction to Head and Neck Anatomy

●●● LEARNING OBJECTIVES

1. Define and pronounce the **key terms** and **anatomic terms** in this chapter.
2. Discuss the clinical applications of head and neck anatomy by dental professionals.
3. Discuss anatomic variation and how it applies to head and neck structures.
4. Correctly complete the review questions and activities for this chapter.
5. Apply the correct anatomic nomenclature during dental clinical procedures.

●●● KEY TERMS

Anatomic nomenclature (an-uh-tom-ik no-muhn-klay-chuhr) System of names for anatomic structures.

Anatomic position Erect position, arms at sides, palms and toes directed forward, with eyes looking forward.

Anterior Front of area.

Apex/Apices (ay-peks, ay-pih-sees) Pointed end(s) of conical structure.

Contralateral (kon-truh-lat-uhr-uhl) Structure on opposite side.

Deep Structure located inwards and away from surface.

Distal (dis-tuhl) Area farther away from median plane.

Dorsal (dor-suhl) Back of area.

External Outer side of wall of hollow structure.

Frontal plane (frun-tuhl) Plane related to imaginary line dividing body

at any level into anterior and posterior parts.

Frontal section Section through any frontal plane.

Horizontal plane Plane related to imaginary line dividing body at any level into superior and inferior parts.

Inferior Area facing away from head and toward feet.

Internal Inner side of wall of hollow structure.

Ipsilateral (ip-see-lat-uhr-uhl) Structure on same side.

Lateral Area farther away from median plane.

Medial (me-dee-uhl) Area closer to median plane; considered mesial within dentition.

Median (me-dee-uhn) Structure at median plane.

Median plane Plane related to imaginary line dividing body into right and left halves.

Midsagittal section (mid-saj-i-tuhl) Section through median plane.

Posterior Back of area.

Proximal (prok-si-muhl) Area closer to median plane.

Sagittal plane (saj-i-tuhl) Planes of body related to any imaginary plane parallel to median plane.

Superficial Structure located toward surface.

Superior Area facing toward head and away from feet.

Transverse section (tranz-vurs) Section through any horizontal plane.

Ventral (ven-truhl) Front of area.

CLINICAL APPLICATIONS

The dental professional must have a thorough understanding of head and neck anatomy when performing patient examination procedures, both extraoral and intraoral procedures (Figure 1-1). This will help determine whether any abnormalities or pathologic lesions exist and possibly indicate their cause and degree of involvement. This will also provide a basis for the description of the lesion and its location for record-keeping purposes.

During examination of the patient, the dental professional may specifically note the presence of dental (or odontogenic) infection. It is important to know the source of the infection as well as the areas to which it could spread by way of certain anatomic features of the head and neck. This background in anatomy will help the dental professional understand the spread of dental infection to reduce its risk.

A patient may also present with features of a temporomandibular joint disorder. A dental professional must understand the anatomy of the joint to understand the various disorders associated with it.

When taking radiographs, the dental professional uses surface landmarks for film placement and consistency. In addition to these landmarks, an understanding of anatomy is important in the mounting and analysis of the films.

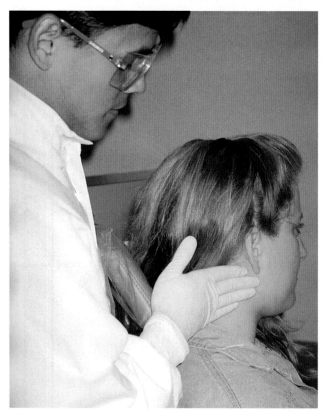

FIGURE 1-1 Examination of the patient is based on an understanding of head and neck anatomy. *(Courtesy of Margaret J. Fehrenbach, RDH, MS.)*

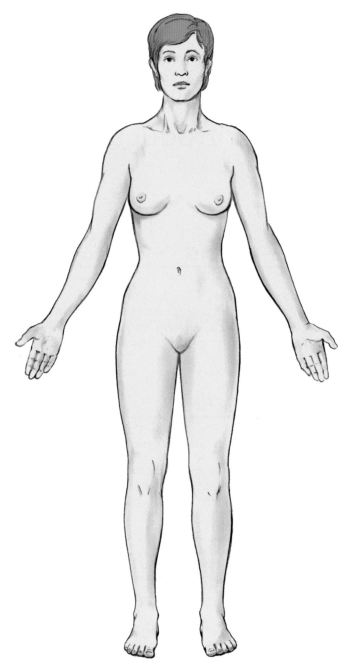

FIGURE 1-2 Body in anatomic position.

The administration of local anesthesia is also based on landmarks of the head and neck. Knowledge of anatomy helps the dental professional plan for use of a local anesthetic to reduce pain levels during various dental procedures. This knowledge also allows for correct placement of the syringe and its anesthetic agent, potentially avoiding complications.

To initially consider patient care through anatomic study, this text takes mainly a systemic approach to the study of head and neck anatomy after its two initial background chapters, Chapters 1 and 2. Through most of its chapters, Chapters 3 to 10, this approach takes a look at each system separately (e.g., skeletal, muscular). Another way to study anatomy for patient care integration is the regional approach, which is taken up later within Chapter 11, since it focuses on the fasciae and fascial spaces of the head and neck. Both approaches, when used in the order presented in this text, are complementary and effective ways to study head and neck anatomy and prepare for patient care considerations.

To reinforce the material already presented and make it readily useful for clinicians, Chapter 9 also has an expanded clinical emphasis covering the anatomy of local anesthesia. The final chapter, Chapter 12, also emphasizes this important clinical approach to head and neck anatomy during the consideration of the spread of infection. In addition, all the other chapters include important clinical considerations when appropriate, such as related pathology.

ANATOMIC NOMENCLATURE

Before beginning the study of head and neck anatomy, the dental professional may need to review anatomic nomenclature, which is the system of names for anatomic structures. This review will allow for easy application of these terms to the head and neck area when examining a patient, for use in the patient's record, or during related clinical procedures.

The nomenclature of anatomy is based on the body being in anatomic position (Figure 1-2). In anatomic position, the body can be standing erect. The arms are at the sides with the palms and toes directed forward and the eyes looking forward. This position is assumed even when the body may be supine (on the back) or prone (on the front) or even with respect to the position of the patient's head and neck when sitting upright in a dental chair.

When studying the body in anatomic position, certain terms are used to refer to areas in relationship to other areas (Figure 1-3). The front of an area in relationship to the entire body is its anterior part.

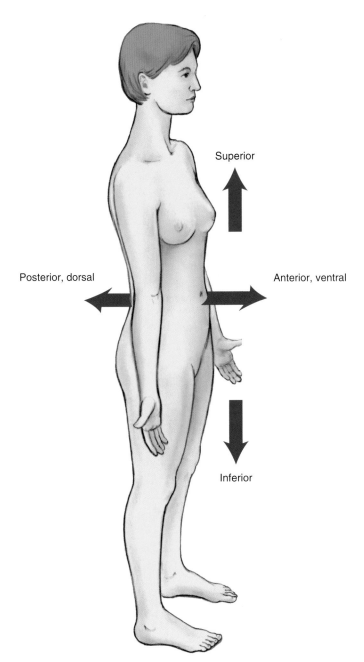

FIGURE 1-3 Body in anatomic position with the anterior (or ventral), posterior (or dorsal), superior, and inferior areas noted.

The back of an area is its **posterior** part. The **ventral** part is directed toward the anterior and is the opposite of the **dorsal** part or part directed toward the posterior when considering the entire body.

Other terms can be used to refer to areas in relationship to other areas of the body. An area that faces toward the head and away from the feet is its **superior** part. An area that faces away from the head and toward the feet is its **inferior** part. As an example, the face is on the anterior side of the head, and the hair is superior and posterior to the face. The **apex** or tip is the pointed end of a conical structure such as the apex or tip of the tongue.

The body in anatomic position can be divided into areas by planes or flat surfaces (Figure 1-4). The **median plane** or *midsagittal plane* (mid-**saj**-i-tuhl) is related by an imaginary line dividing the body into equal right and left halves. On the surface of the body, these halves

are generally symmetric, yet the same symmetry does not apply to all internal structures.

Differing imaginary lines related to other planes can divide the body into areas too. A **sagittal plane** is a plane related to any imaginary line dividing the body that is parallel to the median plane just discussed. A **frontal plane** or *coronal plane* (**kor**-o-nuhl) is related to an imaginary line dividing the body at any level into anterior and posterior parts. A **horizontal plane** is related to an imaginary line dividing the body at any level into superior and inferior parts and is always perpendicular to the median plane.

Parts of the body in anatomic position can also be described in relationship to these planes (Figure 1-5). A structure located at the median plane (e.g., the nose) is considered **median**. An area closer to the median plane of the body or structure is considered **medial** or *mesial* within the dentition. An area farther from the median plane of the body or structure is considered **lateral**. For example, the eyes are medial to the ears and the ears are lateral to the eyes.

Terms can be used to describe the relationship of parts of the body in anatomic position. An area closer to the median plane is considered to be **proximal**, and an area farther from the median plane is **distal** even within the dentition. For example, in the upper limb the shoulder is proximal and the same side fingers are distal.

Additional terms can be used to describe relationships between structures. A structure on the same side of the body is considered **ipsilateral**. A structure on the opposite side of the body is considered **contralateral**. For example, the right leg is ipsilateral to the right arm but contralateral to the left arm.

Certain terms can be used to give information about the depth of a structure in relationship to the surface of the body. A structure located toward the surface of the body is **superficial**. A structure located inward, away from the body surface, is **deep**. For example, the skin is superficial and the bones are deep.

Terms also can be used to give information about location in hollow structures such as the braincase of the skull. The inner side of the wall of a hollow structure is referred to as **internal**. The outer side of the wall of a hollow structure is **external**.

The body or parts of it in anatomic position can also be divided into sections along various planes in order to study the specific anatomy of a region (Figure 1-6). The **midsagittal section** or *median section* is a division through the median plane. The **frontal section** or *coronal section* is a division through any frontal plane. The **transverse section** or *horizontal section* is a division through a horizontal plane.

It is important to keep in mind when studying diagrams or associated photographs especially those of dissections, to first note any overall descriptions (e.g., view, section) as well as any nearby directional pointers. Then note any familiar structures (e.g., apex of tongue or nose, maxilla, or mandible) to allow for basic orientation. Next look to the areas highlighted, if noted, and of course those structures that are labeled. This process will help overall in the study of the head and neck.

ANATOMIC VARIATION

When studying anatomy, the dental professional must understand that there can be anatomic variations of head and neck structures. The number of bones and muscles in the head and neck is usually constant, but specific details of these structures can vary from patient to patient. Bones may have different sizes of processes. Muscles may differ in size and details of their attachments. Joints, vessels, nerves, glands, lymph nodes, fasciae, and spaces of an individual can vary in size, location, and even presence. The most common variations of the head and neck that affect dental treatment are discussed in this text.

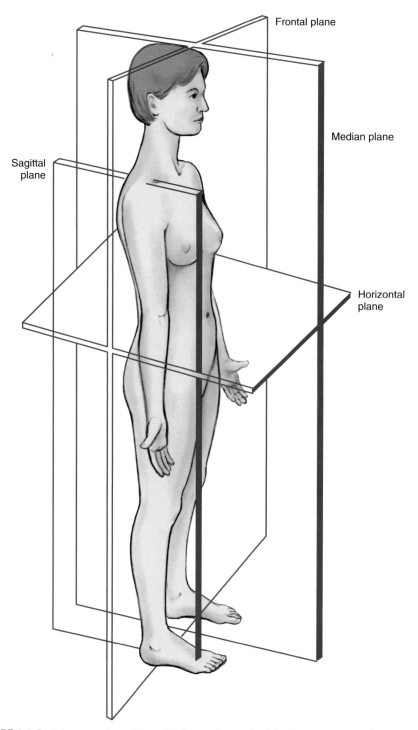

FIGURE 1-4 Body in anatomic position with the median, sagittal, horizontal, and frontal planes noted.

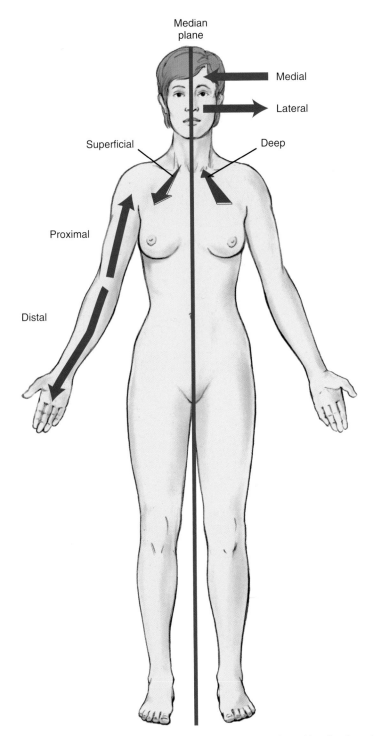

FIGURE 1-5 Body in anatomic position with the medial (or proximal), lateral (or distal), and superficial (or deep) areas noted.

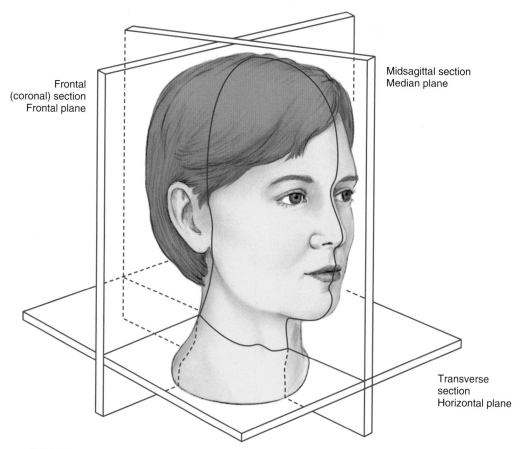

FIGURE 1-6 Head and neck in anatomic position with the midsagittal, transverse, and frontal sections as well as related planes noted.

REVIEW QUESTIONS

1. Which of the following planes divides the body in anatomic position into right and left halves?
   A. Horizontal plane
   B. Median plane
   C. Coronal plane
   D. Frontal plane
2. Which of the following terms is used to describe an area of the body that is farther from the median plane?
   A. Proximal
   B. Lateral
   C. Medial
   D. Ipsilateral
   E. Contralateral
3. Structures on the same side of the body are considered
   A. proximal.
   B. lateral.
   C. medial.
   D. ipsilateral.
   E. contralateral.
4. An area of the body in anatomic position that faces toward the head is considered
   A. inferior.
   B. superior.
   C. proximal.
   D. distal.
   E. dorsal.

5. Through which plane of the body in anatomic position is a midsagittal section taken?
   A. Horizontal plane
   B. Median plane
   C. Coronal plane
   D. Frontal plane
6. Which of the following statements concerning anatomic position is CORRECT?
   A. Body is erect with eyes looking forward.
   B. Arms are at sides with palms directed backward.
   C. Arms are behind the head with toes directed forward.
   D. Body is supine with eyes closed.
7. Which of the following sections is considered also a horizontal section?
   A. Midsagittal section
   B. Transverse section
   C. Frontal section
   D. Median section
8. Structures that are located inward, away from the body surface, are considered
   A. distal.
   B. superficial.
   C. deep.
   D. contralateral.
   E. external.

9. Which of the following planes divides any part of the body further into anterior and posterior parts?
   A. Sagittal plane
   B. Horizontal plane
   C. Frontal plane
   D. Median plane

10. Which of the following is a CORRECT statement concerning human anatomy?
    A. Apex of a conical structure is the flat base.
    B. Two halves of the body are always symmetric.
    C. External surface is the inner wall of a hollow structure.
    D. Joints, vessels, nerves, glands, and nodes vary in size.

11. Which of the following is a CORRECT statement when considering facial features?
    A. Ears are medial to the nose.
    B. Ears are lateral to the nose.
    C. Ears are medial to the eyes.
    D. Mouth is lateral to the nose.

12. Proximal refers to a body part that is
    A. closer to the medial plane of the body than another part.
    B. farther from the medial plane of the body than another part.
    C. farther from the point of attachment to the body than another part.
    D. closer to the point of attachment to the body than another part.

13. The median plane placed through the body will divide the right arm and the
    A. right leg.
    B. brain.
    C. nose.
    D. left leg.

14. A frontal plane placed through the body will ALWAYS bisect the
    A. nose.
    B. mouth.
    C. arms.
    D. eyes.

15. If a transverse plane occurs through the navel, which of the following statements is CORRECT?
    A. Chest and ears will be on different parts of the body.
    B. Chest and knees will be on the same part of the body.
    C. Feet and knees will be on different parts of the body.
    D. Thighs and feet will be on the same part of the body.

16. Which of the following statements is CORRECT concerning anatomic variation within the head and neck?
    A. Number of bones and muscles usually varies.
    B. Bones can vary in the size of processes.
    C. Lymph nodes never vary in placement.
    D. Variations of anatomy do not impact dental treatment.

17. If the shoulder of the upper limb is considered proximal, then the ipsilateral fingers are considered
    A. proximal.
    B. medial.
    C. distal.
    D. superficial.

18. If the skin in a region is considered superficial, then the related bones in the same region are considered
    A. deep.
    B. superficial.
    C. superior.
    D. inferior.

19. Which of the following sections is considered also a coronal section?
    A. Sagittal plane
    B. Horizontal plane
    C. Frontal plane
    D. Median plane

20. The outer side of the wall of a hollow structure is
    A. external.
    B. exterior.
    C. internal.
    D. interior.

Identification Exercises

Identify the structures on the following diagrams by filling in each blank with the correct anatomic term. You can check your answers by looking back at the figure indicated in parentheses for each identification diagram.

1. (Figure 1-3)

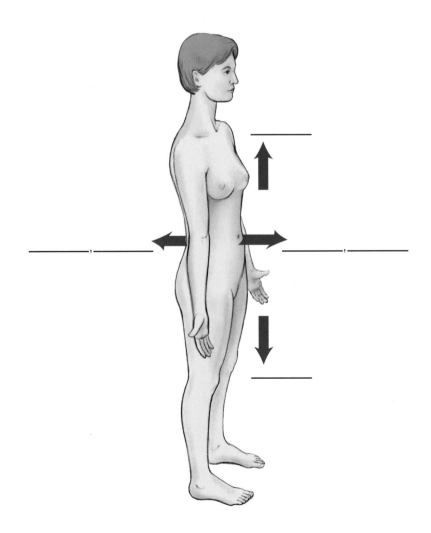

2. (Figure 1-4)

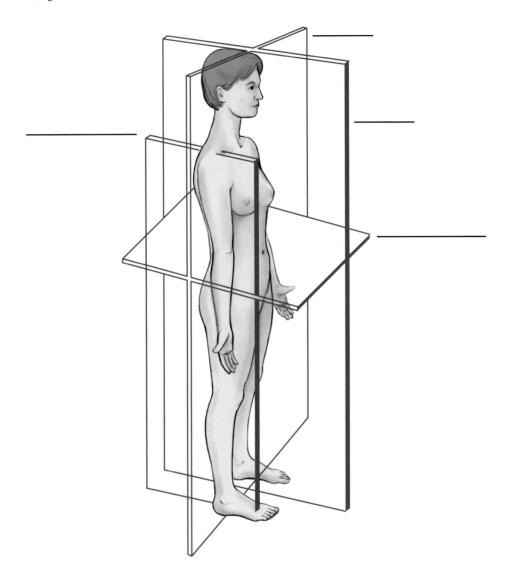

3. (Figure 1-5)

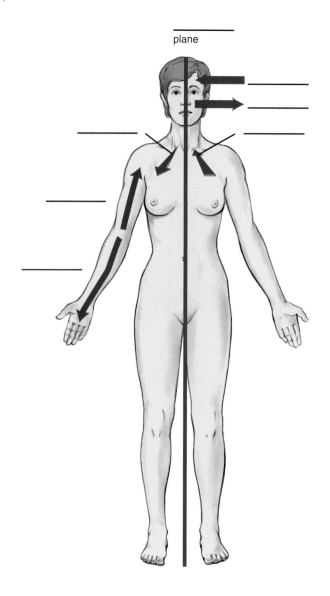

_____ plane

4. (Figure 1-6)

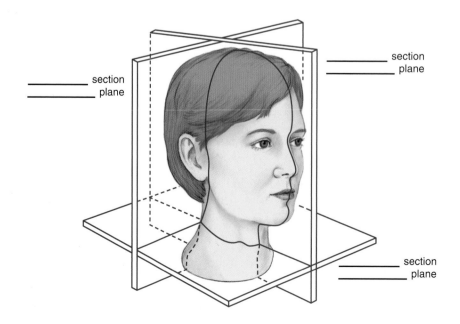

_____ section plane

_____ section plane

_____ section plane

_____ section plane

Surface Anatomy

●●● LEARNING OBJECTIVES

1. Define and pronounce the **key terms** and **anatomic terms** in this chapter.
2. Discuss how the surface anatomy of the face and neck may impact dental clinical procedures.
3. Locate and identify the regions and associated surface landmarks of the head and neck on a diagram and a patient.

4. Correctly complete the review questions and activities for this chapter.
5. Integrate an understanding of surface anatomy into the clinical practice of dental procedures.

●●● KEY TERMS

Buccal (buk-uhl) Structures closest to inner cheek.
Facial Structure closest to facial surface.
Golden Proportions Guidelines for considering vertical dimensions of face to create pleasing proportion.

Labial (lay-be-uhl) Structures closest to lips.
Lingual (ling-gwuhl) Structures closest to tongue.
Palatal (pal-uh-tuhl) Structures closest to palate.

Surface anatomy Study of structural relationships of external features to internal organs and parts.
Vertical dimension of the face Face divided into thirds.

SURFACE ANATOMY OVERVIEW

The dental professional must be comfortably familiar with the surface anatomy of the head and neck in order to examine patients. Surface anatomy is the study of the structural relationships of the external features of the body to the internal organs and parts. The features of the surface anatomy provide essential landmarks for the deeper anatomic structures that will be examined and discussed in subsequent chapters. Thus the examination of these accessible surface features by visualization and palpation can give vital information about the health of deeper tissue (Appendix B). In addition, procedures in dental practice are related to the anatomic features of the head and neck (see Chapter 1).

Some degree of variation in surface features can be possible as was discussed in the last chapter. However, a change in surface features in a given person may signal a condition of clinical significance and must be noted in the patient record, as well as thoroughly followed up by the examining dental professional. Thus it is not variations among individuals but changes in a particular individual that should be noted. In addition, the underlying histologic and embryologic concerns may also help when examining a patient's head and neck; therefore, related reference materials may need to be reviewed (Appendix A).

The study of anatomy of the head and neck begins with the division of the surface into regions. Within each region are certain surface landmarks. To improve the skills of examination, practice finding these surface landmarks in each region of the face and neck using a mirror. Later, locating them on peers and then on patients in a clinical setting adds a real world level of competence.

In this text, the illustrations of the head and neck, as well as any structures associated with them, are oriented to show the patient's head and neck in anatomic position unless otherwise noted (see Chapter 1). This is the same as if the patient is viewed straight on while sitting upright in the dental chair.

Within each of these various regions are certain significant underlying structures for the dental professional. The underlying bony structure of the head and neck is covered in Chapter 3. The underlying muscles of the head and neck are covered in Chapter 4. In addition, Chapter 5 discusses the temporomandibular joint. The underlying glandular tissue, such as the lacrimal, salivary, and thyroid glands, is covered in Chapter 7. Lymph nodes that are within the tissue of the head and neck are covered in Chapter 10, with the related vascular and nervous systems covered in Chapters 6 and 8, respectively.

REGIONS OF HEAD

The **regions of the head** include: the frontal, parietal, occipital, temporal, auricular, orbital, nasal, infraorbital, zygomatic, buccal, oral, and mental regions (Figure 2-1). These regions are used as a basis for

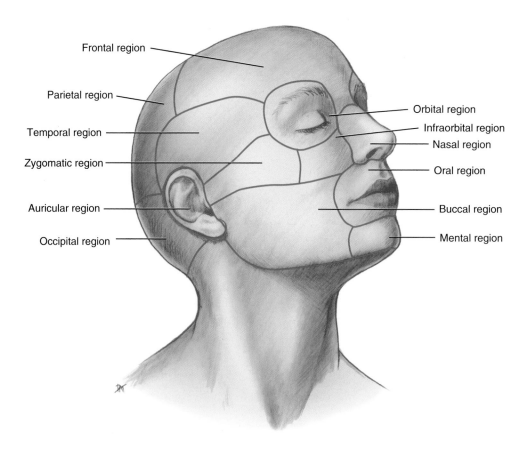

FIGURE 2-1 Regions of the head noted that include the frontal, parietal, occipital, temporal, auricular, orbital, nasal, infraorbital, zygomatic, buccal, oral, and mental regions.

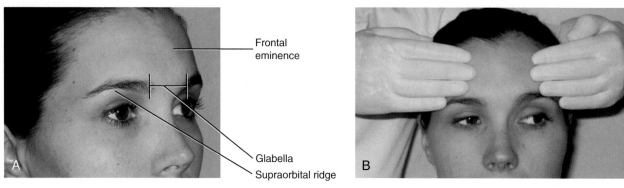

FIGURE 2-2 Frontal view of the head with the associated landmarks of the frontal region noted **(A),** and the demonstration of bilateral palpation of the forehead during an extraoral examination **(B).** *(B Courtesy of Margaret J. Fehrenbach, RDH, MS.)*

the process of an overall evaluation of the head (see Appendix B). During an extraoral examination, seat the patient upright and in a relaxed manner, while noting the symmetry and coloration of the surface. It is important to note that the superficial to deep relationships of the head are relatively simple over most of its posterior and superior surfaces but are more difficult in the region of the face.

FRONTAL REGION

The **frontal region** (**frun**-tuhl) of the head includes the forehead and the area superior to the eyes and is defined by the deeper skull bone (Figure 2-2). Directly inferior to each eyebrow is the **supraorbital ridge** (**soo**-pruh-**or**-bi-tuhl). The smooth elevated area between the eyebrows

is the **glabella** (gluh-**bell**-uh), which tends to be flat in children and adult females and to form a rounded prominence in adult males. The prominence of the forehead, the **frontal eminence** (**em**-i-nuhns), is also evident. In contrast, the frontal eminence is usually more pronounced in children and adult females, and the supraorbital ridge is more prominent in adult males. During an extraoral examination, visually inspect the forehead and bilaterally palpate it (Figure 2-2, *B*).

PARIETAL AND OCCIPITAL REGIONS

The **parietal region** (puh-**ri**-uh-tuhl) and **occipital region** (ok-**sip**-i-tuhl) of the head are both covered by the scalp and defined by the deeper skull bones. The scalp consists of layers of soft tissue overlying

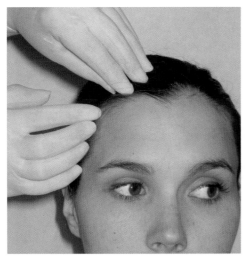

FIGURE 2-3 Demonstration of the visual inspection of the scalp during an extraoral examination. *(Courtesy of Margaret J. Fehrenbach, RDH, MS.)*

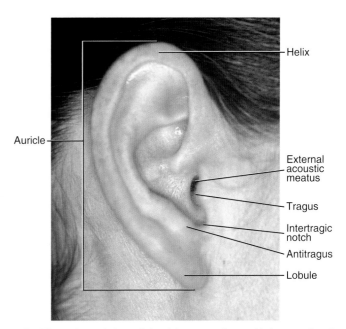

FIGURE 2-4 Lateral view of the right external ear with its associated landmarks within the auricular region noted during an extraoral examination.

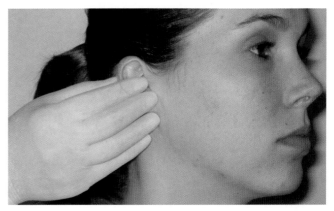

FIGURE 2-5 Demonstration of palpation of the external ear during an extraoral examination. *(Courtesy of Margaret J. Fehrenbach, RDH, MS.)*

the bones of the braincase. Large areas of the scalp may be additionally covered by hair. Trying to fully survey these areas during an extraoral examination is important because any lesions present may be hidden visually from the clinician as well as the patient. During an extraoral examination, visually inspect the scalp by moving the hair, especially around the hairline, starting from around one ear and proceeding to the other ear (Figure 2-3).

TEMPORAL AND AURICULAR REGIONS

Within the **temporal region** (**tem**-puh-ruhl) is the **temple**, the superficial side of the head posterior to each eye, which is defined by the deeper skull bone.

The **auricular region** (aw-**rik**-u-luhr) of each side of the head has the **external ear** as a prominent feature (Figure 2-4). The external ear is composed of an **auricle** (**aw**-ri-kuhl) or oval flap of the ear and the centrally placed **external acoustic meatus** (uh-**koos**-tik me-**ay**-tuhs). The auricle collects sound waves. The external acoustic meatus is a tube through which sound waves are transmitted to the middle ear within the skull.

The superior and posterior free margin of the auricle is the **helix** (**he**-liks), which ends inferiorly at the **lobule** (**lob**-yule), the fleshy protuberance of the earlobe. The upper apex of the helix is usually level with the eyebrows and the glabella, and the lobule is approximately at the level of the apex of the nose.

The **tragus** (**tray**-guhs) is the smaller flap of tissue of the auricle anterior to the external acoustic meatus. The tragus, as well as the rest of the auricle, is flexible when palpated due to its underlying cartilage. The other flap of tissue opposite the tragus is the **antitragus** (an-te-**tray**-guhs). Between the tragus and antitragus is a small groove, the **intertragic notch** (in-tuhr-**tray**-jic). The external acoustic meatus and tragus are important landmarks when taking certain radiographs and administering certain local anesthesia blocks. During an extraoral examination, visually inspect and manually palpate the external ear, as well as the scalp and face around each ear (Figure 2-5).

ORBITAL REGION

In the **orbital region** (**or**-bi-tuhl) of each side of the head, the eyeball and all its supporting structures are contained within the bony socket or **orbit** (**or**-bit), which is formed by various skull bones (Figure 2-6). The eyes are usually near the midpoint of the vertical height of the head. The width of each eye is usually the same as the distance between the eyes. On the eyeball is the white area or **sclera** (**skleer**-uh) with its central area of coloration, the circular **iris** (**eye**-ris). The opening in the center of the iris is the **pupil** (**pu**-pil), which appears black and changes size as the iris responds to changing light conditions.

Two movable eyelids, upper and lower, cover and protect each eyeball. Behind each upper eyelid and deep within the orbit are the lacrimal glands that produce **lacrimal fluid** (**lak**-ri-muhl) or tears.

The **conjunctiva** (kuhn-junk-**ti**-vuh) is the delicate and thin membrane lining the inside of the eyelids and the front of the eyeball. The outer corner(s) where the upper and lower eyelids meet is the **lateral canthus** (plural, **canthi**) (**kan**-thus, **kan**-thy) or *outer canthus*. The inner angle(s) of the eye is the **medial canthus** or *inner canthus*. These canthi are important landmarks when taking extraoral radiographs.

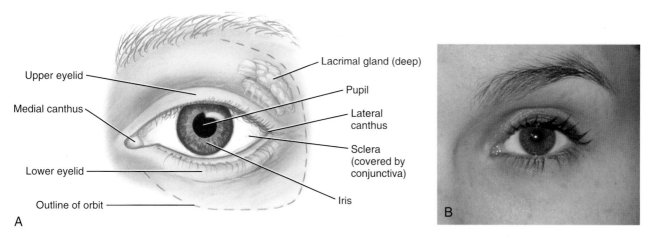

FIGURE 2-6 Frontal view of the left eye with the associated landmarks of the orbital region noted **(A)**, and visualization of the eye during an extraoral examination **(B).**

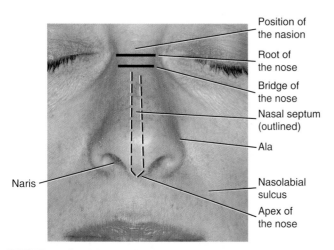

FIGURE 2-7 Frontal view of the face with the landmarks of the nasal region noted during an extraoral examination.

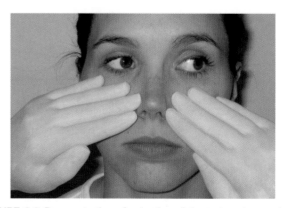

FIGURE 2-8 Demonstration of palpation of the external nose during an extraoral examination starting at the root and proceeding to its apex. *(Courtesy of Margaret J. Fehrenbach, RDH, MS.)*

During an extraoral examination, visually inspect the eyes with their movements and responses to light and action (see Figure 2-6).

NASAL REGION

The main feature of the **nasal region** (**nay**-zuhl) of the head is the **external nose** (Figure 2-7). The **root of the nose** is located between the eyes. Inferior to the glabella is a midpoint cephalometric landmark of the nasal region that corresponds with the junction between the underlying bones, the **nasion** (**nay**-ze-on). Inferior to the nasion is the bony structure of the skull that forms the **bridge of the nose**. The tip or **apex of the nose** is flexible when palpated because it is formed from cartilage.

Inferior to the apex on each side of the nose is a nostril(s) or **naris** (plural, **nares**) (**nay**-ris, **nay**-reez). The nares are separated by the midline **nasal septum** (**sep**-tum), which is formed by various skull bones and the adjoining **nasal septal cartilage** (**sep**-tuhl). The nares are bordered laterally on each side by a winglike cartilaginous structure(s), the **ala** (plural, **alae**) (**ah**-luh, ah-**lee**) of the nose. The width between the alae should be approximately the same width as one eye or the space between the eyes. Both the nasion and the alae

of the nose are landmarks when taking extraoral radiographs. During an extraoral examination, visually inspect the external nose and palpate it by starting at the root of the nose and proceeding to its apex (Figure 2-8).

INFRAORBITAL, ZYGOMATIC, AND BUCCAL REGIONS

The infraorbital, zygomatic, and buccal regions of each side of the head are all located on the facial aspect (Figure 2-9). The **infraorbital region** (in-fruh-**or**-bi-tuhl) of the head is located inferior to the orbital region and lateral to the nasal region. Farther laterally is the **zygomatic region** (zy-go-**mat**-ik), which overlies the cheekbone, the **zygomatic arch**. The zygomatic arch is formed from various skull bones and extends from just inferior to the lateral margin of the eye toward the middle part of the ear.

Inferior to the zygomatic arch and just anterior to the external ear is the **temporomandibular joint (TMJ)** (tem-poh-roh-man-**dib**-u-luhr). This is the location where the upper skull forms a joint with the lower jaw. The movements of the joint can be felt when opening and closing the mouth or when moving the lower jaw to the right or left. After palpating the joint during various movements, feel the lower

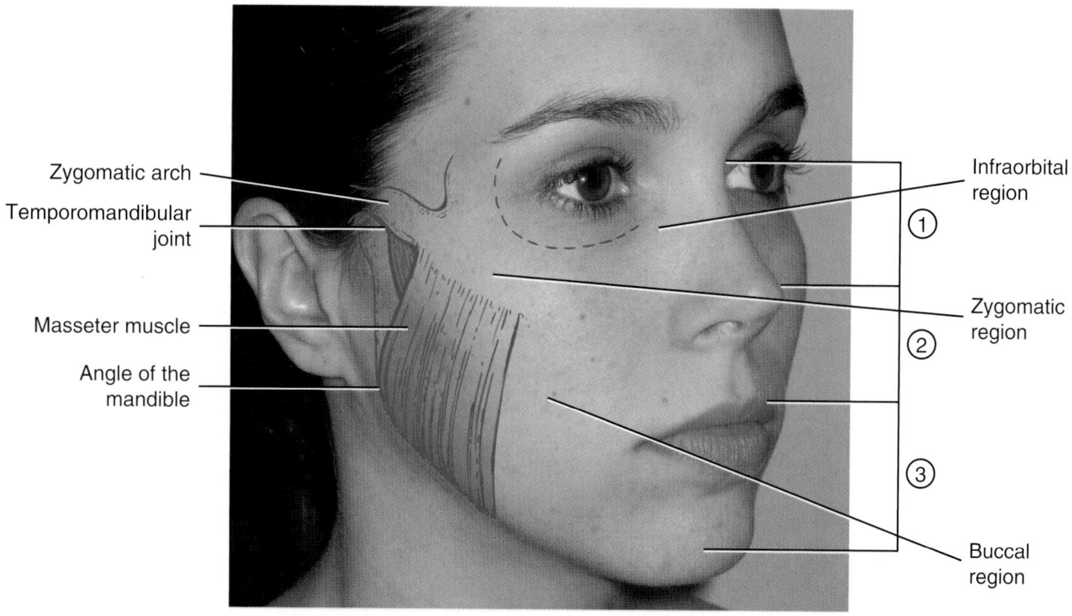

FIGURE 2-9 Lateral view of the face with landmarks of the zygomatic and buccal regions noted as well as the vertical dimension of the face, with the face divided into thirds. This division allows a comparison of the three parts of the face for functional and esthetic purposes using the guidelines of the Golden Proportions.

jaw moving at the temporomandibular joint on a patient by gently placing a finger into the outer part of the external acoustic meatus.

The **buccal region** of the head is composed of the soft tissue of the cheek. The cheek forms the side of the face and is the broad area between the nose, mouth, and ear. Most of the upper cheek is fleshy and is mainly formed by a mass of fat and muscles. One of these is the strong **masseter muscle** (mass-**see**-tuhr), which is felt when a patient clenches the teeth. Also during an extraoral examination, visually inspect and palpate bilaterally the infraorbital, zygomatic, and buccal regions, as well as specifically the temporomandibular joint.

The face can be divided into thirds, and this perspective is the vertical dimension of the face. A discussion of vertical dimension allows a comparison of the three parts of the face for functional and esthetic purposes using the Golden Proportions, which is a set of guidelines. Loss of height in the lower third of the face, which contains the teeth and jaws, can occur in certain circumstances such as with increased aging and severe chronic periodontal disease. These negative clinical ramifications cause pronounced changes in the functions as well as esthetics of the orofacial structures.

ORAL REGION

The **oral region** of the head contains significant structures to the dental professional within it such as the lips, oral cavity, palate, tongue, floor of the mouth, and parts of the throat or pharynx. The lips are the gateway of the oral region, and each lip's **vermilion zone** (vuhr-**mil**-yon) has a darker appearance than the surrounding skin (Figure 2-10). The lips are outlined from the surrounding skin by the transition of the **mucocutaneous junction** (mu-ko-ku-tay-nee-uhs) at the vermilion border. Both lips are covered externally by skin and internally by the same mucous membranes that line the oral cavity (see discussion next). The width of the lips at rest should be approximately the same distance as that between the irises of the eyes.

Superior to the midline of the upper lip, extending downward from the nasal septum, is a vertical groove on the skin, the **philtrum**

(**fil**-truhm). Inferior to the philtrum, the midline of the upper lip terminates in a thicker area or **tubercle of the upper lip** (**too**-buhr-kuhl). The upper and lower lips meet at each corner of the mouth or **labial commissure** (**kom**-uh-shur).

The groove running upward between each labial commissure and each ala of the nose is the **nasolabial sulcus** (nay-zo-**lay**-be-uhl **sul**-kuhs) (see Figure 2-7). The lower lip extends to the horizontally placed **labiomental groove** (lay-be-o-**men**-tuhl), which separates the lower lip from the chin in the mental region (see Figure 2-22). During intraoral examination, bidigitally palpate the lips and visually inspect them in a systematic manner starting on the upper lip from one labial commissure to the one on the other side and then completing the lower lip in the same manner (see Figure 2-10, B).

ORAL CAVITY

The inside of the mouth is considered the **oral cavity**. The jaws are within the oral cavity and deep to the lips (Figure 2-11). Underlying the upper lip is the upper jaw or **maxilla(e)** (mak-**sil**-uh, mak-**sil**-lee); the bone underlying the lower lip is the lower jaw or **mandible** (**man**-di-buhl) (see Figure 3-4). The sharp bent of the lower jaw inferior to the ear's lobule is the **angle of the mandible**.

An understanding of the divisions of the oral cavity is aided by knowing its borders; certain structures of the face and oral cavity mark the borders of the oral cavity (see Figure 2-1). The lips of the face mark the anterior border of the oral cavity, and the throat or pharynx is the posterior border. The cheeks of the face mark the lateral borders, and the roof of the mouth or palate marks the superior border. The floor of the mouth is the inferior border of the oral cavity.

Specific areas within the oral cavity are identified with orientational terms based on their relationship to other orofacial structures such as the facial surface, lips, cheeks, palate, and tongue. Structures closest to the facial surface are termed facial. Those facial structures that are also closer to the lips are termed labial. Facial structures closest to the inner cheek are termed buccal. Structures closest to the tongue

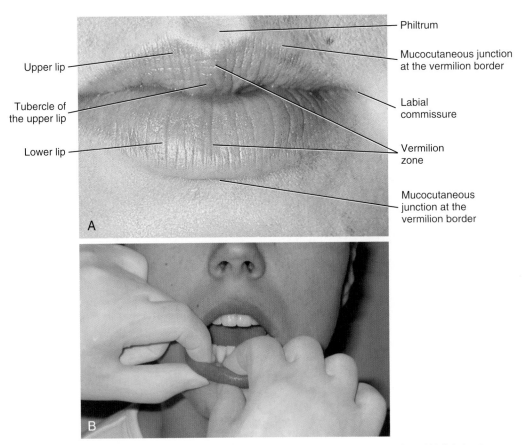

FIGURE 2-10 Frontal view of the lips within the oral region **(A),** and demonstration of bidigital palpation of the lips during an intraoral examination **(B).** *(B Courtesy of Margaret J. Fehrenbach, RDH, MS.)*

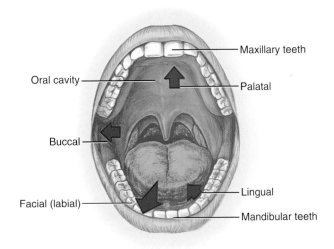

FIGURE 2-11 Oral cavity and jaws with the designation of the terms lingual, palatal, buccal, facial, and labial within the oral cavity. *(From Fehrenbach MJ and Popowics T. Illustrated dental embryology, histology, and anatomy. Elsevier, St. Louis, 2016.)*

are termed **lingual**. Those lingual structures that are also closest to the palate are termed **palatal**.

The oral cavity is lined by a mucous membrane or **oral mucosa** (mu-**ko**-suh) (Figure 2-12). The inner parts of the lips are lined by a pink and thick **labial mucosa**. The labial mucosa is continuous with the equally pink and thick **buccal mucosa** that lines the inner cheek.

However, both the labial and buccal mucosa may vary in coloration, as do other regions of healthy oral mucosa, in individuals with pigmented skin. The buccal mucosa covers a dense pad of inner tissue, the **buccal fat pad**.

Further landmarks can be noted in the oral cavity. On the inner part of the buccal mucosa, just opposite the maxillary second molar, the **parotid papilla** (puh-**rot**-id puh-**pil**-uh) is a small elevation of tissue that protects the ductal opening of the parotid salivary gland. During an intraoral examination, observe the salivary flow from each duct near the parotid papillae after drying it with gauze. A tissue-covered elevation on the posterior aspects of the maxilla just posterior to the most distal maxillary molar is the **maxillary tuberosity** (mak-sil-lare-ee too-buh-**ros**-i-tee). A similar feature on the mandible just posterior to the most distal mandibular molar is a dense pad of tissue, the **retromolar pad** (ret-ro-**moh**-luhr).

In order to examine the labial mucosa during an intraoral examination, ask the patient to open the mouth slightly and gently pull the lips away from the teeth so as to be able to visually inspect and then bidigitally palpate the inner lips. Then gently pull the buccal mucosa slightly away from the teeth so as to be able to visually inspect and then bidigitally palpate the inner cheek on each side using circular compression.

The upper and lower horseshoe-shaped spaces in the open area of the oral cavity between the lips and cheeks anteriorly and laterally and the teeth and their soft tissue medially and posteriorly are considered the maxillary and mandibular **vestibules** (**ves**-ti-bules). Deep within each vestibule is the **vestibular fornix** (**for**-niks), where the pink and thick labial or buccal mucosa meets the redder and thinner **alveolar mucosa** (al-**vee**-uh-luhr) at the **mucobuccal fold**

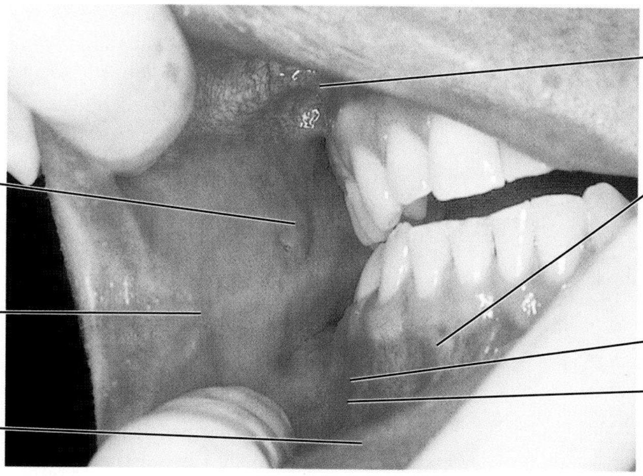

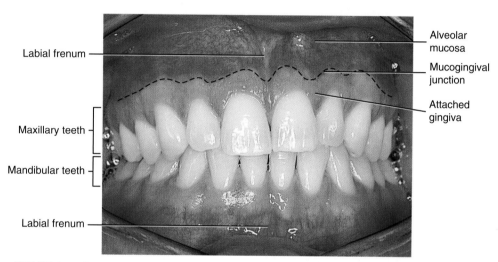

FIGURE 2-12 Oral view of the buccal mucosa and labial mucosa of the oral cavity with associated landmarks noted during an intraoral examination.

FIGURE 2-13 Frontal view of the oral cavity with its associated landmarks noted during an intraoral examination.

(mu-**ko**-buk-uhl). The **labial frenum** (plural, **frena**) (**free**-nuhm, **free**-nuh) is a fold(s) of tissue located at the midline between the labial mucosa and the alveolar mucosa on both the maxilla and mandible (Figure 2-13).

Teeth are located within the upper and lower jaws of the oral cavity within each tooth socket or **alveolus** (plural, **alveoli**) (al-**vee**-lus, al-vee-uh-ly). The teeth of the maxilla are the **maxillary teeth**, and the teeth of the mandible are the **mandibular teeth** (man-**dib**-u-luhr). The maxillary anterior teeth overlap the mandibular anterior teeth, and posteriorly, the maxillary buccal cusps overlap the mandibular buccal cusps. Both dental arches in the adult have permanent teeth that include the **incisors** (in-**sy**-zuhrs), **canines** (**kay**-nines), **premolars** (pre-**moh**-luhrs), and **molars** (**moh**-luhrs).

Surrounding both the maxillary and mandibular teeth are the gums or **gingiva** (jin-**ji**-vuh) or more accurately referred to, but not commonly by the dental community by its plural form, *gingivae* (jin-ji-vee). The gingiva is composed of a firm pink oral mucosa (Figure 2-14 and see Figure 2-13). The gingiva that tightly adheres to the bone around the roots of the teeth is the **attached gingiva**. The attached gingiva may also have localized areas of pigmentation. The line of demarcation between the firmer and pinker attached gingiva and the movable and redder alveolar mucosa is the scallop-shaped **mucogingival junction** (mu-ko-**jin**-ji-vuhl).

At the gingival margin of each tooth is the nonattached or **marginal gingiva** (**mar**-ji-nuhl) or *free gingiva*. The inner surface of the marginal gingiva faces a space(s) or **gingival sulcus** (plural, **sulci**) (**sul**-kuhs, **sul**-ky). The **interdental gingiva** (in-tuhr-**den**-tuhl) is the gingival tissue between adjacent teeth adjoining attached gingiva, with each individual extension being an *interdental papilla*. During an intraoral examination, retract both the buccal mucosa and labial mucosa in order to visually inspect and bidigitally palpate the vestibular area and the gingival tissue using circular compression, including the maxillary tuberosity and retromolar pad on each side.

PALATE

The **palate** (**pal**-uht) or roof of the mouth has two parts: the hard and soft palates (Figure 2-15). The firmer whiter anterior part is the **hard palate**. A small bulge of tissue at the most anterior part of the hard palate, lingual to the anterior teeth, is the **incisive papilla** (in-**sy**-siv). Directly posterior to this papilla are **palatine rugae** (**roo**-gee), which are firm irregular ridges of tissue.

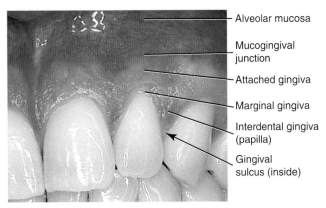

FIGURE 2-14 Close-up of the gingiva with its associated landmarks noted during an intraoral examination.

— Alveolar mucosa

— Mucogingival junction

— Attached gingiva

— Marginal gingiva

— Interdental gingiva (papilla)

— Gingival sulcus (inside)

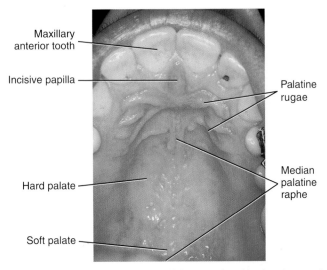

Maxillary anterior tooth

Incisive papilla

Palatine rugae

Median palatine raphe

Hard palate

Soft palate

FIGURE 2-15 View of the palate with its associated landmarks noted during an intraoral examination.

The yellower and looser posterior part of the palate is the **soft palate**; it is the smaller part of the palate since it only comprises approximately 15% of the total palatal surface (see Figures 2-15 and 2-21). The soft palate is connected to the hard palate but it can be separately elevated and depressed by muscles (see Chapter 4).

A midline muscular structure, the **uvula of the palate** (u-vu-luh), hangs from the posterior margin of the soft palate. A midline ridge of tissue on the palate is the **median palatine raphe** (me-dee-uhn pal-uh-tine ray-fe), which runs from the incisive papilla to the uvula (see Figure 2-21).

The **pterygomandibular fold** (ter-i-go-man-dib-u-luhr) is a fold of tissue that extends from the junction of the hard and soft palates on each side down to the mandible, just posterior to the most distal mandibular molar and the nearby retromolar pad, and stretches when the patient opens the mouth wider. This fold covers a deeper tendinous band that separates the cheek from the throat (or pharynx).

During an intraoral examination, have the patient tilt his or her head back slightly and extend the tongue to visually inspect the soft palate and throat or pharynx. Use the mouth mirror to intensify the light source. Then, gently place the mouth mirror with the mirror side down on the middle of the top surface of the tongue and ask the patient to say "*ah*" (see Figure 4-31). As this is done, visually observe the soft palate with uvula and any visible parts of the throat or pharynx. Then, compress the hard palate with the first or second finger of one hand, avoiding circular compression. It is also recommended not to palpate the nearby soft palate so as to prevent initiating the gag reflex.

TONGUE

The **tongue** is a prominent feature of the oral region (Figure 2-16). The posterior one-third is the pharyngeal part of the tongue or **base of the tongue**. The base of the tongue attaches to the floor of the mouth. The base of the tongue does not lie within the oral cavity but within the oral part of the throat or pharynx. The anterior two-thirds of the tongue is the **body of the tongue** or oral part since it lies within the oral cavity. The tip of the tongue is the **apex of the tongue**. Certain surfaces of the tongue have elevated small structures of specialized

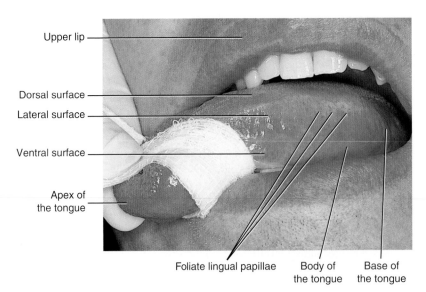

Upper lip

Dorsal surface

Lateral surface

Ventral surface

Apex of the tongue

Foliate lingual papillae   Body of the tongue   Base of the tongue

FIGURE 2-16 Lateral view of the tongue with its associated landmarks noted during an intraoral examination.

mucosa, the **lingual papillae** (puh-**pil**-ee), some of which are associated with taste buds.

The side or **lateral surface of the tongue** is noted for its vertical ridges, the **foliate lingual papillae** (**fo**-lee-uht), which contain taste buds. These lingual papillae are more prominent in children.

The top surface or **dorsal surface of the tongue** (**dor**-suhl) has a midline depression, the **median lingual sulcus**, corresponding with the position of a midline tendinous band deep within the tongue (Figure 2-17). In relationship to the tongue, *dorsal* and *posterior* are not truly equivalent terms, nor are *ventral* and *anterior* the same either as discussed later. Instead, they are four different locations. This is because the human tongue still has the same orientation as the tongue of four-footed animals, in which anterior and posterior originally meant toward the nose and tail, respectively, and *dorsal* and *ventral* refer to the back and belly, respectively (see Chapter 1). Our upright posture on our two feet is the reason that *dorsal* and *posterior* have become synonyms in the rest of the body and now are used in that manner when referring anatomically to these surfaces.

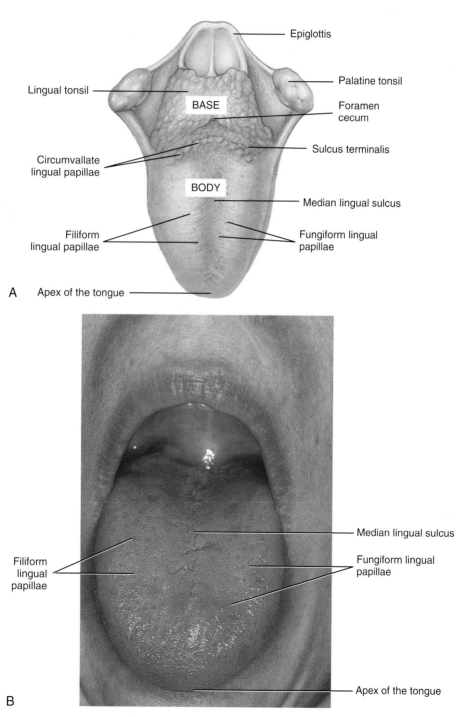

FIGURE 2-17 Dorsal view of the tongue with its associated landmarks noted **(A)** and during an intra-oral examination **(B)**. *(From Fehrenbach MJ and Popowics T. Illustrated dental embryology, histology, and anatomy. Elsevier, St. Louis, 2016.)*

The dorsal surface of the tongue also has varying forms of lingual papillae. The slender, threadlike lingual papillae are the **filiform lingual papillae** (**fil**-i-form), which give the dorsal surface its velvety texture. The red mushroom-shaped dots are the **fungiform lingual papillae** (**fun**-ji-form). The fungiform are found in lesser numbers than are the filiform on the body of the dorsal surface of the tongue and contain taste buds.

Farther posteriorly on the dorsal surface of the tongue and more difficult to see clinically is a "V"-shaped groove, the **sulcus terminalis** (tur-**mi**-nuhl-is). The sulcus terminalis separates the base from the body of the tongue. Where the sulcus terminalis points backward toward the throat or pharynx is a small pitlike depression, the **foramen cecum** (fo-**ray**-men **see**-kuhm). The **circumvallate lingual papillae** (ser-kuhm-**val**-ate), which are approximately 10 to 14 in number, line up along the anterior side of the sulcus terminalis on the body. These large mushroom-shaped lingual papillae have taste buds at their bases. Even farther posteriorly on the dorsal surface of the tongue base on each side is an irregular mass of lymphoid tissue, the **lingual tonsil** (**ton**-sil).

The underside or **ventral surface of the tongue** (**ven**-truhl) is noted for its visibly large blue blood vessel branches of the deep lingual vein that are close to the surface (Figure 2-18). Again, the term used for the underside of the tongue, *ventral*, referred originally to four-footed animals in anatomic position and now is used for that surface for our upright position on our two feet. Lateral to the deep lingual veins on each side is the **plica fimbriata** (plural, **plicae fimbriatae**) (**pli**-kuh fim-bree-**ay**-tuh, pli-kay fim-bree-**ay**-tee), a fold(s) with fringelike projections.

To examine the dorsal and lateral surfaces of the tongue, have the patient slightly extend the tongue and wrap gauze around the anterior third of the tongue in order to obtain a firm grasp (see Figure 2-16). First, visually inspect and then digitally palpate the dorsal surface. Then, turn the tongue slightly on its side to visually inspect its base and bidigitally palpate its lateral borders. To examine the ventral

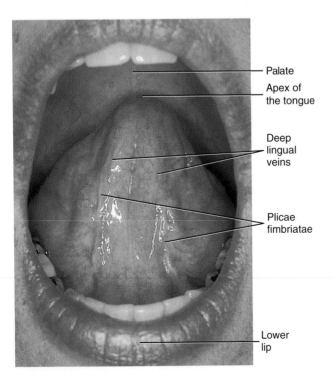

FIGURE 2-18 Ventral surface of the tongue with its associated landmarks noted during an intraoral examination.

Labels in figure:
- Palate
- Apex of the tongue
- Deep lingual veins
- Plicae fimbriatae
- Lower lip

surface, have the patient slightly lift the tongue to visually inspect and digitally palpate its surface.

FLOOR OF THE MOUTH

The **floor of the mouth** is located inferior to the ventral surface of the tongue (Figure 2-19). The **lingual frenum** is a midline fold of tissue between the ventral surface of the tongue and the floor of the mouth.

A ridge of tissue also exists on each side of the floor of the mouth, the **sublingual fold** (sub-**ling**-gwuhl). Together these folds are arranged in a "V"-shaped configuration from the lingual frenum to the base of the tongue. The sublingual folds contain duct openings from the sublingual salivary gland. The small papilla or **sublingual caruncle** (**kar**-ung-uhl) at the anterior end of each sublingual fold contains the duct openings from both the submandibular and sublingual salivary glands.

While the patient lifts the tongue to the palate during an extraoral examination, visually inspect the mucosa of the floor of the mouth using the mouth mirror to intensify the light source and check the lingual frenum at the midline as well. Dry each sublingual caruncle with gauze to observe salivary flow from the ducts. Bimanually palpate the sublingual area by placing an index finger intraorally and the fingertips of the opposite hand extraorally under the chin, compressing the tissue between the fingers (see Figure 7-10).

PHARYNX

The oral cavity also provides the entrance into the throat or **pharynx** (**fare**-inks). The pharynx is a muscular tube that serves both the respiratory and digestive systems. The pharynx consists of three parts: the nasopharynx, oropharynx, and laryngopharynx (Figure 2-20). The **laryngopharynx** (luh-ring-go-**fare**-inks) is located more inferior, close to the laryngeal opening, and thus is not visible during an intraoral examination.

The part of the pharynx that is superior to the level of the soft palate is the **nasopharynx** (nay-zo-**fare**-inks). The nasopharynx is continuous with the nasal cavity. The part of the pharynx that is between the soft palate and the opening of the larynx is the **oropharynx** (or-o-**fare**-inks) (Figure 2-21). Parts of the nasopharynx and oropharynx are visible during an intraoral examination when examining the palate as discussed earlier.

Behind the base of the tongue and in front of the oropharynx is the **epiglottis** (ep-i-**glot**-tis), a flap of cartilage (see Figures 2-17, 2-20, 4-30). At rest, the epiglottis is upright and allows air to pass through the larynx and into the rest of the respiratory system. During swallowing, it folds back to cover the entrance to the larynx, preventing food and liquid from entering the deeper still trachea and then entering the lungs.

The opening from the oral region into the oropharynx is the **fauces** (**faw**-seez) or *faucial isthmus*. The fauces are formed laterally on each side by folds of tissue, both the **anterior faucial pillar** (**faw**-shuhl **pil**-uhr) and the **posterior faucial pillar**. Tonsillar tissue, the **palatine tonsils**, is located between each of these pillars created by underlying muscles (Figure 2-21 and see Figure 4-31). The palatine tonsils are the tonsillar tissue that patients call their "tonsils."

MENTAL REGION

The chin is the major feature of the **mental region** (**men**-tuhl) of the head (Figure 2-22). The **mental protuberance** (pro-**too**-buhr-uhns) is the prominence of the chin. The mental protuberance is often more pronounced in adult males. The labiomental groove, a horizontal

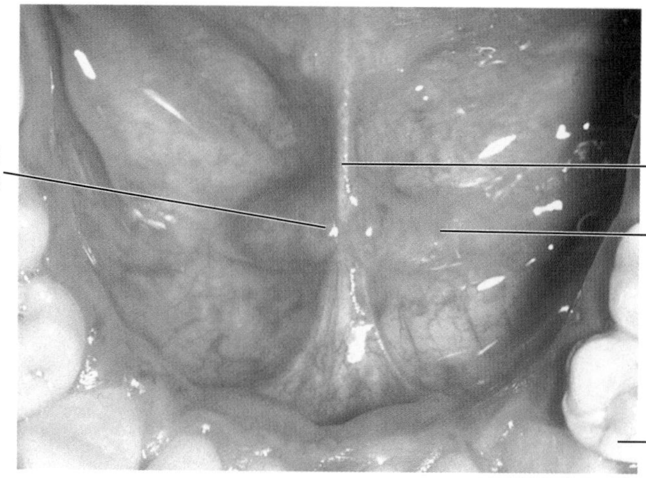

Sublingual
caruncle

Lingual
frenum

Sublingual
fold

Mandibular
teeth

FIGURE 2-19 View of the floor of the mouth with its associated landmarks noted during an intraoral examination.

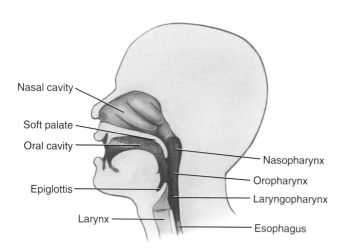

Nasal cavity

Soft palate

Oral cavity

Epiglottis

Larynx

Nasopharynx

Oropharynx

Laryngopharynx

Esophagus

FIGURE 2-20 Midsagittal section of the head and neck with the divisions of the pharynx noted.

groove between the lower lip and the chin mentioned in the description of the oral region, should be approximately midway between the apex of the nose and the chin and level with the angle of the mandible.

Also present on the chin in some individuals is a midline depression or dimple that marks the underlying bony fusion of the lower jaw. Visually inspect and bilaterally palpate the chin during an extraoral examination (see Figure 2-22).

REGIONS OF NECK

The neck extends from the skull and mandible down to the clavicles and sternum. However, the posterior neck is at a higher level than the anterior neck so as to connect the cervical internal organs with the posterior openings of the nasal and oral cavities. The **regions of the neck** can be divided into different cervical triangles on the basis of the large bones and muscles in the area, with each triangle containing structures that are palpated during an extraoral examination (Figure 2-23 and Chapters 3 and 4).

The large strap muscle, the **sternocleidomastoid (SCM) muscle** (stir-no-kli-doh-**mass**-toid), divides each side of the neck diagonally into an **anterior cervical triangle** and **posterior cervical triangle**.

The SCM muscle is palpated during an extraoral examination, as are the regions anterior and posterior to it (see Figure 4-2).

The anterior region of the neck corresponds with the two anterior cervical triangles, which are separated by a midline. Major structures that pass between the head and thorax or chest can be accessed through the anterior cervical triangle. The lateral region of the neck that is posterior to the SCM muscle is considered the posterior cervical triangle on each side.

At the anterior midline, the largest of the larynx's cartilages, the **thyroid cartilage** (**thy**-roid), is visible as the laryngeal prominence or "Adam's apple," especially in adult males. This cartilage is superior to the thyroid gland, which is also palpated during an extraoral examination (Figure 2-24 and see Figure 7-10; discussed in detail in Chapter 7). The **superior thyroid notch** of the thyroid cartilage is just superior to the laryngeal prominence and is also a palpable landmark of the neck. The vocal cords or ligaments of the **larynx** (**lare**-inks) or "voice box" are attached to the posterior surface of the thyroid cartilage.

The **hyoid bone** (**hi**-oid) is also located in the anterior midline and is suspended in the neck without any bony articulations, superior to the thyroid cartilage (see Figure 2-24). Instead, muscles are attached to the hyoid bone that control the tongue and pharynx, assist the muscles of mastication, as well as those muscles involved in swallowing. This bone is also palpated along with the larynx during an extraoral examination.

The anterior cervical triangle on each side can be further subdivided into smaller triangular regions by area muscles that are not as prominent as those of the SCM muscle (Figure 2-25 and see Figures 4-25 and 4-27). Thus, the superior part of each anterior cervical triangle is demarcated by two parts of the digastric muscle (both anterior and posterior bellies), with the mandible forming a **submandibular triangle** (sub-man-**dib**-u-luhr) on each side. The inferior part of each anterior cervical triangle is further subdivided by the omohyoid muscle (superior belly) into a **carotid triangle** (kuh-**rot**-id) superior to it and a **muscular triangle** inferior to it. A single midline **submental triangle** (sub-**men**-tuhl) is also formed by the two parts of both digastric muscles (both right and left anterior bellies) as well as the hyoid bone.

Each posterior cervical triangle can also be further subdivided into smaller triangular regions on each side by area muscles (Figure 2-26). The omohyoid muscle (inferior belly) divides the posterior cervical triangle into the **occipital triangle** (ok-**sip**-i-tuhl) superior to it and the **subclavian triangle** (sub-**klay**-vee-uhn) inferior to it on each side.

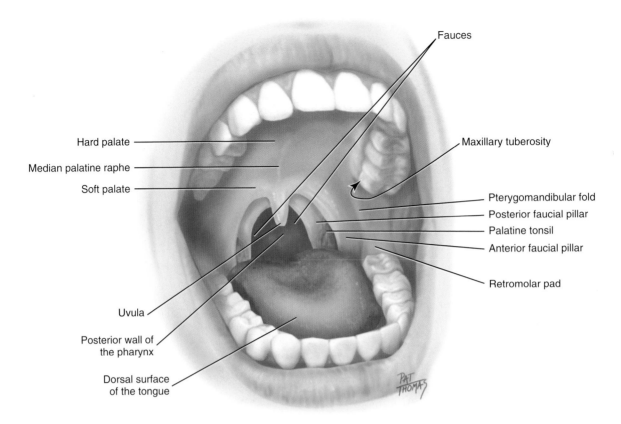

FIGURE 2-21 Oral view of the oral cavity and oropharynx with associated landmarks noted.

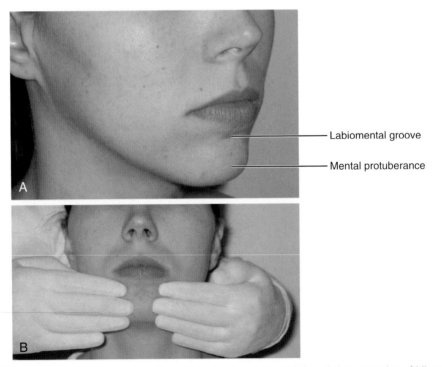

FIGURE 2-22 View of the mental region with its landmarks noted **(A)**, and demonstration of bilateral palpation of the mental region during an intraoral examination **(B)**. (*B Courtesy of Margaret J. Fehrenbach, RDH, MS.*)

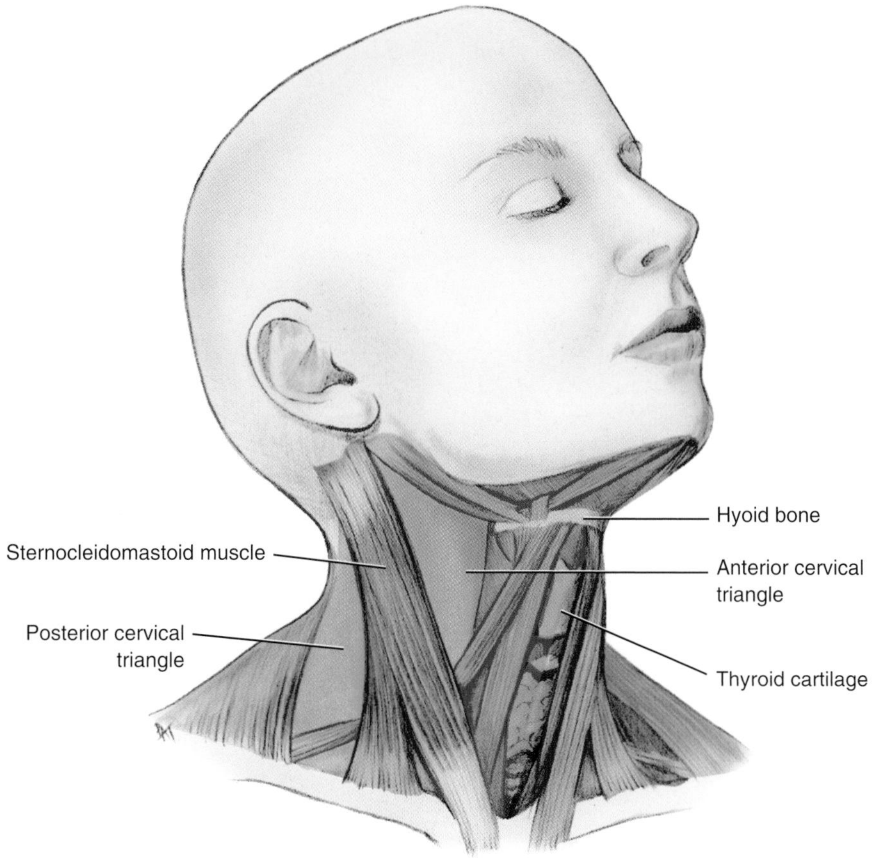

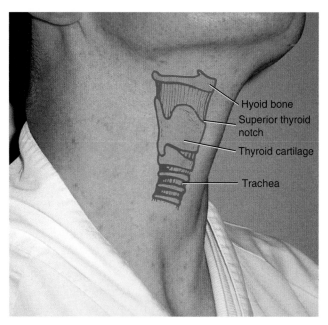

Sternocleidomastoid muscle

Posterior cervical triangle

Hyoid bone

Anterior cervical triangle

Thyroid cartilage

FIGURE 2-23 Division of neck region by the sternocleidomastoid muscle into the anterior cervical and posterior cervical triangles.

Hyoid bone

Superior thyroid notch

Thyroid cartilage

Trachea

FIGURE 2-24 Lateral view of the neck with the skeletal landmarks of the anterior cervical triangle superimposed.

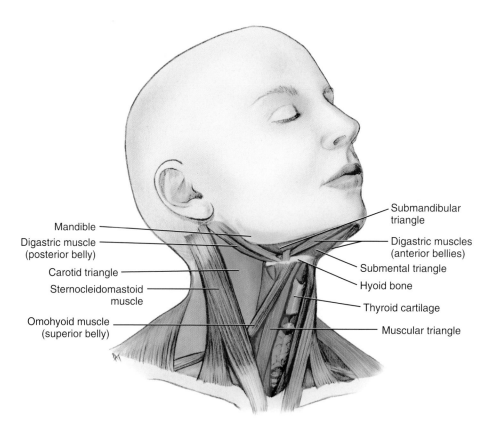

Mandible

Digastric muscle
(posterior belly)

Carotid triangle

Sternocleidomastoid
muscle

Omohyoid muscle
(superior belly)

Submandibular
triangle

Digastric muscles
(anterior bellies)

Submental triangle

Hyoid bone

Thyroid cartilage

Muscular triangle

FIGURE 2-25 Division of the anterior cervical triangle by area muscles into the submandibular, submental, carotid, and muscular triangles.

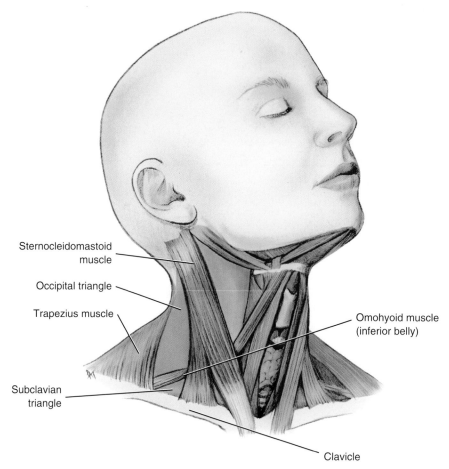

Sternocleidomastoid
muscle

Occipital triangle

Trapezius muscle

Omohyoid muscle
(inferior belly)

Subclavian
triangle

Clavicle

FIGURE 2-26 Division of the posterior cervical triangle by area muscles into the occipital and subclavian triangles.

REVIEW QUESTIONS

1. Those structures in the oral region that are closest to the tongue are considered
   A. buccal.
   B. facial.
   C. lingual.
   D. pharyngeal.
   E. palatal.
2. Which of the following terms is used to describe the smooth, elevated area between the eyebrows in the frontal region?
   A. Supraorbital ridge
   B. Medial canthus
   C. Glabella
   D. Alae
   E. Auricular region
3. In which region of the head and neck is the tragus located?
   A. Frontal region
   B. Nasal region
   C. Auricular region
   D. Anterior cervical triangle
   E. Submandibular triangle
4. The tissue at the junction between the labial or buccal mucosa and the alveolar mucosa is the
   A. mucogingival junction.
   B. mucobuccal fold.
   C. vermilion zone.
   D. labial frenum.
   E. labiomental groove.
5. Into which of the following cervical triangles does the sterno-cleidomastoid muscle divide the neck region?
   A. Superior and inferior triangles
   B. Medial and lateral triangles
   C. Anterior and posterior triangles
   D. Proximal and distal triangles
6. The parietal and occipital regions are covered by the
   A. temporal region.
   B. layers of scalp.
   C. eyelids with their tear ducts.
   D. external acoustic meatus.
7. Which of the following statements concerning the location of the medial canthus is CORRECT when comparing it with the lateral canthus?
   A. Nearer to the nose
   B. Nearer to the ear
   C. Where the upper and lower eyelid meet
   D. Where the upper and lower lip meet
8. Which of the following structures extends from just inferior to the lateral margin of the eye toward the ear?
   A. Pterygomandibular fold
   B. Zygomatic arch
   C. Sulcus terminalis
   D. Sternocleidomastoid muscle
9. The opening from the oral region into the oropharynx is the
   A. fauces.
   B. palatine tonsils.
   C. pterygomandibular fold.
   D. nasopharynx.
10. Which of the following terms is used for the small papilla at the anterior end of each sublingual fold?
    A. Lingual frenum
    B. Plica fimbriata
    C. Foliate papillae
    D. Sublingual caruncle
    E. Incisive papilla
11. Which of the following structures is the opening in the center of the iris?
    A. Sclera
    B. Pupil
    C. Orbit
    D. Iris
12. Which of the following structures is located between the tragus and the antitragus?
    A. Orbit of the eye
    B. Intertragic notch
    C. Angle of the mandible
    D. Helix of the ear
    E. Labial commissure
13. Which of the following structures separates the lower lip from the chin?
    A. Vermilion zone
    B. Tubercle of upper lip
    C. Labial commissure
    D. Labiomental groove
    E. Nasolabial sulcus
14. Which of the following structures is located on the dorsal surface of the tongue?
    A. Labiomental groove
    B. Mucobuccal fold
    C. Median lingual sulcus
    D. Pterygomandibular fold
    E. Median palatine raphe
15. Which of the following structures is located directly posterior to the incisive papilla?
    A. Palatine rugae
    B. Mucogingival junction
    C. Vermilion zone
    D. Labial frenum
16. The root of the nose is located
    A. midline between the nares.
    B. between the eyes.
    C. at the tip of the nose.
    D. at the lateral part of each naris.

17. Which of the following is suspended within the neck without any bony articulations?
    A. Maxillae
    B. Mandible
    C. Hyoid bone
    D. Mandible and hyoid bone
18. The maxillary tuberosity is located on the _____ aspect of each maxilla.
    A. Anterior
    B. Posterior
    C. Medial
    D. Lateral

19. Which of the following are noted on the lateral surface of the tongue?
    A. Median lingual sulcus
    B. Fungiform lingual papillae
    C. Sulcus terminalis
    D. Foliate lingual papillae
20. Where is the labial frenum located?
    A. Floor of the mouth lined by oral mucosa
    B. Near parotid papillae on buccal mucosa
    C. Midline between labial mucosa and alveolar mucosa
    D. Attached to the marginal gingiva on both dental arches

Identify the structures on the following diagrams by filling in each blank with the correct anatomic term. You can check your answers by looking back at the figure indicated in parentheses for each identification diagram.

1. (Figures 2-1, 2-2, A, 2-4, 2-6, 2-7, and 2-9)

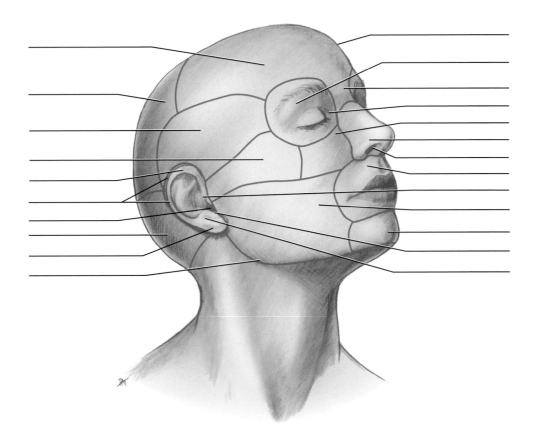

2. (Figure 2-6, *A*)

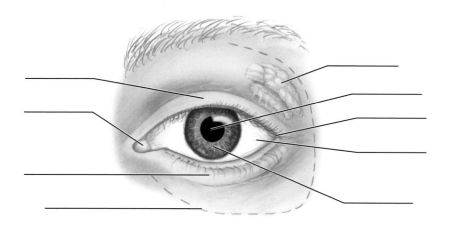

3. (Figure 2-11)

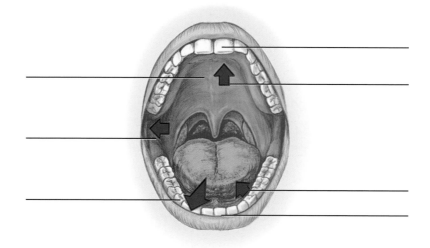

4. (Figure 2-17, *A*)

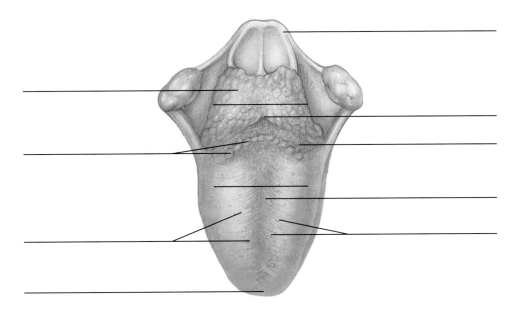

5. (Figure 2-20)

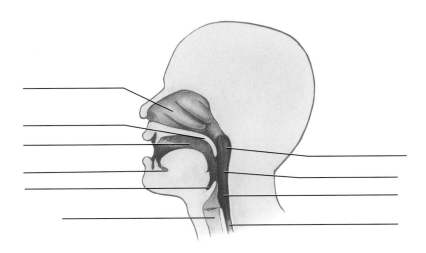

6. (Figure 2-21)

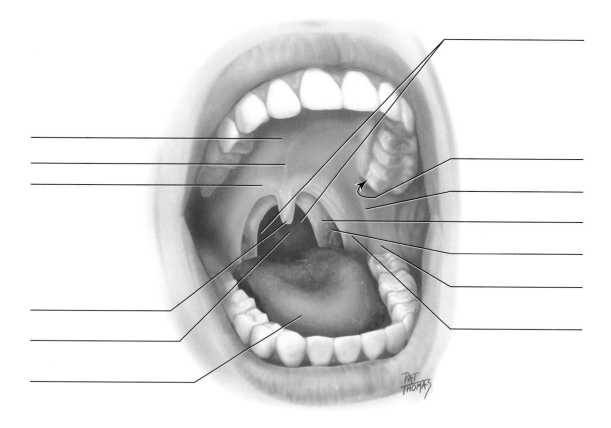

7. (Figure 2-23)

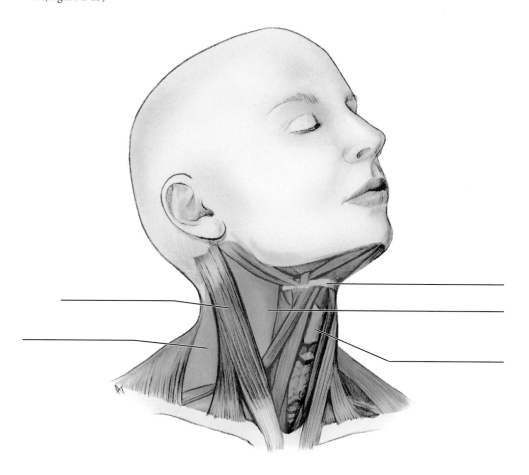

8. (Figure 2-25)

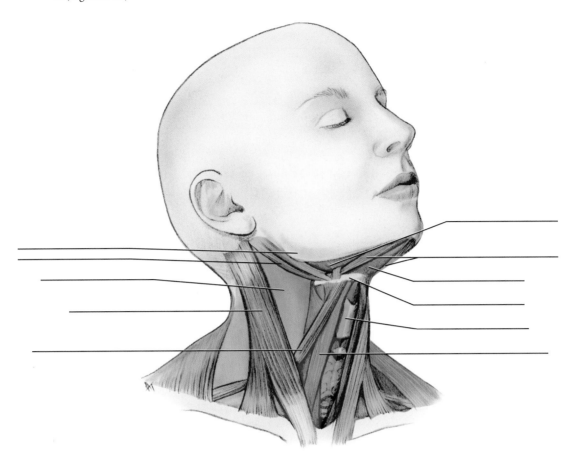

9. (Figure 2-26)

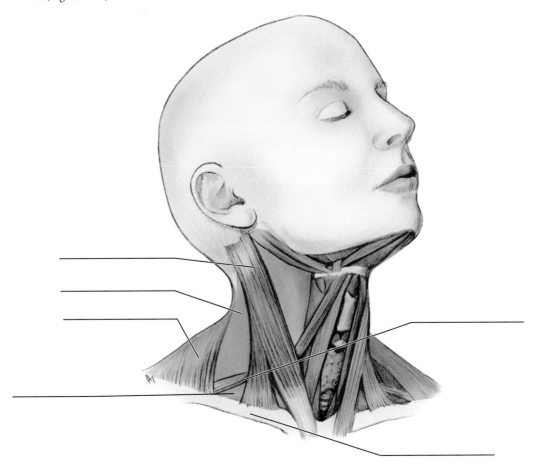

CHAPTER 3

Skeletal System

●●● LEARNING OBJECTIVES

1. Define and pronounce the **key terms** and **anatomic terms** in this chapter.
2. Locate and identify the bones of the head and neck and their landmarks on a diagram, skull, and patient.
3. Describe in detail the landmarks of the maxilla and mandible.
4. Discuss the skeletal system pathology associated with the head and neck.
5. Correctly complete the review questions and activities for this chapter.
6. Integrate an understanding of the skeletal system into the overall study of the head and neck anatomy and clinical dental practice.

●●● KEY TERMS

Aperture (ap-uhr-chuhr) Narrow opening in a bone.

Arch Prominent bridgelike bony structure.

Articulation (ahr-tik-u-lay-shuhn) Area where bones are joined to each other.

Bones Mineralized structures protecting internal soft tissue and serving as biomechanic basis for movement.

Canal Longer narrow, and tubelike opening in a bone.

Condyle (kon-dyl) Oval bony prominence usually involved in joints.

Cornu (kor-noo) Small hornlike prominence of a bone.

Crest Roughened border or ridge on bony surface.

Eminence (em-i-nuhns) Tubercle or small rounded elevation on bony surface.

Epicondyle (ep-i-kon-dyl) Small prominence located superior to or upon a condyle.

Fissure (fish-uhr) Narrow cleftlike opening in a bone.

Foramen/Foramina (fo-ray-muhn, fo-ram-i-nuh) Short windowlike opening(s) in a bone.

Fossa/Fossae (fos-uh, fos-ee) Deeper depression(s) on bony surface.

Head Rounded structure projecting from a bony surface by a neck.

Incisura (in-si-su-ruh) Indentation or notch at the edge of a bone.

Joint Site of a junction or union between two or more bones.

Line Small straight ridge of a bone.

Meatus (me-ay-tuhs) Opening or canal in a bone.

Notch Indentation at edge of bone.

Ostium/Ostia (os-tee-uhm, os-tee-uh) Smaller opening(s) in a bone.

Perforation (pur-fuh-ray-shuhn) Abnormal hole in a hollow organ such as in the wall of a sinus.

Plate Flat structure of a bone.

Primary sinusitis (sy-nuhs-i-tis) Inflammation of sinus.

Process General term for any prominence on bony surface.

Secondary sinusitis Inflammation of the sinus related to another source.

Skeletal system Consists of bones, associated cartilage, and joints.

Spine Abrupt small prominence of a bone.

Sulcus/Sulci (sul-kuhs, sul-ke) Shallow depression(s) or groove(s) on a bony surface.

Suture (soo-chuhr) Generally immovable articulation joining bones by fibrous tissue.

Tubercle (too-buhr-kuhl) Eminence or small rounded elevation on bony surface.

Tuberosity (too-buh-ros-i-tee) Large, often rough, prominence on bony surface.

SKELETAL SYSTEM OVERVIEW

The skeletal system consists of the bones and their associated cartilage and joints. The bones of the skeletal system are mineralized structures protecting the internal soft tissue. Bones also serve as the biomechanic basis for movement along with muscles, tendons, and ligaments.

The bony prominences and depressions on a bony surface serve as muscle attachments (see Chapter 4). Another feature of a bone are the openings where various nerves and blood vessels travel through (see Chapters 6 and 8). Bones of the skeleton also join together at articulations.

BONY PROMINENCES

A general term for any prominence on a bony surface is a process. One specific type of prominence located on a bony surface is a condyle, an oval prominence usually involved in joints. An epicondyle is a small prominence located superior to or upon a condyle. A rounded structure projecting from a bony surface by a neck is a **head**. Another large, often rough prominence on a bony surface is a tuberosity. Tuberosities are usually attachment sites for muscles or tendons. An **arch** is a prominence shaped like a bridge with a bowlike outline. A cornu is a small hornlike prominence.

Other prominences of bone include tubercles, crests, lines, and spines. These primarily serve as muscle and ligament attachments. A tubercle or eminence is a small rounded elevation on a bony surface. A crest is a prominent, often roughened border or ridge on a bony surface. A line is a small straight ridge. An abrupt small prominence of a bone that may be a blunt or sharply pointed projection is a spine.

BONY DEPRESSIONS

One type of depression on a bony surface is an incisura, or notch, which is an indentation at the edge of a bone. Another depression(s) on a bony surface is a sulcus (plural, sulci), which is a shallow depression or groove that usually marks the course of blood vessels or nerves. A generally deeper depression(s) or concavity on a bony surface is a fossa (plural, fossae). Fossae can be parts of joints or attachment sites for muscles, or they can have other functions.

However, an area on a bony surface that is neither a prominence nor depression is a plate, which is a flat structure of a bone.

BONY OPENINGS

Bones can have openings within them such as a foramen or canal. A foramen (plural, foramina) is a short windowlike opening(s) in a bone. A canal is a longer narrow tubelike opening in a bone. A meatus is a type of canal. Another opening in a bone is a fissure, which is a narrow cleftlike opening. A smaller opening(s), especially as an entrance into a hollow organ or canal, is an ostium (plural, ostia). A narrow opening is an aperture.

SKELETAL ARTICULATIONS

An articulation is an area of the skeleton where the bones are joined to each other. An articulation can be associated with either a movable or immovable joint. A joint is a site of a junction or union between two or more bones. A suture is the union of bones joined by fibrous tissue that appears on the dry skull as a jagged line. Sutures are considered to be generally immovable but may provide biomechanic protection from the force of a blow by moving slightly to absorb the force. They are most flexible in infants, with much of the early growth of the skull occurring at the sutural edges of the cranial bones.

HEAD AND NECK BONES

The bones of the head and neck serve as a base for palpation of the soft tissue during both an intraoral and extraoral examination of a patient (see Appendix B). A dental professional must not only locate each of the head and neck bones but also recognize any abnormalities in the bony surface structure (discussed later).

In order to recognize any bony abnormalities, the dental professional must understand the anatomy of the bones of the head and neck. This includes locating the surface bony prominences, depressions, and articulations as well as the openings in these bones and the nerves and blood vessels that travel through those openings.

The bones of the head and neck are the most complicated bony structures of the body. For effective study of the bones of the head and neck, it is helpful to use both photographs and diagrams of these

bones as well as the skull itself. Unless noted, the skull in these figures is in anatomic position, so that the inferior margins of the orbits and the superior margins of the external acoustic meatuses are within parallel horizontal planes (see Chapter 1). This is similar in respect to the position of the patient's head and neck when sitting upright in a dental chair. Thus, the palpation of the skull of peers, and then later of patients, during both extraoral and intraoral examination adds to the overall study of the skeletal system.

Bones and their associated surface tissue also serve as landmarks when describing the location of a pathologic lesion, taking dental radiographs (see Chapter 2), and administering a local anesthetic injection (see Chapter 9), as well as understanding the spread of dental (or odontogenic) infections (see Chapter 12).

SKULL BONES

The bones of the **skull** or braincase can be divided into the **cranium** (**kray**-nee-uhm), which contains the brain with its outer shell of the **cranial bone** (**kray**-nee-uhl), and into the face with its inner support by the **facial bones**. The bones of the skull, whether cranial or facial, protect the brain, form the facial features, participate in the temporomandibular joint, and serve as a base for the dentition. The bones of the skull can be single or paired. Anatomists may also use the term *neurocranium* for the cranial bones because they enclose the brain, and the term *viscerocranium* for the facial bones. The skull has 22 bones, not including the six auditory ossicles of the middle ear (Table 3-1). Each middle ear contains one *malleus, incus,* and *stapes* (in order from outer to inner). Their function is to transmit and amplify vibrations to the inner ear by way of the tympanic membrane or *eardrum*.

Growth continues to take place in all bones of the skull during early childhood. Growth of the upper face also occurs at the sutures between the maxillae and other bones, as well as at bony surfaces. Growth in the lower face takes place at the bony surfaces of the mandible and at the head of its condyle. Inadequate or disproportionate bone growth of the upper face or mandible may leave inadequate room for the developing dentition and cause occlusal complications. These difficulties with growth involving the dentition can be addressed by orthodontic therapy and osseous surgery, if needed, after ruling out any underlying endocrine disorder.

All skull bones are immovable, except the mandible at its temporomandibular joint. Instead, the articulation of certain of the bones in the skull is by sutures (Table 3-2). In addition, the skull also has a movable articulation with the bony vertebral column in the cervical region.

TABLE 3-1		Cranial Bones and Facial Bones	
CRANIAL BONES	**NUMBER**	**FACIAL BONES***	**NUMBER**
Ethmoid bone	Single	Inferior nasal conchae	Paired
Frontal bone	Single	Lacrimal bones	Paired
Occipital bone	Single	Mandible	Single
Parietal bones	Paired	Maxillae	Paired
Sphenoid bone	Single	Vomer	Single
Temporal bones	Paired	Zygomatic bones	Paired

*Note that the palatine bones are paired bones of the skull that are not included since they are not strictly considered facial bones.

The skull bones have openings for the main nerves and blood vessels of the head and neck (Table 3-3). Skull bones also have associated processes that are involved in prominent structures of the face and head (Table 3-4). For more effective study, this chapter can also be later reviewed after reading the chapters on the vascular and nervous systems (see Chapters 6 and 8), the muscles of the head and neck (see Chapter 4), and the temporomandibular joint (see Chapter 5).

TABLE 3-2		Skull Sutures and Articulations
SUTURE(S)	**NUMBER**	**BONY ARTICULATIONS**
Coronal sutures	Paired	Frontal bone and parietal bones
Frontonasal suture	Single	Frontal bone and nasal bones
Intermaxillary suture	Single	Maxillae
Lambdoidal suture	Single	Occipital bone and parietal bones
Median palatine suture	Single	Anterior part: Maxillae Posterior part: Palatine bones
Sagittal suture	Single	Parietal bones
Squamosal sutures	Paired	Temporal bones and parietal bones
Temporozygomatic sutures	Paired	Temporal bones and zygomatic bones
Transverse palatine suture	Single	Maxillae and palatine bones
Zygomaticomaxillary sutures	Paired	Zygomatic bones and maxillae

This chapter studies the skull by first looking at it externally from different viewpoints: superior, anterior, lateral, and inferior views, and then by examining its internal surface from both superior and inferior viewpoints. This format of first visualizing the entire skull helps to obtain more general information about structures formed by several skull bones. Next, the skull is studied by looking at its individual bones and their various features, using the major categories of the cranial bones, facial bones, and cervical bones. Finally, the more general features of the skull are again studied including the skull fossae and paranasal sinuses.

SUPERIOR VIEW OF EXTERNAL SKULL

To view the external skull, the cap can be removed from the skull and studied. The cranial bones and associated sutures are easily noted from this view.

Cranial Bones From Superior View. When the external skull is viewed from the superior aspect, four cranial bones are noted (Figure 3-1). At the anterior part of the skull is the single **frontal bone** (**frun**-tuhl). At each lateral part of the skull is the paired **parietal bone** (puh-**ri**-uh-tuhl). At the posterior part of the skull is the single **occipital bone** (ok-**sip**-i-tuhl). This main division of the cranial bones of the skull is discussed in detail later.

Skull Sutures From Superior View. Sutures among these four cranial bones as noted from the superior aspect include: the coronal, sagittal, and lambdoidal sutures (Figure 3-2 and see Table 3-2). The suture extending across the skull, between the frontal bone and each parietal bone, is the paired **coronal suture** (**kor**-o-nuhl). This is also the location of the diamond-shaped *anterior fontanelle* (**fon**-tuh-nel) or "soft spot" in a newborn where the frontal bone and both parietal bones join. This site generally remains open until closure at about 2 years of age.

A single suture, the **sagittal suture** (**saj**-i-tuhl)**,** extends from the anterior to the posterior of the skull at the midline between the parietal bones; the sagittal suture is parallel with the sagittal plane of the

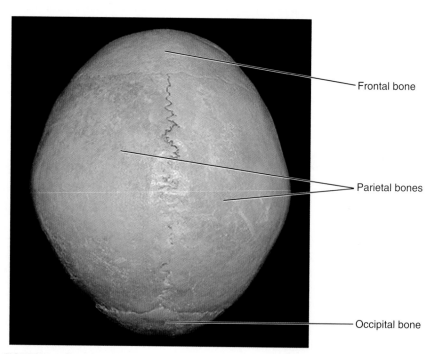

- Frontal bone

- Parietal bones

- Occipital bone

FIGURE 3-1 Superior view of the external skull with its cranial bones noted from this view.

TABLE 3-3	**Skull Bony Openings and Contents***	
BONY OPENING(S)	**LOCATION**	**CONTENTS FOR OPENINGS**
Carotid canals	Temporal bones	Internal carotid arteries and plexuses of nerves
Cribriform plate with foramina	Ethmoid bone	First cranial nerves
External acoustic meatuses	Temporal bones	Canals with tympanic membranes that when intact block entry to tympanic cavities
Foramina lacera	Between sphenoid bone, occipital bone, and temporal bones	Cartilage when intact
Foramen magnum	Occipital bone	Spinal cord, vertebral arteries, and eleventh cranial nerves
Foramina ovales	Sphenoid bone	Mandibular nerves (or third division) of fifth cranial or trigeminal nerve and lesser petrosal nerves and blood vessels
Foramina rotunda	Sphenoid bone	Maxillary nerves (or second division) of fifth cranial or trigeminal nerve and blood vessels
Foramina spinosa	Sphenoid bone	Middle meningeal arteries
Greater palatine foramina	Palatine bones	Greater palatine nerves and blood vessels
Hypoglossal canals	Occipital bone	Twelfth cranial nerves and blood vessels
Incisive foramen	Maxillae	Right and left nasopalatine nerves and branches of the sphenopalatine arteries
Inferior orbital fissures	Between sphenoid bone and maxillae	Infraorbital and zygomatic nerves, infraorbital arteries, and inferior ophthalmic veins
Infraorbital foramina and canals	Maxillae	Infraorbital nerves and blood vessels
Internal acoustic meatuses	Temporal bones	Seventh and eighth cranial nerves
Jugular foramina	Between occipital bone and temporal bones	Internal jugular veins and ninth, tenth, and eleventh cranial nerves
Lesser palatine foramina	Palatine bones	Lesser palatine nerves and blood vessels
Mandibular foramina	Mandible	Inferior alveolar nerves and blood vessels
Mental foramina	Mandible	Mental nerves and blood vessels
Optic canals and foramina	Sphenoid bone	Optic nerves and ophthalmic arteries
Petrotympanic fissures	Temporal bones	Chorda tympani nerves
Posterior superior alveolar foramina	Maxillae	Posterior superior alveolar nerves and blood vessels
Pterygoid canals	Sphenoid bone	Pterygoid nerves and blood vessels
Sphenopalatine foramina	Between palatine bones and sphenoid bone	Sphenopalatine arteries and posterior superior nasal nerves
Stylomastoid foramina	Temporal bones	Seventh cranial nerves
Superior orbital fissures	Sphenoid bone	Third, fourth, and sixth cranial nerves and ophthalmic nerves (or first division) of fifth cranial or trigeminal nerve and blood vessels
Supraorbital notches (foramina)	Frontal bone	Supraorbital nerves and arteries
Zygomaticofacial foramina	Zygomatic bones	Zygomaticofacial nerves and blood vessels
Zygomaticotemporal foramina	Zygomatic bones	Zygomaticotemporal nerves and blood vessels

*Openings of the nasal cavity are not included

skull. The coronal sutures and sagittal suture generally form a right angle with each other. Another single suture located between the occipital bone and each parietal bone is the **lambdoidal** (lam-**doid**-uhl) **suture**, which is far more serrated-looking than the others and resembles an upside down "V".

ANTERIOR VIEW OF EXTERNAL SKULL

When the external skull is viewed from the anterior aspect, certain bones of the skull (or parts of these bones) are noted (Figure 3-3).

These bones include: the single frontal bone, ethmoid bone, vomer, sphenoid bone, mandible, and also the paired lacrimal bones, nasal bones, inferior nasal conchae, and zygomatic bones as well as the maxillae. The facial bones as a group that form the facial features, the orbit, and the nasal cavity are also noted from this view.

Facial Bones From Anterior View. The facial bones noted on the anterior aspect of the skull include: the **lacrimal bone** (lak-ri-muhl), **nasal bone** (nay-zuhl), **vomer** (vo-muhr), **inferior nasal concha** (plural, **conchae**) (kong-kah, kong-kee), **zygomatic bone**

TABLE 3-4	**Skull Processes**	
PROCESS(ES) OF SKULL	**SKULL BONE**	**ASSOCIATED STRUCTURES**
Alveolar process	Mandible	Contains roots of mandibular teeth within alveoli
Alveolar process	Maxillae	Contains roots of maxillary teeth within alveoli
Condyloid processes	Mandible	Consist of mandibular condyles and necks
Coronoid processes	Mandible	Parts of mandibular rami
Frontal processes	Maxillae	Articulate with frontal bone
Frontal processes	Zygomatic bones	Form anterior lateral orbital walls
Lesser wings	Sphenoid bone	Anterior processes to body of sphenoid bone and form bases of orbital apices
Greater wings	Sphenoid bone	Posterolateral processes to body of sphenoid bone
Hamuli	Sphenoid bone	Inferior terminations of medial pterygoid plates
Mastoid processes	Temporal bones	Composed of mastoid air cells
Maxillary processes	Zygomatic bones	Form lateral part of infraorbital rims and parts of anterior lateral orbital walls
Orbital processes	Palatine bone	Small inferior parts of orbital apices
Palatine processes	Maxillae	Form anterior hard palate
Postglenoid processes	Temporal bones	Posterior structures to temporomandibular joints
Pterygoid processes	Sphenoid bone	Consists of medial and lateral pterygoid plates
Pyramidal processes	Palatine bones	On vertical plates that project posteriorly and lateralward
Styloid processes	Temporal bone	Serve as attachments for muscles and ligaments
Temporal processes	Zygomatic bones	Form parts of zygomatic arches
Zygomatic processes	Frontal bone	Lateral to orbits
Zygomatic processes	Maxillae	Form medial parts of infraorbital rims
Zygomatic processes	Temporal bones	Form parts of zygomatic arches

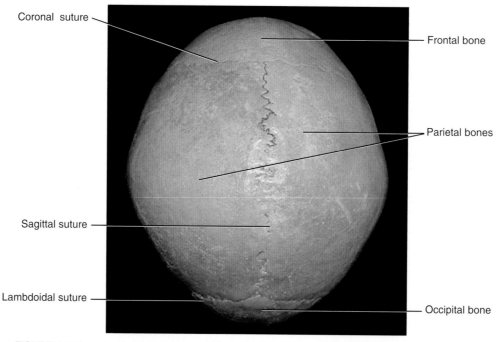

FIGURE 3-2 Superior view of the external skull with its cranial bones and associated sutures noted from this view.

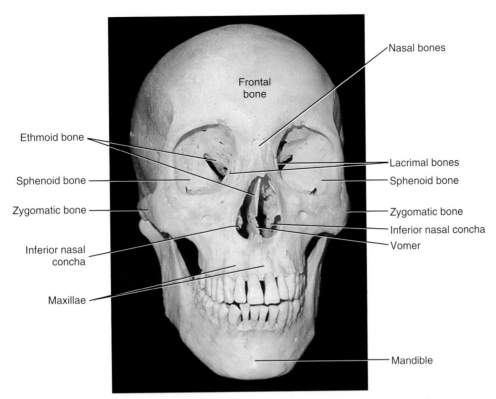

FIGURE 3-3 Anterior view of the external skull with its bones noted from this view.

TABLE 3-5	Orbital Bones
PART OF EACH ORBIT	**SKULL BONES**
Roof or superior wall	Frontal bone
Medial wall	Ethmoid bone and lacrimal bone
Lateral wall	Zygomatic bone and sphenoid bone
Apex or base	Sphenoid bone, maxilla, and palatine bone

(zy-go-**mat**-ik), maxilla (mak-**sil**-uh), and mandible (**man**-di-buhl) (Figure 3-4). However, the paired **palatine bone** (**pal**-ah-tine) is not noted from this view. In fact, the palatine bone is not considered to be a facial bone by anatomists, but for ease of learning it is included under the general heading of facial bones. This main division of the facial bones of the skull is discussed in detail later.

Orbit and Associated Structures From Anterior View. The orbit (**or**-bit), which contains and protects the eyeball, is a prominent feature of the anterior part of the skull (Figure 3-5 and see Figure 2-6). Certain skull bones form both the four walls and apex of each of the orbits (Table 3-5). The larger **orbital walls** (**or**-bi-tuhl) are composed of the orbital plates of the frontal bone (the roof or superior wall), the ethmoid bone (the greatest part of the medial wall), the lacrimal bone (at the anterior medial corner of the orbit and orbital surfaces of the maxilla, the floor or inferior wall), and the zygomatic bone (the anterior part of the lateral wall). The orbital surface of the greater wing of the sphenoid bone is also included (the posterior part of the lateral wall).

The **orbital apex** (plural, **apices**) is the deepest part of the orbit and is composed of both the lesser wing of the sphenoid bone (the base) and the palatine bone (a small inferior part) (Figure 3-6 and see Table 3-5). The round opening in the orbital apex is the **optic canal** (**op**-tik), which lies between the two roots of the lesser wing of the sphenoid bone (see Table 3-3). The second cranial or optic nerve passes through the optic canal to reach the eyeball. The ophthalmic artery also extends through the optic canal to reach the eye.

Two orbital fissures are noted on the anterior aspect: the superior and inferior orbital fissures (Figure 3-7 and see Table 3-3). Lateral to the optic canal is the curved and slitlike **superior orbital fissure**, located between the greater wing and lesser wing of the sphenoid bone. Similar to the optic canal, the superior orbital fissure connects the orbit with the cranial cavity. The third cranial or oculomotor nerve, the fourth cranial or trochlear nerve, the sixth cranial or abducens nerve, and the ophthalmic nerve (or first division from the fifth cranial or trigeminal nerve) and vein travel through this fissure (see Figures 8-8 and 8-9).

The **inferior orbital fissure** can also be noted between the greater wing of the sphenoid bone and the maxilla. The inferior orbital fissure connects the orbit with both the infratemporal fossa and pterygopalatine fossa (discussed later). Both the infraorbital and zygomatic nerves, which are branches of the maxillary nerve, and the infraorbital artery enter the orbit through this fissure. The inferior ophthalmic vein also travels through this fissure to join the pterygoid plexus of veins (see Figure 6-12).

The mostly sharp edge of the orbital opening or orbital rim (or margin) is the peripheral border of the base of the pyramid-shaped orbit. The orbital rim is rectangular-shaped with rounded corners; its margin is discontinuous at the lacrimal fossa. The superior half of the orbital rim is the **supraorbital rim** (**soo**-pruh-**or**-bi-tuhl) (or margin), and the inferior half is the **infraorbital rim** (**in**-fruh-**or**-bi-tuhl) (or margin) (see Figure 3-7). The frontal bone and zygomatic bones as well as the maxilla contribute to the orbital rim, which is generally

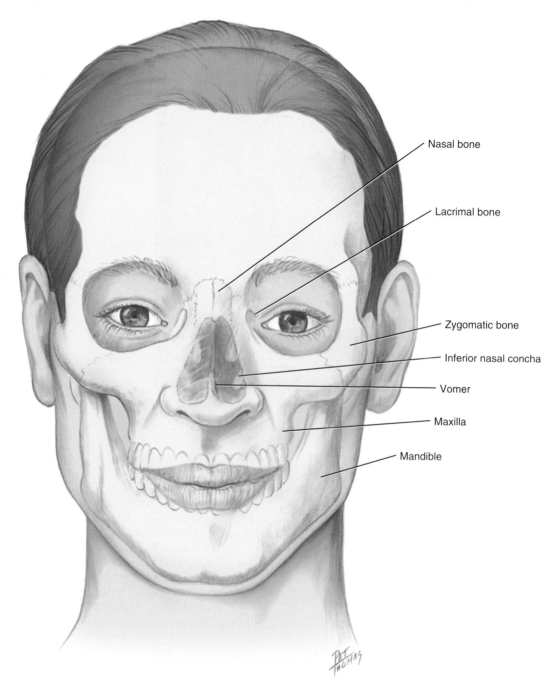

Nasal bone

Lacrimal bone

Zygomatic bone

Inferior nasal concha

Vomer

Maxilla

Mandible

FIGURE 3-4 Anterior view of the facial bones superimposed over the corresponding facial features formed from them.

strong to protect the orbital contents (also discussed later in the chapter with each of the bones).

A "notch", or more correctly described as a depression, in the midpoint of the infraorbital rim (or margin) can be palpated on a patient that is formed by the more vertical paired **zygomaticomaxillary suture** (zy-go-**mat**-i-ko-**mak**-sil-lare-ee). This suture is located between the two bones that form the infraorbital rim (or margin): the zygomatic bone with its maxillary process (lateral part) and maxilla with its zygomatic process (medial part).

Nasal Cavity and Associated Structures From Anterior View. The **nasal cavity** or *nasal fossa* can also be viewed on the skull from the anterior (Figure 3-8 and see Figures 2-7, 3-39, and 3-56).

The nasal cavity is the superior part of the respiratory tract and is located between the orbits. It has lateral walls and a floor with anterior and posterior openings, and it is mainly composed of bone and cartilage.

The bridge of the nose is formed from the paired nasal bones (see Figures 2-7 and 3-40). The nasion, a midpoint cephalometric landmark, is located at the junction of the frontal bone and nasal bones. The prominent anterior opening of the nasal cavity on the skull, the **piriform aperture** (**pir**-i-form), is large and triangular. And the large deeper posterior openings are the posterior nasal apertures or *choanae* (ko-**uh**-nee) (discussed later). The piriform aperture anchors the cartilaginous midline part of the nose, the

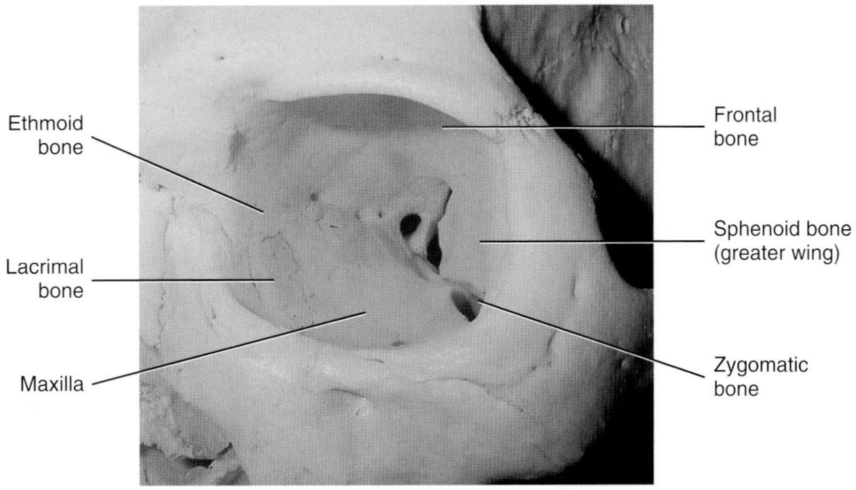

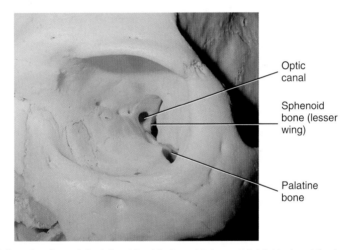

Ethmoid
bone

Frontal
bone

Lacrimal
bone

Sphenoid bone
(greater wing)

Maxilla

Zygomatic
bone

FIGURE 3-5 Anterior view of the left orbit of the skull with the orbital walls highlighted and the bones that form them noted.

Optic
canal

Sphenoid
bone (lesser
wing)

Palatine
bone

FIGURE 3-6 Anterior view of the left orbit with the orbital apex highlighted and the bones that form it noted.

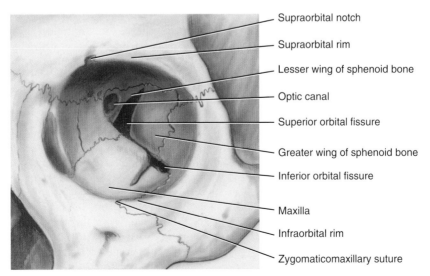

Supraorbital notch

Supraorbital rim

Lesser wing of sphenoid bone

Optic canal

Superior orbital fissure

Greater wing of sphenoid bone

Inferior orbital fissure

Maxilla

Infraorbital rim

Zygomaticomaxillary suture

FIGURE 3-7 Anterior view of the left orbit with the orbital fissures and the bones associated with them noted along with parts of the orbital rim.

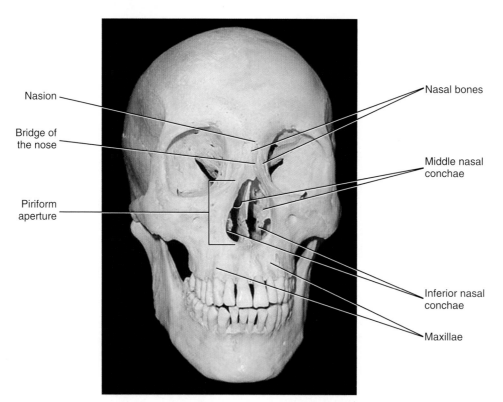

FIGURE 3-8 Anterior view of the external skull and nasal cavity with its features and associated bones noted.

nasal septal cartilage, in the intact state. Also when intact, the anterior openings to the nasal cavities are the nares, bordered laterally by the cartilaginous alae.

The floor of the nasal cavity is formed from the two separate bones of the hard palate: the palatine processes of the maxillae anteriorly and the horizontal plates of the palatine bones posteriorly (see Figure 3-16). The lateral walls of the nasal cavity are mainly formed by the maxillae. In addition, each lateral wall of the nasal cavity has three projecting structures that extend inward, which are the nasal conchae or *turbinates* (**tur**-bi-nates).

These nasal conchae are divided into: the superior, middle, and inferior nasal conchae. Each nasal concha projects into the nasal cavity. By projecting into the nasal cavity, the medial surface of these bony structures assists in increasing the surface area of the cavity by directing and deflecting airflow of inspired air. Protected by each nasal concha is a channel, the **nasal meatus** (see Figure 3-38). Each nasal meatus has openings through which the paranasal sinuses or nasolacrimal duct communicates with the nasal cavity. The superior nasal concha and middle nasal concha are bony projections from the ethmoid bone; the inferior nasal concha is a separate facial bone.

The vertical partition or fin, the nasal septum, divides the nasal cavity into two parts (Figure 3-9 and see Figures 2-7 and 3-39). Although it is frequently deflected slightly to the left or right, in general the septum is aligned perpendicularly. Anteriorly, the nasal septum is formed by both the perpendicular plate of the ethmoid bone superiorly and the nasal septal cartilage inferiorly; the posterior parts of the nasal septum are formed by the vomer.

LATERAL VIEW OF EXTERNAL SKULL

When the external skull is viewed from the lateral aspect, the division between the cranial bones and facial bones can be noted. This division

between the bones of the skull can be reinforced by making an imaginary diagonal line that passes inferior and posterior from the supraorbital ridge of the frontal bone to the tip of the mastoid process of the temporal bone (Figure 3-10). These two main divisions of the bones of the skull are discussed in more detail later.

Cranial Bones From Lateral View. Parts of the cranium are noted on the lateral aspect and include the following cranial bones: the occipital, frontal, parietal, temporal bones, as well as the **sphenoid bone** (**sfe**-noid) and **ethmoid bone** (**eth**-moid) (Figure 3-11). This main division of the bones of the skull is discussed in detail later.

Skull Sutures From Lateral View. Also noted on the lateral surface of the skull are the associated sutures of the cranial bones (see Figure 3-11 and Table 3-2). These sutures include: the coronal suture, an articulation between the frontal bone and each parietal bone, and the lambdoidal suture, an articulation between the occipital bone and each parietal bone. Also present is the arched paired **squamosal suture** (**skway**-moh-suhl), which is located between the temporal bone and parietal bone on each side.

Skull Lines From Lateral View. On the lateral surface of the skull are two separate parallel ridges, the temporal lines, crossing both the frontal bone and each parietal bone (Figure 3-12). The superior ridge is the **superior temporal line** (**tem**-puh-ruhl). The inferior ridge is the **inferior temporal line**, which is the superior border of the temporal fossa where the fan-shaped temporalis muscle originates (see Figure 4-22).

Skull Fossae From Lateral View. The **temporal fossa** is noted on the lateral surface of the skull (Figure 3-13). The temporal fossa is formed by parts of several bones of the skull and contains the body of the temporalis muscle. Inferior to the temporal fossa is the **infratemporal fossa** (in-fruh-**tem**-puh-ruhl). Deep to the infratemporal fossa and more difficult to see is the **pterygopalatine fossa** (**ter**-i-go-**pal**-uh-tine). The temporal, infratemporal, and pterygopalatine fossae

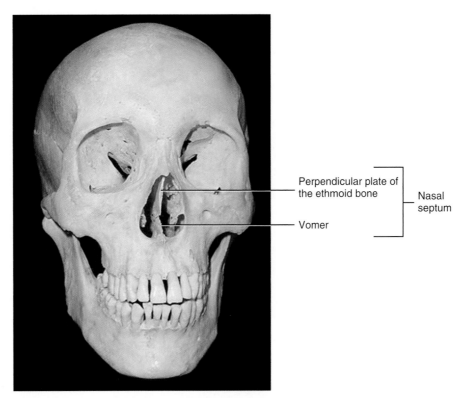

FIGURE 3-9 Anterior view of the external skull with the nasal septum and the bones that form it noted.

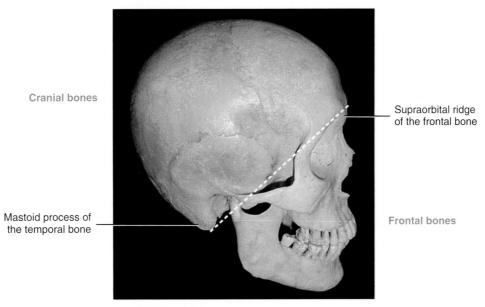

FIGURE 3-10 Lateral view of the external skull with an imaginary diagonal line (*dashed*) that divides the cranial bones and facial bones. The line passes inferior and posterior from the supraorbital ridge of the frontal bone to the tip of the mastoid process of the temporal bone. The cranium is formed from the cranial bones, with the facial features formed from the facial bones.

are discussed in detail later, including the head and neck structures that travel through them.

Zygomatic Arch and Temporomandibular Joint From Lateral View. Farther inferior on the lateral aspect of the skull are prominent landmarks (Figure 3-14). The zygomatic arch or cheekbone is noted, which is formed by the union of the slender zygomatic process of the temporal bone and the broad temporal process of the zygomatic bone (see Table 3-4 and Figure 2-9). The suture between these two bones is the paired **temporozygomatic suture** (**tem**-puh-roh-zi-go-**mat**-ik) (see Table 3-2). The zygomatic arch serves as the origin for the prominent masseter muscle (see Figure 4-21).

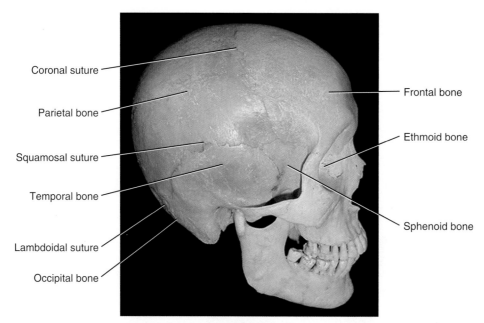

FIGURE 3-11 Lateral view of the external skull with the cranial bones highlighted and noted along with the associated suture lines.

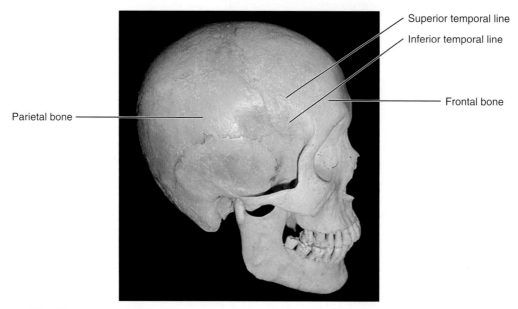

FIGURE 3-12 Lateral view of the external skull with the superior and inferior temporal lines and associated bones noted.

Also noted is the nearby temporomandibular joint (TMJ), a movable articulation between the temporal bone and the mandible on each side of the skull (see Chapter 5). More specific landmarks of each of these bones are discussed later.

INFERIOR VIEW OF EXTERNAL SKULL

Most of the structures of the inferior view of the external skull are noted on the skull when the mandible is removed. The zygomatic bones, vomer, temporal bones, sphenoid bone, occipital bones, and palatine bones, as well as the maxillae are noted on the inferior view of the skull's external surface (Figure 3-15).

Hard Palate From Inferior View. At the anterior part of the skull's inferior surface is the hard palate, which is bordered by the **alveolar process of the maxilla** (al-**vee**-uh-luhr) (**mak**-sil-uh) that usually contains the roots of the maxillary teeth within the alveoli (Figure 3-16 and see Figure 2-15 and Table 3-4). The hard palate is formed from two separate bones: the two palatine processes of the maxillae anteriorly and the two horizontal plates of the palatine bones posteriorly, with an articulation at the prominent median palatine suture that underlies the median palatine raphe (see Figure 2-15 and Table 3-2). The other nearby suture is the **transverse palatine suture** (tranz-**vurs**), an articulation located between the two palatine processes of the maxillae and the two horizontal plates of the palatine bones.

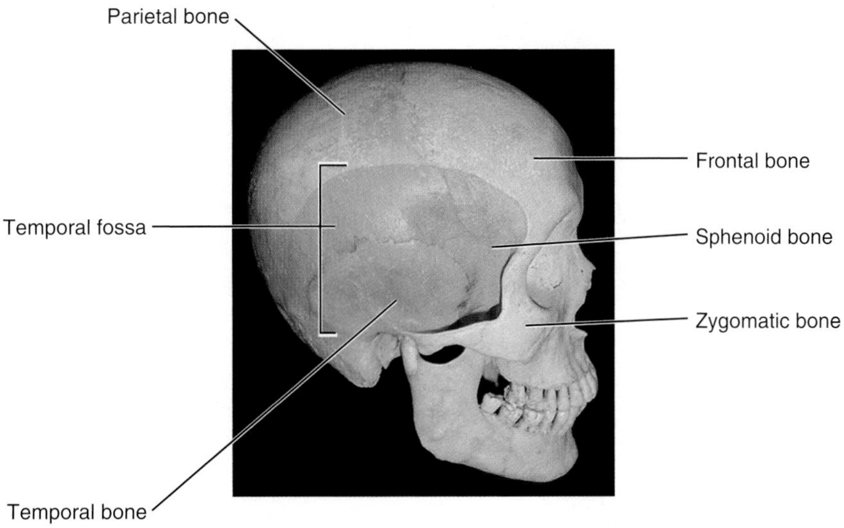

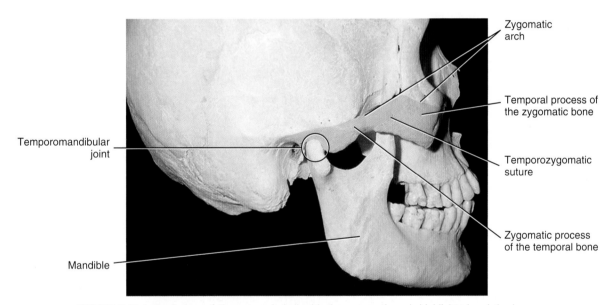

FIGURE 3-13 Lateral view of the external skull with the temporal fossa highlighted and the bones that form it noted.

FIGURE 3-14 Lateral view of the external skull with the zygomatic arch highlighted and the bones that form it noted along with the nearby temporomandibular joint (*circle*).

The hard palate forms the floor of the nasal cavity as well as the roof of the mouth. The posterior edge of the hard palate forms the inferior border of two funnel-shaped cavities, the **posterior nasal apertures** or *choanae* as discussed earlier with the nasal cavity (see Figure 3-16). These apertures serve as the posterior openings of the nasal cavity. Each posterior nasal aperture is bordered medially by the vomer, inferiorly by the horizontal plate of the palatine bone, laterally by the medial pterygoid plate of the sphenoid bone, and superiorly by the body of the sphenoid bone. Thus the posterior nasal apertures are located between the nasal cavity and the nasopharynx, allowing for communication.

Near the superior border of each posterior nasal aperture is a small canal, the **pterygoid canal** (**ter**-i-goid) (see Figure 3-16 and Table 3-3). The pterygoid canal runs through the medial pterygoid plate of the sphenoid bone (discussed next) to the posterior border of the pterygopalatine fossa. Thus the pterygoid canal extends to open into the pterygopalatine fossa and carries the pterygoid nerve and blood vessels (discussed later).

Middle Part of Skull From Inferior View. The middle part of the skull from the inferior view also has prominent landmarks (Figure 3-17). The lateral borders of the posterior nasal apertures are formed on each side by the **pterygoid process** of the sphenoid bone (see Table 3-4).

Each pterygoid process consists of a thin **medial pterygoid plate** and a flattened **lateral pterygoid plate**. The depression located between the medial plate and lateral plate is the **pterygoid fossa**. At the inferior part of the medial plate of the pterygoid process is a thin curved process, the **hamulus** (plural, **hamuli**) (**ham**-u-lis, **ham**-u-ly). The sphenoid bone and its structure are discussed in detail later.

External Skull Foramina From Inferior View. The inferior surface of the external skull has a large number of foramina (Figure 3-18 and see Table 3-3). These openings provide entrances and exits for the arteries and veins that supply the brain and facial tissue (see Chapter 6). They also allow the cranial nerves to pass to and from the brain (see Figure 8-5).

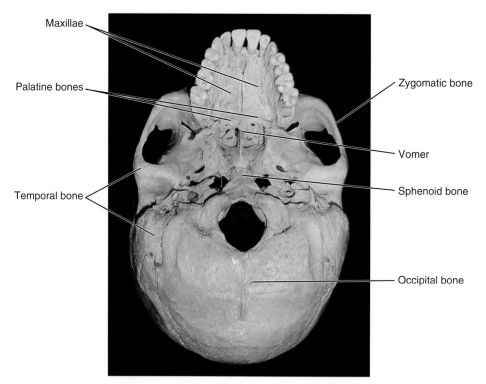

Maxillae

Palatine bones

Temporal bone

Zygomatic bone

Vomer

Sphenoid bone

Occipital bone

FIGURE 3-15 Inferior view of the external surface of the skull with its bones noted from this view.

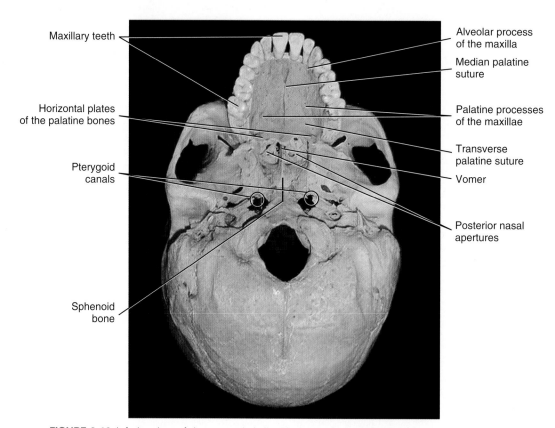

Maxillary teeth

Horizontal plates
of the palatine bones

Pterygoid
canals

Sphenoid
bone

Alveolar process
of the maxilla

Median palatine
suture

Palatine processes
of the maxillae

Transverse
palatine suture

Vomer

Posterior nasal
apertures

FIGURE 3-16 Inferior view of the external skull with the hard palate highlighted and the bones that form it noted along with other features noted. Note the pterygoid canals (*circles*).

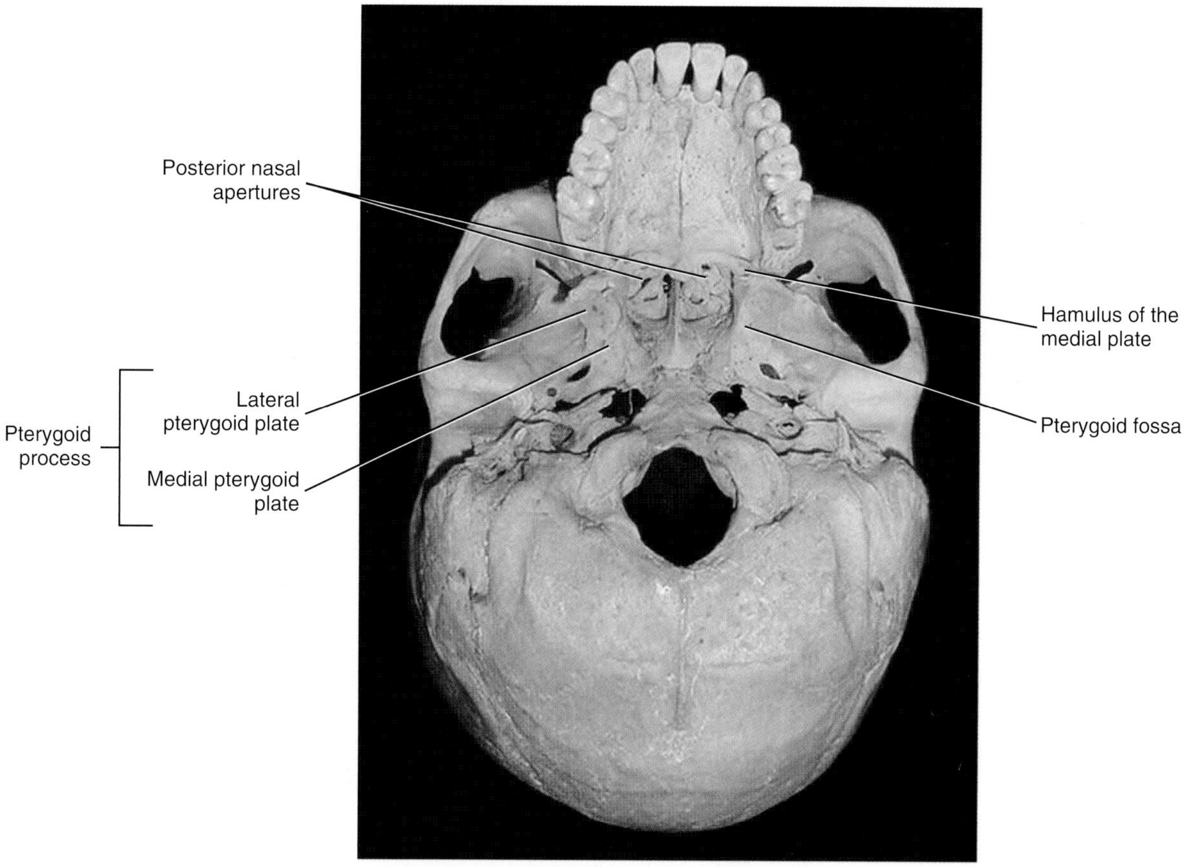

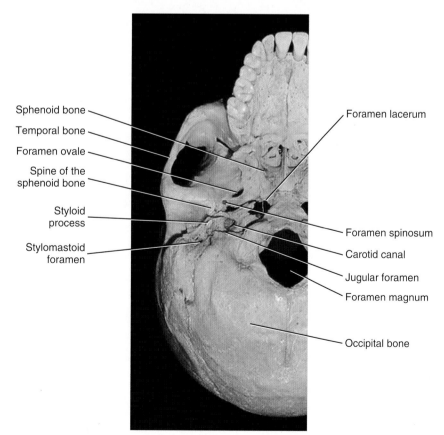

Posterior nasal apertures

Hamulus of the medial plate

Pterygoid process

Lateral pterygoid plate

Medial pterygoid plate

Pterygoid fossa

FIGURE 3-17 Inferior view of the external skull with its features of the middle section noted.

Sphenoid bone

Temporal bone

Foramen ovale

Spine of the sphenoid bone

Styloid process

Stylomastoid foramen

Foramen lacerum

Foramen spinosum

Carotid canal

Jugular foramen

Foramen magnum

Occipital bone

FIGURE 3-18 Inferior view of the external skull with its foramina and associated structures noted.

The larger anterior oval opening on the sphenoid bone, the **foramen ovale** (o-**vuh**-lee), is for the mandibular nerve (or third division) of the fifth cranial or trigeminal nerve (see Figure 8-7). The adjacent smaller and more posterior opening is the **foramen spinosum** (spine-o-sum), which carries the middle meningeal artery into the cranial cavity. The foramen spinosum receives its name from the nearby (angular) **spine of the sphenoid bone**, which is at the posterior extremity of the sphenoid bone.

Also on the external surface of the skull is the large, irregularly shaped **foramen lacerum** (**las**-er-uhm), which when intact is filled with cartilage. This foramen is located between the sphenoid bone, apex of petrous part of the temporal bone, and basilar part of occipital bone (discussed later). Posterolateral to the foramen lacerum is a round opening in the petrous part of the temporal bone, the **carotid canal** (kuh-**rot**-id). The carotid canal carries the internal carotid artery and carotid plexus of nerves. The carotid plexus of nerves is a network of intersecting sympathetic nerves that run parallel to the carotid artery into the head. A pointed bony projection, the **styloid process** (**sty**-loid) of the temporal bone, is noted lateral and posterior to the carotid canal (see Table 3-4). Immediately posterior to the

styloid process is the **stylomastoid foramen** (sty-lo-**mass**-toid), an opening through which the seventh cranial or facial nerve exits from the skull to the face.

The **jugular foramen** (**jug**-u-luhr), just medial to the styloid process, is visible if the skull is tilted to one side. The jugular foramen is the opening through which pass the internal jugular vein and three cranial nerves: the ninth cranial or glossopharyngeal nerve, the tenth cranial or vagus nerve, and the eleventh cranial or accessory nerve.

The largest opening on the inferior view is the **foramen magnum** (**mag**-nuhm) of the occipital bone, through which the spinal cord, vertebral arteries, and eleventh cranial or accessory nerve pass.

SUPERIOR VIEW OF INTERNAL SKULL

For a superior view of the internal skull, again remove the cap of the skull. The frontal bone, ethmoid bone, sphenoid bone, temporal bones, occipital bone, and parietal bones are noted from this view of the internal surface of the skull (Figure 3-19).

Internal Skull Foramina From Superior View. Also present on the superior surface of the internal skull are the inner openings of

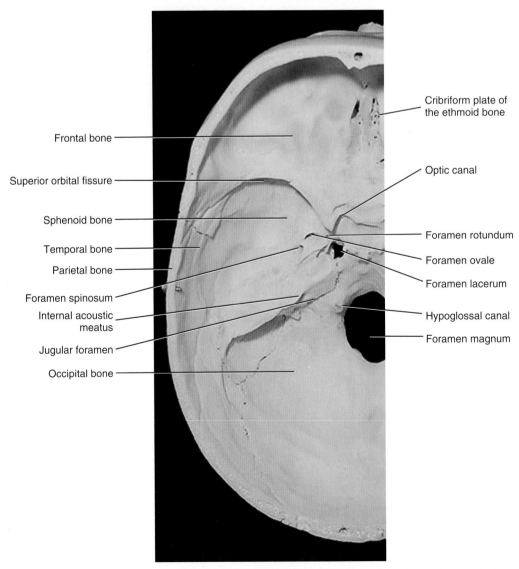

FIGURE 3-19 Superior view of the internal surface of the skull with its foramina and associated structures noted.

the optic canal, superior orbital fissure, foramen ovale, foramen spinosum, foramen lacerum, jugular foramen, and foramen magnum, as discussed before when viewing the external skull surface (see Figure 3-19 and Table 3-3). Additionally, other foramina are present on the internal surface of the skull. The perforated **cribriform plate (krib-ri-form),** with numerous foramina for the first cranial or olfactory nerve, and the **foramen rotundum** (roh-**tun**-dum) for the maxillary nerve (or second division) of the fifth cranial or trigeminal nerve are also noted from this view (see Figure 8-7).

Finally, also present are the **hypoglossal canal** (hi-poh-**gloss**-uhl) for the twelfth cranial or hypoglossal nerve and the **internal acoustic meatus** (uh-**koos**-tik) for the seventh cranial or facial nerve and the eighth cranial or vestibulocochlear nerve.

CRANIAL BONES

The cranium is formed from the eight cranial bones. The cranial bones include: the single occipital bone, frontal bone, sphenoid bone, and ethmoid bone as well as the paired parietal bones and temporal bones (Figure 3-20).

OCCIPITAL BONE

The occipital bone is a single cranial bone that forms the posterior part of the skull and the base of the cranium (Figure 3-21). It is an irregular four-sided bone that is somewhat curved. It can be divided into four parts: the single squamous part, single basilar part, and

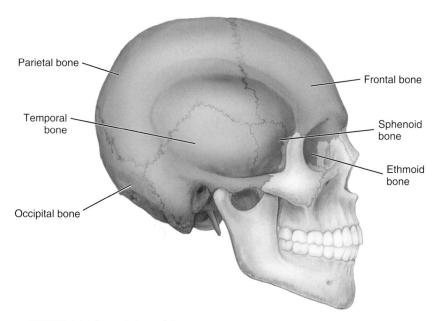

FIGURE 3-20 Lateral view of the external skull with the cranial bones highlighted.

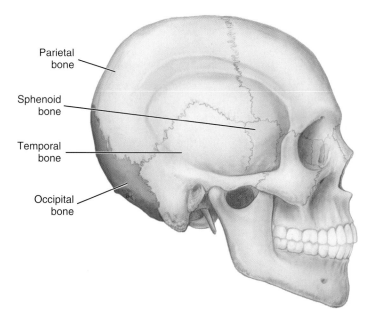

FIGURE 3-21 Lateral view of the external skull with the occipital bone highlighted and its bony articulations noted.

paired lateral parts. The occipital bone articulates with the parietal bones, temporal bones, and sphenoid bone of the skull. The occipital bone also articulates with the first cervical vertebra or atlas (see Figure 3-62). The occipital bone can be additionally studied from an inferior view as well as a posterior view of its external surface.

Occipital Bone From Inferior View. On the external surface of the occipital bone from an inferior view, it can be noted that the

foramen magnum is completely formed by the occipital bone (Figure 3-22 and see Table 3-3).

On the lateral part of the occipital bone and anterior to the foramen magnum are the paired **occipital condyles**, which are curved and smooth projections. The occipital condyles have a movable articulation with the atlas, the first cervical vertebra of the vertebral column (discussed later). On the stout **basilar part of the occipital**

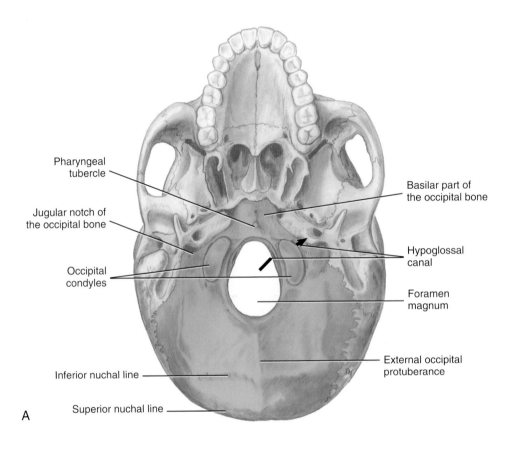

Pharyngeal tubercle

Jugular notch of the occipital bone

Occipital condyles

Inferior nuchal line

Superior nuchal line

A

Basilar part of the occipital bone

Hypoglossal canal

Foramen magnum

External occipital protuberance

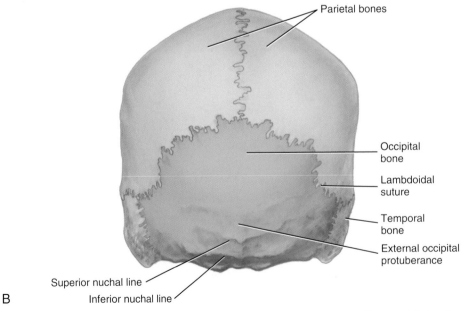

Parietal bones

Occipital bone

Lambdoidal suture

Temporal bone

External occipital protuberance

Superior nuchal line

Inferior nuchal line

B

FIGURE 3-22 External surface of the skull with the occipital bone highlighted. From an inferior view, its features are noted including the passageway of the hypoglossal canal (*arrow*) **(A),** and also from a posterior view **(B).**

bone (**bay**-si-luhr), which is a four-sided plate anterior to the foramen magnum, with a midline projection, the **pharyngeal tubercle** (fuh-**rin**-je-uhl).

When tilting the skull, prominent openings anterior and lateral to the foramen magnum are noted on the inferior view of the occipital bone (see Table 3-3). These openings are the paired hypoglossal canals (see Figure 3-22, *A*). The twelfth cranial or hypoglossal nerve is transmitted through the hypoglossal canal. Also present is the **jugular notch of the occipital bone**, which forms the medial part of the jugular foramen (the lateral part is from the temporal bone).

Occipital Bone From Posterior View. On the external surface of the occipital bone from a posterior view, the horizontally placed nuchal lines can be noted that mark the superior limit of the neck. The most raised of the nuchal lines includes the **superior nuchal line** (**noo**-kuhl) and the **inferior nuchal line** (see Figure 3-22, *B*). These curved ridges on the external surface of the occipital bone serve as sites for muscle attachments; the originations of the sternocleidomastoid, trapezius, and occipitalis muscles are from the superior nuchal line (see Figures 4-1 and 4-3). Another ridge on the midline of the bone's posterior surface is the **external occipital protuberance** (pro-**too**-buhr-uhns) that runs vertically, intersecting with the nuchal lines.

FRONTAL BONE

The frontal bone is a single cranial bone that forms the anterior part of the skull superior to the eyes in the frontal region. It includes the majority of the forehead as well as the roof of each orbit (Figure 3-23 and see Figures 2-2 and 2-6). It develops as two bones, which are usually fused together by 5 or 6 years of age.

The frontal bone's part of the superior temporal line and inferior temporal line is noted when the bone is viewed from the lateral aspect as discussed earlier. The frontal bone articulates with the parietal bones, sphenoid bone, lacrimal bones, nasal bones, ethmoid bone, and zygomatic bones, as well as the maxillae. Internally, the frontal bone contains the paired paranasal sinuses, the frontal sinuses (discussed later). The frontal bone can also be studied from both anterior and inferior viewpoints.

Frontal Bone From Anterior View. On the anterior aspect, landmarks are noted on the frontal bone (Figure 3-24 and see Figures 2-2 and 2-6). The orbital plate of the frontal bone forms the superior wall or orbital roof. The curved elevations over the superior part of the orbit are the supraorbital ridges, subjacent to the eyebrows, with these ridges more prominent in adult males.

Located between the supraorbital ridges is the glabella, the smooth elevated area also between the eyebrows, which tends to be flat in children and adult females, but forms a rounded prominence in adult males. The prominence of the forehead, the frontal eminence, is also evident. In contrast, the frontal eminence is usually more pronounced in children and adult females. Lateral to the orbit is a projection, the orbital surface of the **zygomatic process of the frontal bone** (see Table 3-4).

The **supraorbital notch** (or supraorbital foramen) is located on the medial part of the more inferiorly located supraorbital rim, where the supraorbital nerve and artery travel from the orbit to the frontal region. Due to the presence of the nerve, palpation of this indentation in the supraorbital rim in a patient can produce transient soreness during an extraoral examination.

The frontal bone articulates with the nasal bones and the frontal processes of the maxillae to form the root of the nose (see Figure 2-7).

Frontal Bone From Inferior View. From the inferior view of the frontal bone, each **lacrimal fossa** is noted (Figure 3-25 and see Figure 2-6). The lacrimal fossa is located just internal to the lateral part of the supraorbital rim. This fossa contains the lacrimal gland, which produces lacrimal fluid or tears (see Chapter 7). After lubricating the eye, the lacrimal fluid empties into the nasal cavity through the nasolacrimal duct.

PARIETAL BONES

The parietal bones are paired cranial bones that articulate with each other at the sagittal suture (Figure 3-26 and see Table 3-2). Each bone is relatively square, like a curved plate, and has four borders. These bones are located posterior to the frontal bone, forming the greater part of the right and left lateral walls and the roof of the skull. The

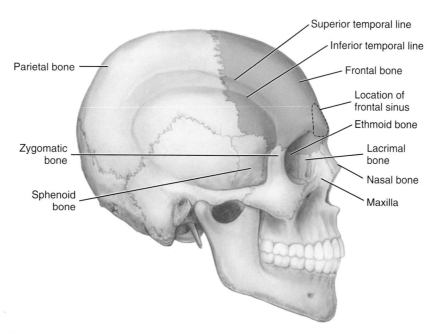

FIGURE 3-23 Lateral view of the skull with the frontal bone highlighted and its bony articulations and features noted including the location of the frontal sinuses (*dashed lines*).

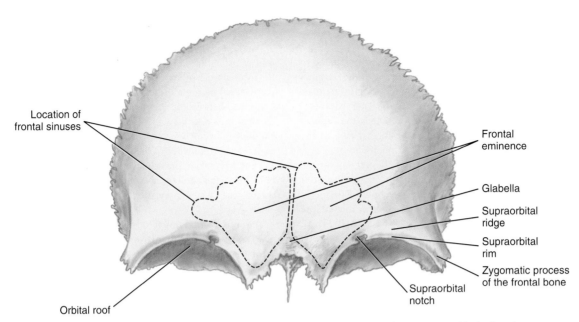

FIGURE 3-24 Anterior view of the disarticulated frontal bone with its features noted including the location of the frontal sinuses (*dashed lines*).

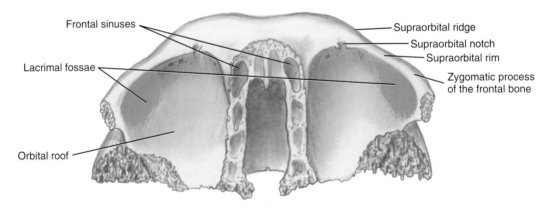

FIGURE 3-25 Inferior view of the disarticulated frontal bone with the lacrimal fossae highlighted and other features noted.

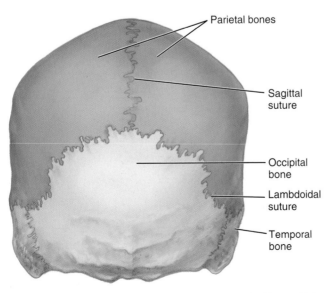

FIGURE 3-26 Posterior view of the skull with the parietal bones highlighted and some of its bony articulations noted.

parietal bones also articulate with the occipital bone, frontal bone, temporal bones, and sphenoid bone; the parietal bones articulate with the occipital bone at the lambdoidal suture.

TEMPORAL BONES

The **temporal bones** are paired cranial bones that form the lateral walls of the skull in the temporal region and part of the base of the skull in the auricular region. Each bone is deep to the temple, the superficial side of the head posterior to each eye (Figure 3-27). Each temporal bone articulates with the zygomatic bone and parietal bone as well as the occipital bone, sphenoid bone, and the mandible. Each temporal bone is composed of three parts: the squamous, tympanic, and petrous parts.

These three parts of the temporal bone can be best viewed all at one time from the lateral aspect of the skull (Figure 3-28). The large, fan-shaped, flat part on each of the temporal bones is the **squamous part of the temporal bone** (**skway**-muhs). The second part is the small, irregularly shaped **tympanic part of the temporal bone** (tim-**pan**-ik), which is associated with the ear canal. The third part is the **petrous part of the temporal bone** (**pet**-ruhs), which is inferiorly located and helps form the cranial floor.

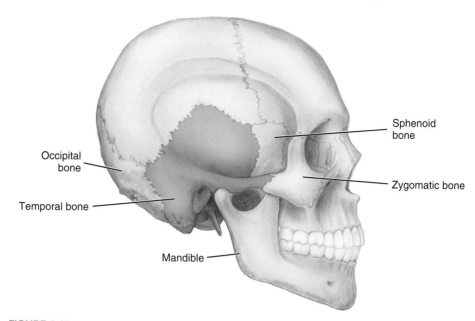

FIGURE 3-27 Lateral view of the skull with the temporal bone highlighted and its bony articulations noted.

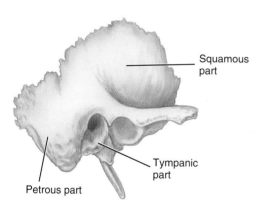

FIGURE 3-28 Lateral view of disarticulated temporal bone and its three parts noted: the squamous, tympanic, and petrous parts.

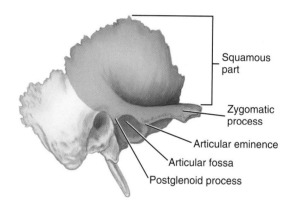

FIGURE 3-29 Lateral view of the disarticulated temporal bone with its squamous part highlighted.

Squamous Part of the Temporal Bone. In addition to helping form the braincase, the squamous part of the temporal bone forms the **zygomatic process of the temporal bone**, which consequentially goes on to be a part of the zygomatic arch (Figure 3-29 and see Table 3-4). This part of the temporal bone also forms the cranial part of the temporomandibular joint with its own complex structures (see Chapter 5). On the inferior surface of the zygomatic process of the temporal bone is the **articular fossa** (ahr-**tik**-u-luhr) (see Figures 5-2 and 5-4). Anterior to the articular fossa is the **articular eminence** and posterior to it is the **postglenoid process** (post-**gle**-noid) (see Table 3-4).

Tympanic Part of the Temporal Bone. The tympanic part of the temporal bone forms most of the **external acoustic meatus**, a short canal leading to the tympanic membrane when intact, located posterior to the articular fossa (Figure 3-30 and see Figure 2-4 and Table 3-3). Also, posterior to the articular fossa, the tympanic part is separated from the petrous part by the **petrotympanic fissure** (pet-roh-tim-**pan**-ik), through which the chorda tympani nerve emerges.

Petrous Part of the Temporal Bone. On the inferior aspect of the petrous part of the temporal bone and posterior to the external

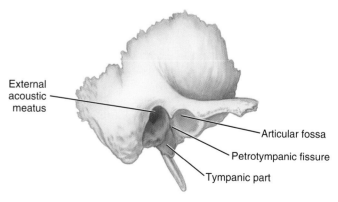

FIGURE 3-30 Lateral view of the temporal bone with its tympanic part highlighted.

acoustic meatus is a large roughened projection, the **mastoid process** (**mass**-toid) (Figure 3-31 and see Table 3-4). The mastoid process is composed of air spaces or **mastoid air cells** that communicate with the middle ear and also serves as the site for attachment of the large cervical muscles including the sternocleidomastoid muscle (see

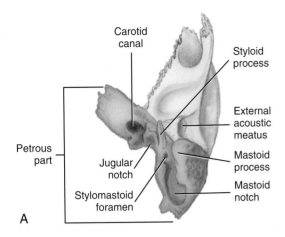

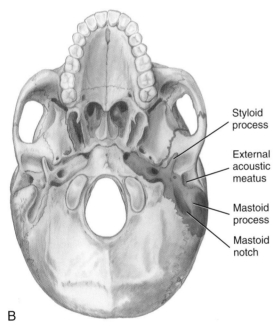

FIGURE 3-31 Inferior view of the disarticulated temporal bone with its petrous part highlighted and its features noted **(A)**, and also an inferior view of the external skull surface with the petrous part of the temporal bone highlighted **(B)**.

Figure 4-1). Medial to the mastoid process is the deep groove of the **mastoid notch** (see Figure 3-31).

Inferior and medial to the external acoustic meatus is a long, pointed bony projection, the styloid process, which is a structure that serves as a site for muscle attachments of the tongue as well as the pharynx (see Table 3-4). The nearby stylomastoid foramen carries the seventh cranial or facial nerve and is named for its location between the styloid process and mastoid process (see Table 3-3).

Also noted is the large circular aperture of the carotid canal, which first ascends vertically, and then making a bend, runs horizontally and anteriorly medialward. The carotid canal transmits the internal carotid artery and the carotid plexus of nerves into the cranium. When the skull is tilted, the **jugular notch of the temporal bone** is visible (see Table 3-3), which forms the lateral part of the jugular foramen (the medial part is from the occipital bone).

On the intracranial surface of the petrous part of the temporal bone is the internal acoustic meatus, which carries the eighth cranial or

vestibulocochlear nerve and the seventh cranial or facial nerve (see Figure 3-19 and Table 3-3). The size of the internal acoustic meatus varies considerably; its margins are smooth and rounded. The internal acoustic meatus leads into a canal approximately 1 cm in length, which then runs lateralward. Both of these cranial nerves enter the skull at the internal acoustic meatus from the brain. The vestibulocochlear nerve remains within the petrous part of the temporal bone, which contains the inner ear. In contrast, the facial nerve takes a convoluted path through the bone, eventually emerging at the stylomastoid foramen.

SPHENOID BONE

The sphenoid bone is a single cranial bone that somewhat resembles a bat with its wings extended; others see a butterfly taking wing (Figures 3-32 to 3-34). The sphenoid is a midline bone that runs through the midsagittal plane and thus is internally wedged between several other bones in the anterior part of the cranium. This bone assists with the formation of the base of the cranium and the lateral borders of the skull, as well as the floors and walls of each of the orbits. The sphenoid bone articulates with the frontal bone, parietal bones, ethmoid bone, temporal bones, zygomatic bones, palatine bones, vomer, and occipital bones as well as the maxillae. Thus the sphenoid helps to connect the cranial skeleton to the facial skeleton.

Since this bone is complex and centrally located, parts of the sphenoid are encountered in almost every significant juncture of the skull. The bone itself consists of a body and its processes along with a number of features and openings. Both of these factors allow the sphenoid bone to be noted from various viewpoints of the skull. Thus it is one of the more difficult bones of the skull to describe and visualize. The sphenoid bone is also important to dental professionals because it is the attachment site for certain muscles of mastication and also provides passage by way of its foramina for the branches of the fifth cranial or trigeminal nerve that serves the oral cavity.

Body of the Sphenoid Bone. In the center of the sphenoid is the **body of the sphenoid bone,** which articulates on its anterior surface with the ethmoid bone and posteriorly with the basilar part of the occipital bone (see Figures 3-24, 3-32, and 3-33). The body contains the paranasal sinuses, the **sphenoidal sinuses (sfe-**noid-uhl) (discussed in detail later).

On the superior surface of the body is a deep saddle-shaped depression, the **sella turcica (sell-**uh **tur-**ki-kuh) or pituitary fossa. Its deepest part is the **hypophyseal fossa** (hi-**pof-**i-zee-uhl), which contains the pituitary gland (or hypophysis). It is a pea-sized gland that controls the function of the endocrine glands. Posterior to this fossa is the **dorsum sellae (dor-**suhm **sell-**ee), a square part of the bone; anterior to the fossa is a slight elevation, the **tuberculum sellae** (too-**bur-**ku-luhm). Additionally, this part of the sphenoid bone presents a prominent **ethmoidal spine** for articulation with the cribriform plate of the ethmoid bone. The anterior part of the body of the sphenoid bone helps form part of the nasal cavity. The paired cavernous sinus covers each of the lateral surfaces of the body; this venous sinus is important to dental care since it can be involved in the serious spread of dental (or odontogenic) infection (see Figure 6-12 and Chapter 12).

Processes of the Sphenoid Bone. The body of the sphenoid bone has three paired processes that project from it: the lesser wing, greater wing, and pterygoid process (see Figures 3-32 to 3-34 and Table 3-4). The **lesser wing** of the sphenoid bone is an anterior process that forms the base of the orbital apex.

The **greater wing** of the sphenoid bone is a posterolateral process (see Figures 3-5 and 3-6). Each greater wing is divided into two

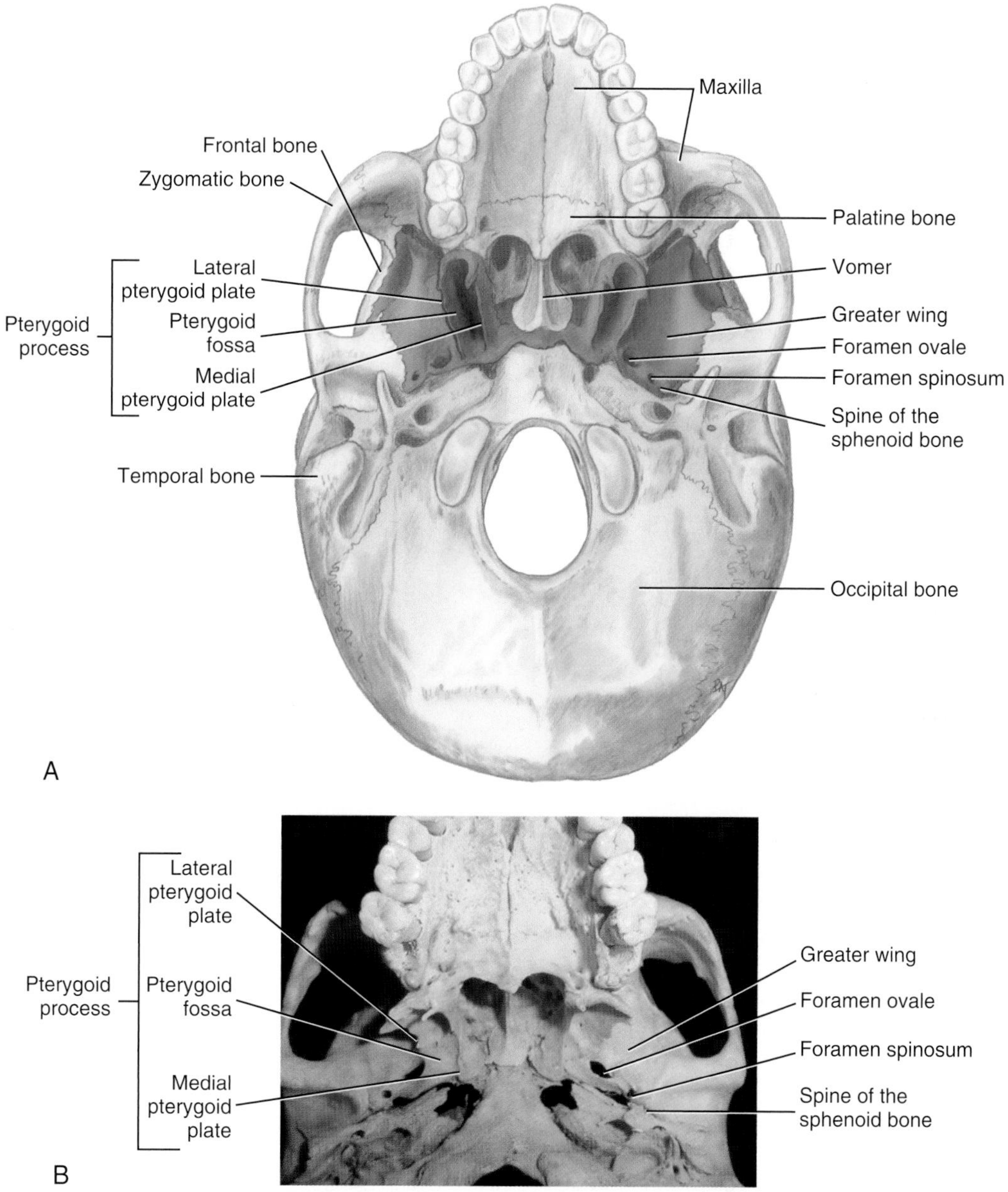

FIGURE 3-32 Inferior view of the external surface of the skull with the sphenoid bone highlighted with its bony articulations and features noted **(A)**, and also a close-up of the sphenoid bone **(B).**

smaller surfaces by the infratemporal crest: the temporal and infratemporal surfaces. A sharp pointed structure, the (angular) spine of the sphenoid bone, is located at the posterior corner of each greater wing of the sphenoid bone.

Inferior to the greater wing of the sphenoid bone is the pterygoid process, a site of attachment for certain muscles of mastication. The pterygoid process consists of two plates that project inferiorly, the flattened lateral pterygoid plate and thinner medial pterygoid plate; the pterygoid fossa lies between the two plates (see Figure 3-17). The infratemporal fossa is located lateral to the lateral pterygoid plate. The hamulus, a thin curved process, is the inferior termination of the medial pterygoid plate. The pterygomaxillary fissure is located between the pterygoid process of the sphenoid bone and the maxillary tuberosity of the maxilla (see Figure 3-61).

Openings of the Sphenoid Bone. Foramina and fissures are located within the sphenoid bone that carry nerves and blood vessels of the head and neck significant to dental professionals. These include the superior orbital fissure (carrying the ophthalmic nerve), foramen rotundum (carrying the maxillary nerve), and foramen ovale (carrying the mandibular nerve) (see Figures 3-32 and 3-33 and Table 3-3). In addition, the sphenoid bone contains the foramen spinosum (with the middle meningeal artery, middle meningeal vein, and the meningeal branch of the mandibular nerve). A part of the foramen lacerum is also noted (other parts are from both the temporal bone and occipital bone).

ETHMOID BONE

The ethmoid bone is a single midline cranial bone of the skull that runs through the midsagittal plane (Figure 3-35). The ethmoid bone is located anterior to the sphenoid bone in the anterior part of the cranium. The ethmoid bone articulates with the frontal bone,

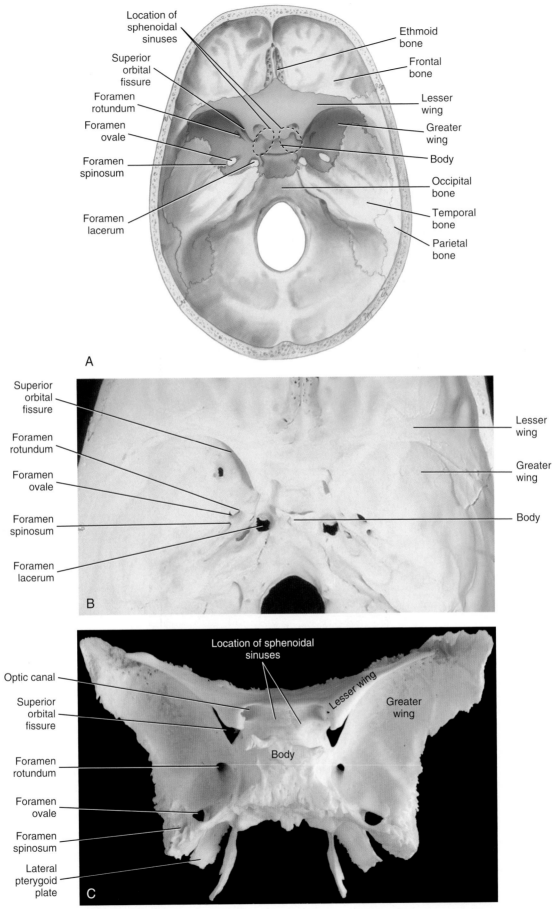

FIGURE 3-33 Superior view of the internal surface of the skull with the sphenoid bone highlighted and its bony articulations and features noted including the location of the sphenoidal sinuses (*dashed lines*) **(A)**, with a close-up of the sphenoid bone **(B)**, and also a superior view of the disarticulated sphenoid bone **(C)**.

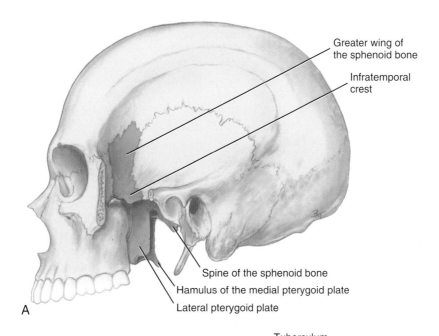

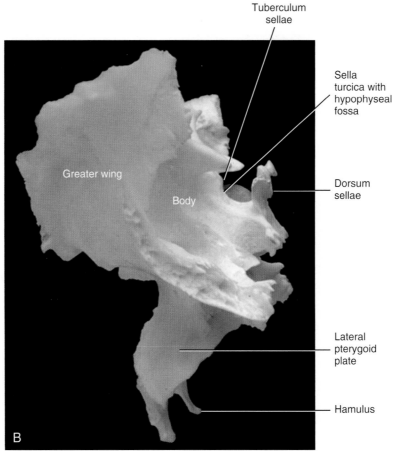

FIGURE 3-34 Lateral cutaway view of the upper part of the skull with the sphenoid bone highlighted and its features noted **(A)**, and also a lateral view of the disarticulated sphenoid bone **(B)**. The sphenoid bone helps to connect the cranial skeleton to the facial skeleton.

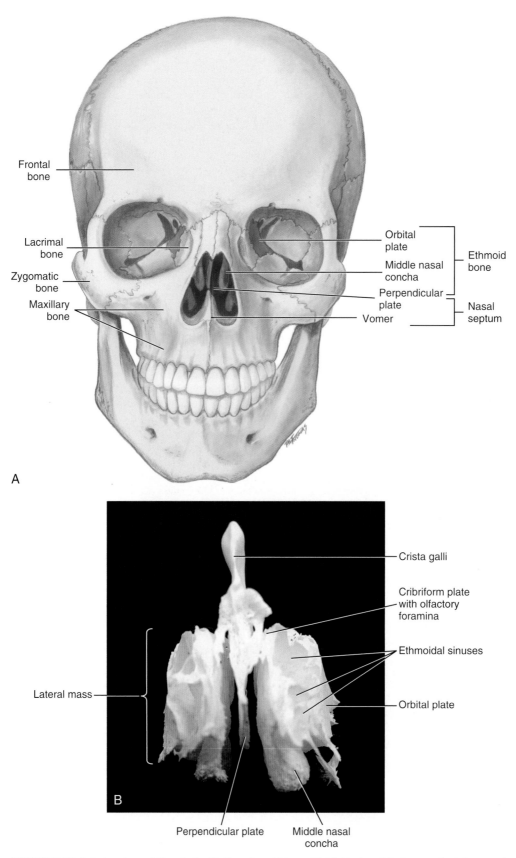

FIGURE 3-35 Anterior view of the skull with the ethmoid bone highlighted and its bony articulations and features noted **(A)**, and also an anterior view of the disarticulated ethmoid bone **(B)**. (***B** courtesy of Neil S. Norton, PhD, Professor of Oral Biology, School of Dentistry, Creighton University, Omaha, NE.)*

sphenoid bone, lacrimal bones, and the maxillae, as well as adjoining the vomer at its inferior and posterior borders. The bone has a number of features, but unlike the sphenoid, the ethmoid cannot be noted from the usual viewpoints of the skull. Because of these factors, if the sphenoid is considered the most difficult cranial bone to describe and then visualize, the more hidden ethmoid is the second most difficult.

Plates and Associated Structures of the Ethmoid Bone. There are two unpaired plates forming the ethmoid bone: the midline vertical **perpendicular plate** (per-pen-**dik**-u-luhr) and the horizontal cribriform plate, which cross over one another. The perpendicular plate is viewed within the structure of the nasal cavity, aiding the nasal septal cartilage and vomer in forming the nasal septum (see Figures 3-35 and 3-39). A vertical midline continuation of the perpendicular plate superiorly into the cranial cavity is the wedge-shaped **crista galli** (**kris**-tuh **gal**-ee), which serves as an attachment for layers covering the brain.

The horizontal cribriform plate is within the inner surface of the cranial cavity and is present on the superior surface of the ethmoid bone surrounding the crista galli. It is perforated by numerous olfactory foramina to allow the passage of the olfactory nerves for the sense of smell (Figures 3-36 and 3-37).

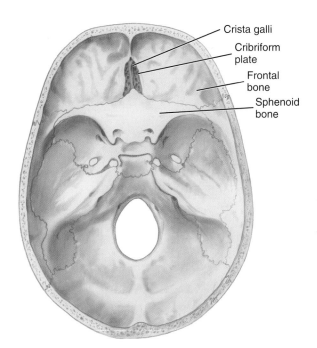

FIGURE 3-36 Superior view of the internal surface of the skull with the ethmoid bone highlighted and its bony articulations and features noted.

Crista galli
Cribriform plate
Frontal bone
Sphenoid bone

The lateral part of the ethmoid bone forms the **superior nasal concha** (plural, **conchae**) and **middle nasal concha** (plural, **conchae**) on each side that projects inward within the nasal cavity (in that order as part of the lateral nasal wall) as well as forming the paired orbital plate (Figure 3-38 and see Figure 3-37). The **orbital plate of the ethmoid bone** forms the medial orbital wall. Located between the orbital plate and each set of these two conchae are the **ethmoidal sinuses** (eth-**moy**-duhl) or *ethmoid air cells*, which are a variable number of small cavities within the **lateral masses of the ethmoid bone**. Each lateral mass forms part of the lateral wall of the nasal cavity (discussed in detail later).

FACIAL BONES

The facial bones form the facial features and serve as a base for the dentition. The facial bones include: the single vomer and mandible as well as the paired lacrimal bones, nasal bones, inferior nasal conchae, zygomatic bones, and maxillae (see Figure 3-4). For ease of learning, the paired palatine bones are considered under the general heading of facial bones but are not strictly considered facial bones by anatomists.

VOMER

The vomer is a thin, flat, single midline facial bone that is almost trapezoidal in shape. The vomer forms the posterior part of the nasal septum, with the anterior part of the nasal septum formed by the ethmoid bone. The bone is located in the midsagittal plane within the nasal cavity, and its articulations are noted on a lateral view of the bone (Figure 3-39).

The vomer has two lateral surfaces and four borders. The vomer articulates with the perpendicular plate of the ethmoid bone on the superior half of its anterior border, with its inferior half grooved for the inferior margin of the nasal septal cartilage. The vomer also articulates with the sphenoid bone on its superior border.

On its inferior border, the vomer articulates with the median palatine suture located between the palatine processes of the maxillae anteriorly and the horizontal plates of the palatine bones posteriorly. The posterior border is free of bony articulation and also has no muscle attachments; the posterior border is concave and separates the posterior nasal apertures or *choanae*. On each lateral surface is the **nasopalatine groove** (nay-zo-**pal**-uh-tine) in which the nasopalatine nerve and branches of the sphenopalatine blood vessels travel.

LACRIMAL BONES, NASAL BONES, AND INFERIOR NASAL CONCHAE

Each paired lacrimal bone is an irregular, thin plate of bone that forms a small part of the anterior medial wall of the orbit (Figure 3-40 and

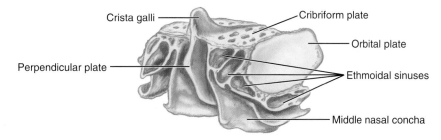

Crista galli
Perpendicular plate
Cribriform plate
Orbital plate
Ethmoidal sinuses
Middle nasal concha

FIGURE 3-37 Oblique view of the disarticulated ethmoid bone with its plates and other features noted.

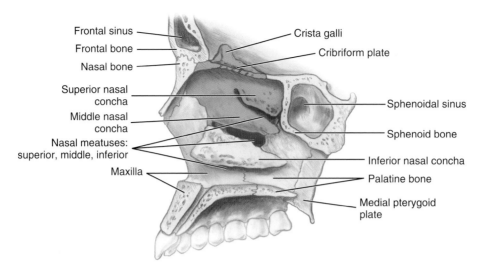

FIGURE 3-38 Lateral wall of the right nasal cavity with the ethmoid bone highlighted and its bony articulations and features noted. Each lateral wall of the nasal cavity is mainly formed by the maxilla; however, it also includes the ethmoid bone with its superior nasal concha and middle nasal concha, as well as the vertical plate of the palatine bone, the medial pterygoid plate of the sphenoid bone, and the inferior nasal concha.

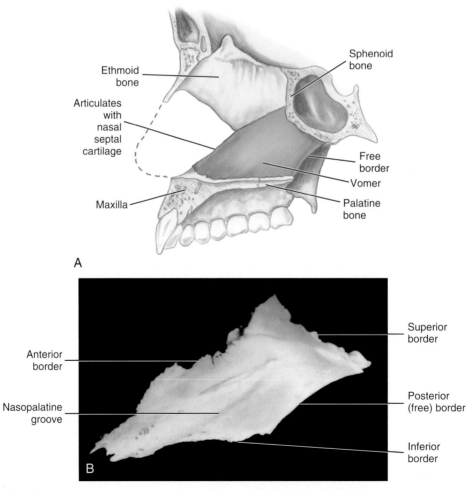

FIGURE 3-39 Medial surface of the left nasal septum with the vomer highlighted with its bony articulations and features noted including the location of the nasal septal cartilage (*dashed line*) **(A)**, and also a lateral view of the disarticulated vomer with its borders noted and nasopalatine groove for the nasopalatine nerve snd branches of the sphenopalatine blood vessels **(B)**. (*B courtesy of Neil S. Norton, PhD, Professor of Oral Biology, School of Dentistry, Creighton University, Omaha, NE.*)

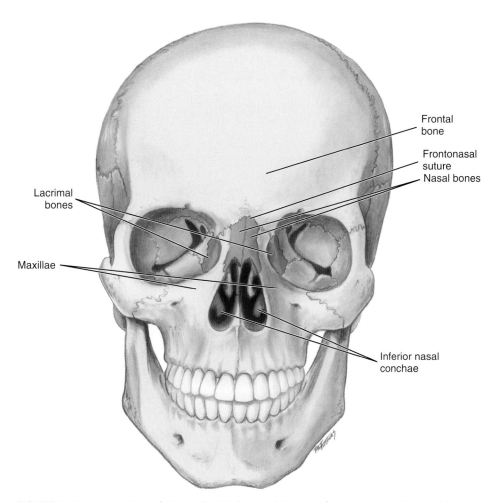

FIGURE 3-40 Anterior view of the skull with the nasal bones, inferior nasal conchae, and lacrimal bones highlighted.

see Figure 3-5). The lacrimal bones are the smallest and most fragile of the facial bones and are located posterior to the frontal processes of the maxillae. Each lacrimal bone articulates with the ethmoid bone and frontal bone as well as the maxilla. The **nasolacrimal duct** (nay-zo-**lak**-ri-muhl) is formed at the junction of the lacrimal bone and the maxilla. Lacrimal fluid or tears from the lacrimal gland are drained through this duct into the inferior nasal meatus (see Figure 2-6 and Chapter 7).

The nasal bones are small oblong paired facial bones that lie side by side, fused to each other to form the bridge of the nose in the midline superior to the piriform aperture (see Figure 2-7). The nasal bones fit between the frontal processes of the maxillae and thus articulate with the maxillae laterally as well as the frontal bone superiorly at the single **frontonasal suture** (frun-toh-**nay**-zuhl) (see Figure 3-40 and Table 3-2).

The inferior nasal conchae are paired facial bones that project from the maxillae to form a part of the lateral walls of the nasal cavity (see Figures 3-38 and 3-40). However, unlike the paired superior and middle nasal conchae from ethmoid bone that project inward off the lateral walls of the nasal cavity, the inferior nasal conchae are separate facial bones. Each inferior nasal concha is composed of a fragile thin and spongy bone curved onto itself like a scroll, similar to the other conchae of the ethmoid. The inferior nasal conchae articulate with the ethmoid bone, lacrimal bones, and palatine bones as well as

the maxillae; yet these bones do not have any associated muscle attachments.

ZYGOMATIC BONES

The zygomatic bone or *zygoma* is a paired facial bone of the skull that forms the majority of the cheekbone or *malar* surface, and also helps to form the lateral wall and floor of the orbit (Figures 3-41 and 3-42 and see Figure 2-9). Each zygomatic bone articulates with the frontal bone, temporal bone, and sphenoid bone as well as the maxilla. Each zygomatic bone is diamond-shaped and composed of three processes with similarly named associated bony articulations: the frontal, temporal, and maxillary processes.

Processes of the Zygomatic Bone. Each of the three processes of the zygomatic bone helps to form structures of the skull (see Figures 3-41 and 3-42 and Table 3-4). The orbital surface of the **frontal process of the zygomatic bone** forms the anterior lateral orbital wall, usually with a paired small **zygomaticofacial foramen** (zy-go-**mat**-i-ko-fay-shuhl) opening onto its lateral surface (see Table 3-3). The **temporal process of the zygomatic bone** forms the zygomatic arch along with the zygomatic process of the temporal bone, with a paired **zygomaticotemporal foramen** (zy-go-**mat**-i-ko-**tem**-puh-ruhl) present on the surface of the bone (see Table 3-3). The orbital surface of the **maxillary process of the zygomatic bone**

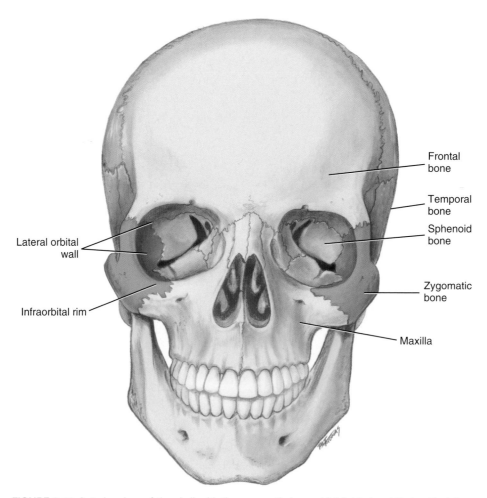

Frontal bone

Temporal bone

Sphenoid bone

Zygomatic bone

Maxilla

Lateral orbital wall

Infraorbital rim

FIGURE 3-41 Anterior view of the skull with the zygomatic bones highlighted and their articulations and features noted.

(**mak**-sil-lare-ee) forms the lateral part of the infraorbital rim and a small part of the anterior part of the lateral orbital wall.

PALATINE BONES

The palatine bones are paired bones of the skull that are not strictly facial bones according to anatomists but are considered under this general heading for ease of learning. Each palatine bone is somewhat "L"-shaped and thus consists of two plates: the horizontal and vertical plates.

Plates and Sutures of the Palatine Bones. Both the horizontal and vertical plates can be noted from a posterior view of the palatine bone (Figure 3-43). The **horizontal plates of the palatine bone** form the posterior hard palate. The **vertical plates of the palatine bone** form a part of the lateral walls of the nasal cavity, and with each plate contributing a small part of bone to the orbital apex. The **pyramidal process of the palatine bone** (pi-**ram**-i-duhl) projects posteriorly and lateralward from the junction of the vertical and horizontal plates.

The palatine bones serve as a link between the maxillae and the sphenoid bone with which they both articulate, in addition to articulating with each other. The two horizontal plates articulate with each other at the posterior part of the median skalatine suture underlying the median palatine raphe, as discussed earlier, and more anteriorly

with the palatine processes of the maxillae at the transverse palatine suture (Figure 3-44 and see Table 3-2 and Figure 2-15).

Foramina of the Palatine Bones. There are two main foramina in the palatine bones: the greater and lesser palatine foramina (see Figure 3-44 and Table 3-3). The larger **greater palatine foramen** is located in the posterolateral region of each horizontal plate of the palatine bones, usually superior to the apices of the maxillary second or third molars. The foramen is approximately 10 mm medial and directly superior to the palatal gingival margin. Thus the depression from the foramen can be palpated on a patient approximately midway between the median palatine raphe overlying the median palatine suture and the palatal gingival margin of the maxillary molar. To locate this foramen, palpate the hard palate starting near the most distal maxillary molar and move anteriorly. The greater palatine foramen transmits the greater palatine nerve and blood vessels, serving as a landmark for the administration of the greater palatine block (see Figure 9-19).

A smaller opening nearby, the **lesser palatine foramen**, transmits the lesser palatine nerve and blood vessels to the soft palate and tonsils. Both the greater and lesser palatine foramina are openings of the pterygopalatine canal that carries the descending palatine nerve and blood vessels from the pterygopalatine fossa to the palate.

The paired **sphenopalatine foramen** (sfe-no-**pal**-uh-tine) is the opening located between the sphenoid bone and orbital processes of

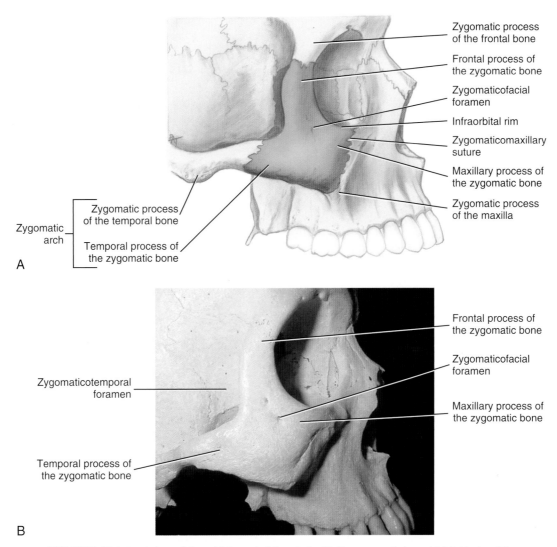

FIGURE 3-42 Lateral view of the middle part of the skull with the zygomatic bone highlighted and its bony articulations and features noted such as the zygomatic arch **(A)**, and close-up of zygomatic bone and its three processes, the frontal, temporal, and maxillary processes as well as associated foramina **(B)**.

the palatine bone; it opens into the nasal cavity and gives passage to branches from the pterygopalatine ganglion and the sphenopalatine artery from the maxillary artery.

MAXILLAE

The upper jaw or maxillae (mak-**sil**-ee) consists of two maxilla fused together at the single **intermaxillary suture** (in-tuhr-**mak**-sil-lare-ee) (Figure 3-45 and see Table 3-2). Each maxilla articulates with the frontal bone, lacrimal bone, nasal bone, inferior nasal concha, vomer, sphenoid bone, ethmoid bone, palatine bone, and zygomatic bone. Each maxilla includes a body and four processes: the frontal, zygomatic, palatine, and alveolar processes.

The **body of the maxilla** is pyramid-shaped and has four surfaces: the orbital, nasal, infratemporal, and facial surfaces. The two bodies contain air-filled spaces or paranasal sinuses, the **maxillary sinuses** (discussed in detail later). Each maxilla can be studied from three viewpoints: the anterior, lateral, and inferior views.

Maxillae From Anterior View. From the anterior view, each **frontal process of the maxilla** articulates with the frontal bone (Figure 3-46 and see Figure 3-45 and Table 3-4). Each maxilla's orbital surface is separated from the sphenoid bone by the inferior orbital fissure (see Figure 3-7 and Table 3-3). The inferior orbital fissure carries the infraorbital and zygomatic nerves, infraorbital artery, and inferior ophthalmic vein. The groove in the floor of the orbital surface is the **infraorbital sulcus**.

The infraorbital sulcus becomes the **infraorbital canal** and then terminates on the facial surface of each maxilla as the **infraorbital foramen** (see Table 3-3). The infraorbital foramen is located approximately 10 mm inferior to the midpoint of the infraorbital rim of the orbit. The infraorbital foramen transmits the infraorbital nerve and blood vessels.

To locate the infraorbital foramen, extraorally palpate on a patient the midpoint of the infraorbital rim and then move slightly inferior while applying pressure until the depression from the infraorbital foramen is felt, surrounded by smoother bone (see Figure 9-16). The

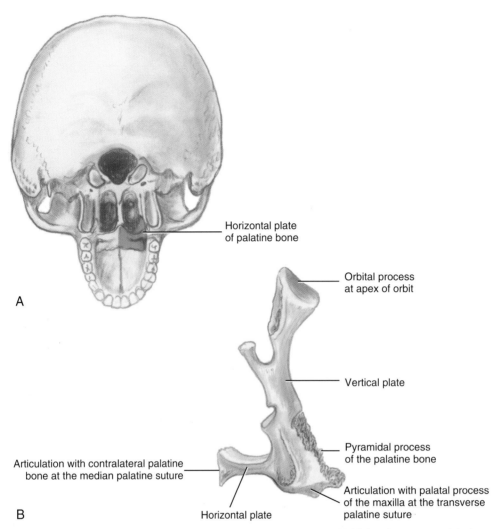

Horizontal plate
of palatine bone

A

Orbital process
at apex of orbit

Vertical plate

Pyramidal process
of the palatine bone

Articulation with contralateral palatine
bone at the median palatine suture

Articulation with palatal process
of the maxilla at the transverse
palatine suture

B

Horizontal plate

FIGURE 3-43 Posterior view of the right palatine bone with its location highlighted on a posteroinferior view of the skull as it articulates with the left palatine bone **(A),** and from the posterior oblique view of the disarticulated bone with its features noted **(B).**

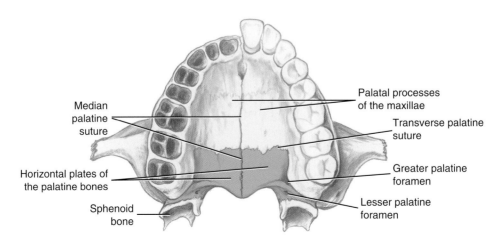

Median
palatine
suture

Palatal processes
of the maxillae

Transverse palatine
suture

Horizontal plates of
the palatine bones

Greater palatine
foramen

Sphenoid
bone

Lesser palatine
foramen

FIGURE 3-44 Inferior view of the hard palate with the horizontal plates of the palatine bones highlighted and features noted.

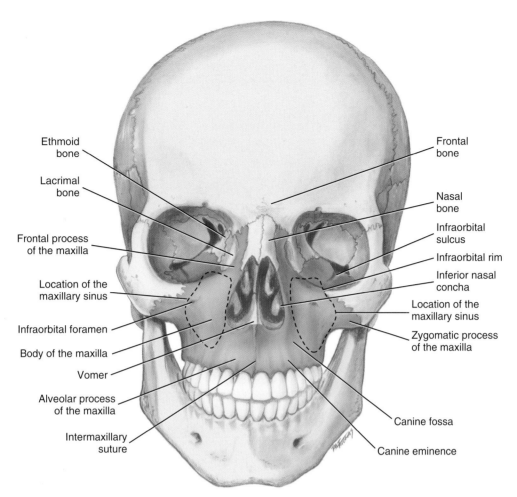

Ethmoid bone

Lacrimal bone

Frontal process of the maxilla

Location of the maxillary sinus

Infraorbital foramen

Body of the maxilla

Vomer

Alveolar process of the maxilla

Intermaxillary suture

Frontal bone

Nasal bone

Infraorbital sulcus

Infraorbital rim

Inferior nasal concha

Location of the maxillary sinus

Zygomatic process of the maxilla

Canine fossa

Canine eminence

FIGURE 3-45 Anterior view of the skull with the maxillae highlighted and its bony articulations and features noted such as the location of the maxillary sinuses (*dashed lines*). Note that the articulation of the maxillae with the pterygoid process of the sphenoid bone and palatine bones is not visible in this view.

patient may feel soreness when pressure is applied due to the presence of the nearby nerve. A "notch" or depression in the midpoint of the infraorbital rim can help with this palpation, which has been formed by the more vertical zygomaticomaxillary suture located between the maxillary process of the zygomatic bone and zygomatic process of the maxilla, forming the infraorbital rim.

The infraorbital foramen also has a linear relationship on the ipsilateral side of the face with the more superiorly located supraorbital notch of the supraorbital rim and midpoint of the infraorbital rim as well as the pupil of the eye and labial commissure. The infraorbital foramen serves as a landmark for the administration of the infraorbital block.

Inferior to the infraorbital foramen is an elongated depression, the **canine fossa** (**kay**-nine), which is just posterosuperior to each of the roots of the maxillary canines. Also present is a facial and palatal cortical plate, which is also part of the alveolar process of the maxilla (see Table 3-4).

The root of each tooth of the maxillary arch is covered by a prominent facial ridge of bone, a part of the alveolar process of the maxilla. The more prominent facial ridge over each of the roots of the maxillary canines, the **canine eminence**, serves as a landmark for the administration of the anterior superior alveolar block (see Figure 9-12).

The alveolar process of the maxilla usually contains the roots of the maxillary teeth within the alveoli. The apices of these roots between both the facial and palatal cortical plates of the alveolar process of the maxilla are landmarks for the administration of the majority of the maxillary local anesthetic injections (see Chapter 9).

In general, the alveolar process of the maxillary teeth is less dense and more porous than the alveolar process of similar mandibular teeth as demonstrated on a panoramic radiograph (see Figures 3-46 and 3-50). These differences in bone density allow a greater incidence of clinically adequate local anesthesia for the maxillary arch when the local anesthetic agent is administered as a supraperiosteal injection than would occur with similar teeth on the mandibular arch (see Chapter 9).

Maxilla From Lateral View. Some of the landmarks noted from the anterior view of the maxilla are also present from the lateral view. From the lateral view, each **zygomatic process of the maxilla** articulates at the zygomaticomaxillary suture with the maxillary process of the zygomatic bone laterally, completing the medial part of the infraorbital rim (Figure 3-47 and see Figure 3-46 and Table 3-4). The infratemporal surface of the maxilla inferior to the temple is convex, directed to the posterior and to the lateral, and forms part of the infratemporal fossa (discussed later); it is separated from the anterior surface by the zygomatic process.

On the posterior part of the body of the maxilla is a rounded, roughened elevation, the maxillary tuberosity, just posterior to the most distal molar of the maxillary arch. It is a landmark for

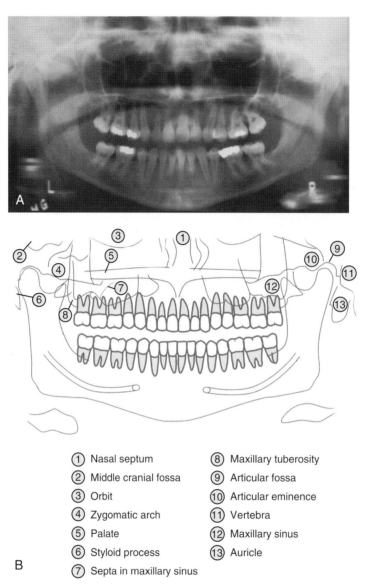

1. Nasal septum
2. Middle cranial fossa
3. Orbit
4. Zygomatic arch
5. Palate
6. Styloid process
7. Septa in maxillary sinus
8. Maxillary tuberosity
9. Articular fossa
10. Articular eminence
11. Vertebra
12. Maxillary sinus
13. Auricle

B

FIGURE 3-46 Panoramic radiograph **(A)** and associated anatomy of the midface **(B)**. *(A, From Feh-renbach MJ, Popowics T:* Illustrated dental embryology, histology, and anatomy, *ed 4, St. Louis, 2016, Elsevier.)*

mounting radiographs and also serves as one of the borders of the infratemporal fossae of the skull (Figure 3-48 and see Figures 2-21, 3-46, 3-47, and 3-61).

Posterosuperior on the maxillary tuberosity are the **posterior superior alveolar foramina** that perforate the infratemporal surface of the maxilla multiple times. These foramina are where the posterior superior alveolar nerve branches and blood vessel branches enter the bone from the posterior and then open up onto the infratemporal surface of the maxilla. Both the maxillary tuberosity and posterior superior alveolar foramina serve as landmarks for the administration of the posterior superior alveolar block (see Figure 9-2). The maxillary tuberosity also serves as a landmark for the administration of the Vazirani-Akinosi mandibular block (see Figure 9-54).

Maxillae From Inferior View. On the inferior aspect, each **palatine process of the maxilla** articulates with the other to form the anterior hard palate (see Figures 3-46 and 3-48 and Table 3-4). On the posterior part of the body of the maxilla, the maxillary tuberosity

is again visible. In addition, a number of small pores in the maxilla of the anterior hard palate allow for the diffusion of local anesthetic agent during the administration of the anterior middle superior alveolar block.

The suture located between these two palatine processes of the maxilla is the anterior part of the median palatine suture (see Table 3-2). In the patient, the suture is covered by the median palatine raphe, which is a midline tendinous band of tissue that serves as one of the landmarks for the administration of both the greater palatine and anterior middle superior alveolar blocks (see Figures 2-15 and 9-28).

In the anterior midline between the articulating palatine processes of the maxillae, just palatal to the maxillary central incisors, is the **incisive foramen** (in-**sy**-siv) (see Table 3-3). This foramen carries the branches of the right and left nasopalatine nerves as well as the sphenopalatine arteries from the nasal cavity to the anterior hard palate. The soft tissue that bulges over the opening of the incisive foramen is the incisive papilla (see Figure 2-15). The incisive foramen and its

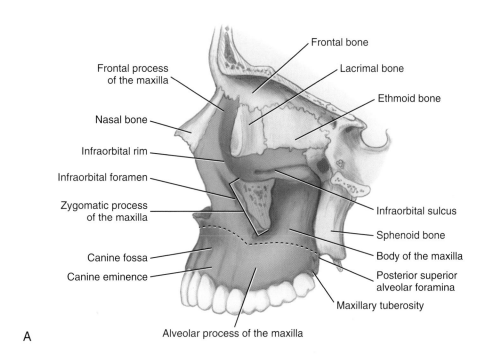

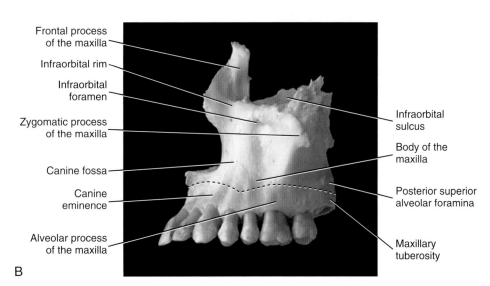

FIGURE 3-47 Cutaway view of the lateral aspect of the skull with the maxilla highlighted with bony articulations and features noted such as the approximate junction between the alveolar process of the maxilla and the body of the maxilla (*dashed line*) **(A),** and the disarticulated bone **(B).**

incisive papilla both serve as landmarks for the administration of the nasopalatine block (see Figure 9-23).

The alveolar process of the maxilla can become resorbed when completely edentulous in the maxillary arch; resorption occurs to a lesser extent in partially edentulous cases. This resorption can possibly lead to problems with the maxillary sinuses (discussed later). However, the more superior body of the maxilla is not resorbed with tooth loss, but its walls may become thinner in this case.

The density of the maxilla within its regions determines the route that a dental (or odontogenic) infection takes with abscess and fistula formation (see Chapter 12). In addition, the differences in alveolar process of the maxilla density also determine the most clinically effective regions for bony fracture if needed during tooth extraction. The

maxillary teeth are surgically best removed by fracturing the thinner facial cortical plate rather than the thicker palatal cortical plate.

MANDIBLE

The mandible is a single facial bone that forms the lower jaw and is the only freely movable bone of the skull. This almost horseshoe shaped bone is also the strongest facial bone, with an upward sloping part at each end. The mandible has its movable articulation with the temporal bones at each temporomandibular joint (Figure 3-49 and see Figure 5-1). The mandible also occludes with the maxillae by way of their contained respective maxillary and mandibular arches of the dentition. The mandible is more effectively studied when it is removed from the skull and then examined from three viewpoints: the anterior, lateral, and medial views.

Mandible From Anterior View. From the anterior view, prominent landmarks are visible such as the mental protuberance, the bony prominence of the chin located inferior to the roots of the mandibular incisors (Figure 3-50 and see Figure 2-22). The mental protuberance is more pronounced in males but can be still be viewed and palpated in females.

In the midline on the anterior surface of the mandible is a faint ridge, an indication of the **mandibular symphysis (sim**-fi-sis),

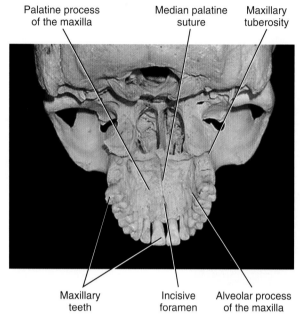

Palatine process of the maxilla

Median palatine suture

Maxillary tuberosity

Maxillary teeth

Incisive foramen

Alveolar process of the maxilla

FIGURE 3-48 Posteroinferior view of the maxillae and hard palate with features noted.

demonstrating the fusion of right and left mandibular processes during the embryologic development of the mandible. Like other symphyses in the body, this is a midline articulation where the bones are joined by fibrocartilage but this articulation between the two processes fuses together in early childhood.

Farther posteriorly on the lateral surface of the mandible is the opening of the **mental foramen (men**-tuhl), which is usually inferior to the apices of the mandibular premolars (Figures 3-51 and 3-52 and see Table 3-3). As mandibular growth proceeds in young children, the direction of the opening of the mental foramen changes from anterior to posterosuperior. The mental foramen allows entry of the mental nerve and blood vessels into the mandibular canal to merge with the incisive nerve and blood vessels (discussed later).

The mental foramen's posterosuperior opening in adults signifies the changed direction of the emerging mental nerve. This opening of the mental foramen onto the lateral surface of the mandible is a landmark to note intraorally and on a radiograph during the administration of both the mental and incisive blocks (see Figure 9-44). It is also important to not confuse the circular radiolucent mental foramen on a radiograph with a periapical lesion related to the adjacent teeth or any other oral radiolucent lesions.

Palpation of the mental foramen on a patient during an examination or during administration of a local anesthetic agent will cause transient soreness in the region due to the presence of the nerve. However, studies show that the mental foramen can be as far posterior as the apex of the mandibular first molar or as far anterior as the apex of the mandibular canine. Thus to locate the mental foramen on a patient, palpate intraorally the depth of the mandibular mucobuccal fold starting out inferior to the apex of the mandibular first molar and moving anteriorly to the apex of the mandibular canine or at a site indicated by a radiograph until a depression from the foramen is felt on the lateral surface of the mandible, surrounded by smoother bone.

The heavy horizontal part of the lower jaw inferior to the mental foramen is the **body of the mandible** or *base* (see Figure 3-51). Superior to this, the part of the lower jaw that usually contains the roots of the mandibular teeth within the alveoli is the **alveolar process of**

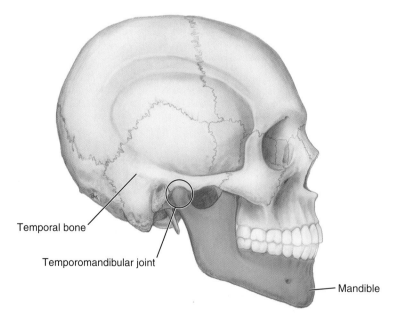

Temporal bone

Temporomandibular joint

Mandible

FIGURE 3-49 Lateral view of the skull with the mandible highlighted and the temporomandibular joint (*circle*) and its articulating bones noted.

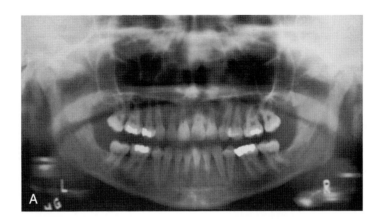

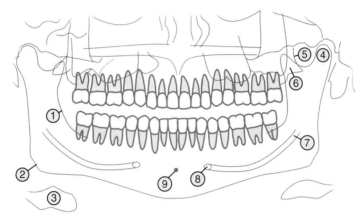

①	External oblique line	⑥	Coronoid process
②	Angle of the mandible	⑦	Mandibular canal
③	Hyoid bone	⑧	Mental foramen
④	Mandibular condyle	⑨	Genial tubercles
⑤	Pterygoid plates		with lingual foramina

FIGURE 3-50 Panoramic radiograph **(A)** and associated anatomy of the lower face **(B)**. *(A, From Fehrenbach MJ, Popowics T: Illustrated dental embryology, histology, and anatomy, ed 4, St. Louis, 2016, Elsevier.)*

the mandible (see Figures 2-13 and 3-52 and Table 3-4). Also present is a facial and lingual cortical plate within the alveolar process of the mandible. However, the slightly more prominent facial ridge over each of the mandibular canines, the canine eminence, is less extensive than its maxillary counterpart. The body of the mandible, along with the alveolar process, elongates posteriorly with growth to provide space for additional permanent teeth as the child nears adulthood.

The alveolar process of the mandible can become resorbed when completely edentulous in the mandibular arch; resorption occurs to a lesser extent in partially edentulous cases. This resorption can occur to such an extent that the mental foramen is virtually on the superior border of the mandible, instead of opening onto the lateral surface, changing its relative position. However, the more inferior body of the mandible is not affected and remains thick and rounded. This resorption can possibly alter the landmarks when administering the mental, incisive, or inferior alveolar blocks (see Chapter 9).

In general, the alveolar process of the mandibular anterior teeth is less dense and more porous than the alveolar process of

the mandibular posterior teeth, as demonstrated on a panoramic radiograph (see Figures 3-46 and 3-50). These differences in bone density allow a supraperiosteal injection of the mandibular anterior teeth by a local anesthetic agent to have a greater incidence of clinically adequate local anesthesia than would occur with the mandibular posterior teeth, but always with less clinically effective overall anesthesia than the maxillary teeth (see Chapter 9).

The density of the mandibular bone with its regions also determines the route that a dental (or odontogenic) infection takes with abscess and fistula formation (see Chapter 12). In addition, the differences in alveolar process of the mandible density determine the most clinically effective regions for bony fracture used during tooth extraction; the mandibular third molar is easier to surgically remove by fracturing the thinner lingual cortical plate (being careful of the nearby lingual nerve) rather than the thicker facial cortical plate, if needed.

Mandible From Lateral View. On the lateral aspect of the mandible, the stout flat plate of the **mandibular ramus** (man-**dib**-u-luhr) (plural, **rami**) (**ray**-muhs, **ray**-my) extends superiorly and

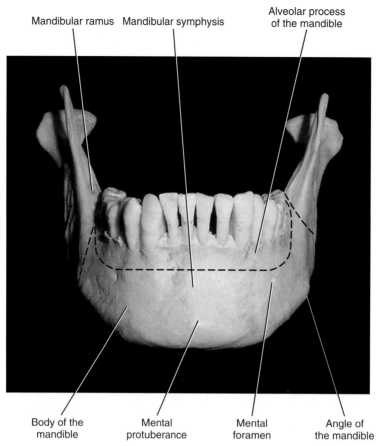

Mandibular ramus   Mandibular symphysis   Alveolar process of the mandible

Body of the mandible   Mental protuberance   Mental foramen   Angle of the mandible

FIGURE 3-51 Anterior view of the disarticulated mandible and its associated features such as the approximate junction between the alveolar process of the maxilla and the body of the mandible (*dashed lines*).

posteriorly from the body of the mandible on each side (see Figure 3-52). Each mandibular ramus serves as the primary site for the attachment for certain muscles of mastication. As adulthood nears, both mandibular rami grow superiorly and posteriorly, displacing the mental protuberance of the chin inferiorly and anteriorly.

The anterior border of the mandibular ramus has a thin sharp margin that terminates in the **coronoid process** (**kor**-uh-noid) (see Table 3-4). The main part of the anterior border of the mandibular ramus forms a concave anterior curve, the **coronoid notch**. The coronoid notch is the greatest depression on the anterior border of the mandibular ramus and serves as a bony landmark for administration of the inferior alveolar block (see Figures 9-35 and 9-37).

Inferior to the coronoid notch, the anterior border of the mandibular ramus becomes the **external oblique line** (o-**bleek**), a crest where the mandibular ramus joins the body of the mandible. On a radiograph, the external oblique line is noted as a radiopaque line superior to the mylohyoid line (discussed next); this may also be palpated intraorally on a patient to help locate the coronoid notch (see Figure 3-50).

The posterior border of the mandibular ramus becomes thicker and extends from the angle of the mandible, which is the juncture between the mandibular ramus and the body of the mandible, to a large and more posterior projection, the **condyloid process** (**kon**-duh-loid). This process consists of two parts: the **mandibular condyle** and the constricted part that supports it, its **neck** (Figure 3-53 and see Figures 3-50 and 3-51 and Table 3-4). The anteromedial border of the neck of the mandibular condyle serves as a bony landmark for the

administration of the Gow-Gates mandibular block (see Figure 9-48). The **articulating surface of the condyle** is an oval head that is involved in the temporomandibular joint (see Figure 5-3). Located between the coronoid process and the condyle is a deep concavity, the **mandibular notch** or *sigmoid notch*.

Mandible From Medial View. Noted on the medial view of the mandible are the body of the mandible, the alveolar process of the mandible (see Table 3-4), and the mandibular ramus (Figure 3-54). In addition, near to its mental symphysis are the **genial tubercles** (juh-**ni**-uhl) or *mental spines*, four small projections that serve as muscle attachments (see Figures 4-26 and 4-54). Also near to the genial tubercles but along the inferior border of the mandible is the **digastric fossa** (di-**gas**-trik) as well as the tiny **lingual foramen** on each side (see Figure 4-25). The anterior belly of the digastric muscle inserts onto this fossa.

At the lateral edge of each alveolar process of the mandible is a rounded, roughened area, the **retromolar triangle** (ret-roh-**moh**-luhr), just posterior to the most distal mandibular molar, if present. The retromolar triangle is a bony landmark for the administration of the buccal block, and when covered with soft tissue, is the retromolar pad (see Figure 2-21).

Along each medial surface of the body of the mandible is the **mylohyoid line** (my-lo-**hi**-oid) or *internal oblique ridge* that extends posteriorly and superiorly, becoming more prominent as it moves superiorly onto the body of the mandible. The mylohyoid line is the point of attachment of the mylohyoid muscle that forms the floor of

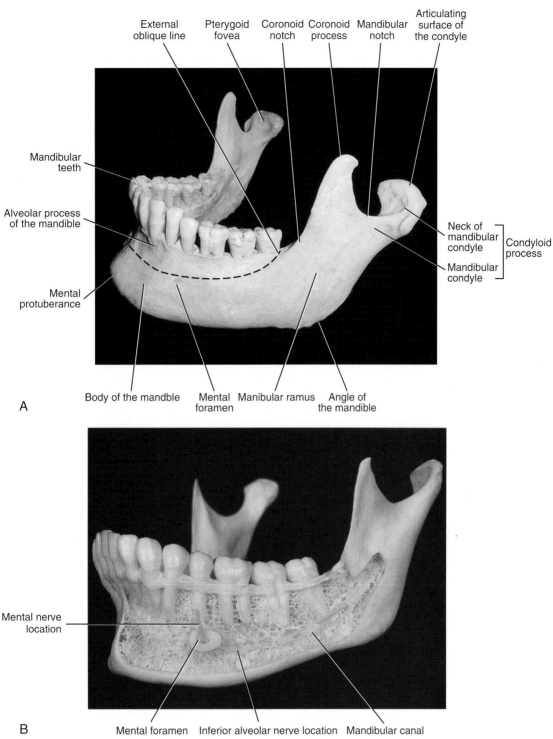

FIGURE 3-52 Slightly oblique lateral view of the disarticulated mandible and its associated features. Note the approximate junction between the alveolar process of the maxilla and the body of the mandible (*dashed line*) **(A),** and with a cutaway view demonstrating the pathway of the inferior alveolar nerve (*yellow marker*) as it forms from a merger of the mental and incisive nerves (not shown here) and travels within the mandibular canal and then exits by way of the mandibular foramen (has been cut away in this view; see instead Figure 3-54, *B*). Note also the mental foramen with the mental nerve; the incisive nerve nor the mandibular incisive canal are not shown in this view **(B).** *(B, Modified from Logan BM, Reynold PA, Hutching RT: McMinn's color atlas of head and neck anatomy, ed 4, London, 2010, Elsevier.)*

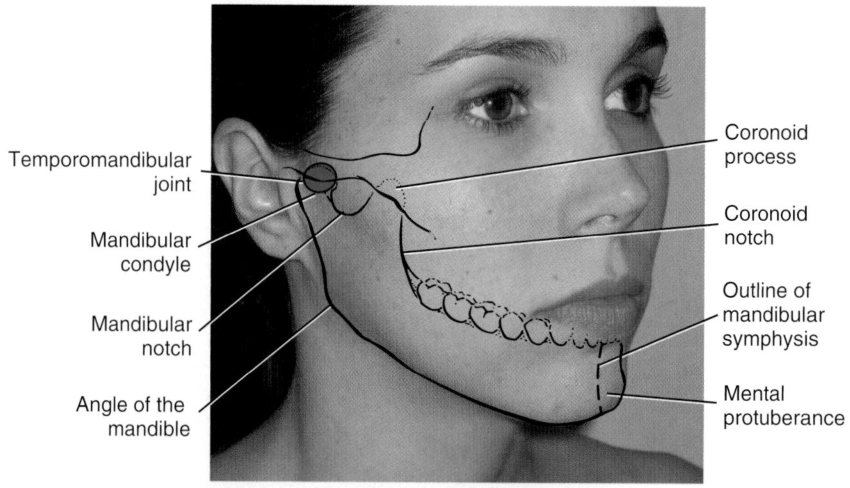

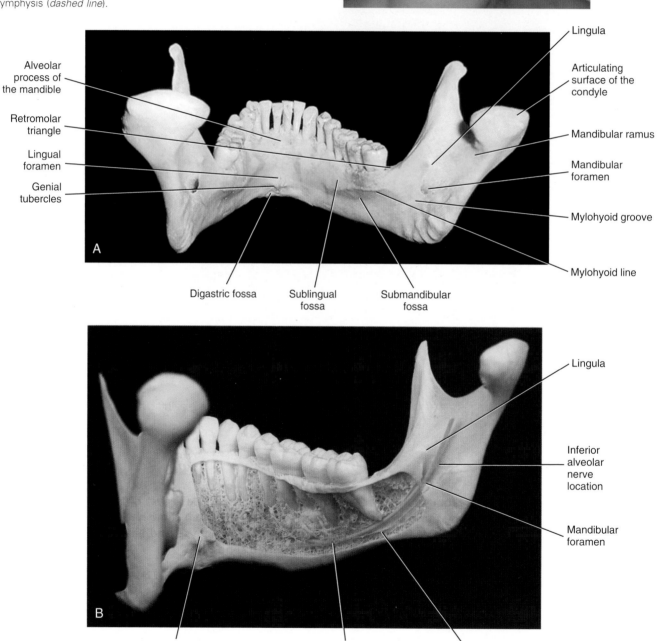

FIGURE 3-53 Lateral view of the face with a superimposition of the associated bony landmarks of the mandible noted, such as the temporomandibular joint (*colored in circle*) and the mandibular symphysis (*dashed line*).

Temporomandibular joint

Mandibular condyle

Mandibular notch

Angle of the mandible

Coronoid process

Coronoid notch

Outline of mandibular symphysis

Mental protuberance

Alveolar process of the mandible

Retromolar triangle

Lingual foramen

Genial tubercles

Lingula

Articulating surface of the condyle

Mandibular ramus

Mandibular foramen

Mylohyoid groove

Mylohyoid line

Digastric fossa

Sublingual fossa

Submandibular fossa

Lingula

Inferior alveolar nerve location

Mandibular foramen

Lingual foramen

Inferior alveolar nerve location

Mandibular canal

FIGURE 3-54 Medial view of the disarticulated mandible and its associated features **(A),** and a cutaway view that demonstrates the pathway of the inferior alveolar nerve (*yellow marker*) within the mandibular canal as it forms from a merger of the mental and incisive nerves (not shown in this view) and exits by way of the mandibular foramen. The mandibular foramen is two-thirds the distance from the coronoid notch to the posterior border of the mandibular ramus. This distance determination is from most recent studies of skulls and not from older sources that quote three-fourths along the ramus **(B).** *(B, From Logan BM, Reynold PA, Hutching RT: McMinn's color atlas of head and neck anatomy, ed 4, London, 2010, Elsevier.)*

the mouth (see Figure 4-24). The posterior border of the mylohyoid line also provides for attachment of the pterygomandibular raphe, which underlies the surface pterygomandibular fold. Additionally, the mylohyoid line helps divide the sublingual fossa from the submandibular fossa. The roots of the mandibular posterior teeth often extend internally inferior to the mylohyoid line, which can be noted on a radiograph as the radiopaque line inferior to the external oblique line (see Figure 3-50).

A shallow depression, the **sublingual fossa** (sub-**ling**-gwuhl), which contains the sublingual salivary gland, is located superior to the anterior part of the mylohyoid line (see Figure 7-7). Inferior to the posterior part of the mylohyoid line as well as the mandibular posterior teeth is a deeper depression, the **submandibular fossa** (sub-man-**dib**-u-luhr), which contains the submandibular salivary gland (see Figure 7-5).

On the medial surface of the mandibular ramus is the **mandibular foramen** (see Figures 3-52, 3-54, 9-35, and Table 3-3). Although older sources give its location as three-fourths along the ramus, most recent studies of skulls show the mandibular foramen position as approximately two-thirds the distance from the coronoid notch to the posterior border of the mandibular ramus. The foramen is a landmark for administering the inferior alveolar and Vazirani-Akinosi mandibular blocks.

The mandibular foramen is the opening of the **mandibular canal.** Thus, the mandibular canal runs horizontally in a posterior direction within the body of the mandible on each side, where it is inferior to the alveoli (or tooth sockets) and communicates with them by small openings. The mandibular canal then runs obliquely in a posterosuperior direction within the mandibular ramus. The inferior alveolar nerve and blood vessels travel within the mandibular canal after the merging of the mental and incisive nerves and blood vessels, and then exits the mandible through the mandibular foramen. The incisive nerve was originally located within the **mandibular incisive canal**, which is an anterior continuation of the mandibular canal bilaterally between the two mental foramina.

With age and tooth loss, the alveolar process of the mandible becomes absorbed as discussed earlier so that the mandibular canal ends up nearer to its superior border. In some of the cases with excessive alveolar process absorption, the mandibular canal disappears entirely and leaves the inferior alveolar nerve without its bony protection, although it is still covered by soft tissue. The height of the mandibular foramen can also seem to be more superior without the presence of teeth in the mandibular posterior sextant.

Rarely, a bifid inferior alveolar nerve may be present, in which case a second more inferiorly placed mandibular foramen is present that can be detected by noting a doubled mandibular canal on a radiograph (see Chapter 8). Keeping this anatomic variant of the mandibular foramen in mind is important when administering an inferior alveolar block as well as any changes due to bony resorption (see Chapter 9).

Overhanging the mandibular foramen is a bony spine, the **lingula** (**ling**-gu-luh), which serves as an attachment for the sphenomandibular ligament associated with the temporomandibular joint (see Figure 5-5, *A*). A small groove, the **mylohyoid groove**, passes anteriorly to and inferiorly from the mandibular foramen. The mylohyoid nerve and blood vessels travel in the mylohyoid groove; the mylohyoid nerve can in some cases have an unusual pathway that may cause difficulty with the administration of an inferior alveolar block (see Chapter 9).

The articulating surface of the condyle can also be noted from the medial view. This is where the mandible articulates with the temporal bone at the temporomandibular joint (see Chapter 5). Inferior to the articular surface of the mandibular condyle on the anterior surface of

the neck is a triangular depression, the **pterygoid fovea** (**fo**-vee-uh), which serves for the attachment of the lateral pterygoid muscle (see Figures 3-52 and 4-23).

PARANASAL SINUSES

The **paranasal sinuses** (pare-uh-**nay**-zuhl) are paired air-filled cavities within the bones of the head that project laterally, superiorly, and posteriorly into surrounding bones (Figures 3-55 and 3-56). These sinuses are lined with mucous membranes that are continuous with the nasal cavities. The sinuses communicate with the nasal cavity through ostia in the lateral nasal wall. The sinuses serve to lighten the skull bones, act as sound resonators, and provide mucus for the nasal cavity. The paranasal sinuses include: the frontal, sphenoidal, ethmoidal, and maxillary sinuses.

FRONTAL SINUSES

The paired frontal sinuses are located within the frontal bone just superior to the nasal cavity (see Figures 3-23 and 3-25). These two paranasal sinuses are approximately 2 to 3 cm in diameter and are asymmetric, with the left and right sinuses always separated by a septum. Each frontal sinus communicates with and drains into the nasal cavity by a constricted canal to the middle nasal meatus, the **frontonasal duct**. During an extraoral examination, visually inspect and bilaterally palpate the frontal sinuses on a patient (Figure 3-57).

SPHENOIDAL SINUSES

The paired sphenoidal sinuses are located deep within the body of the sphenoid bone and thus cannot be palpated on a patient during an extraoral examination (see Figure 3-33). These two paranasal sinuses are approximately 1.5 to 2.5 cm in diameter and are frequently asymmetric due to the lateral displacement of the intervening septum. The sphenoidal sinuses communicate with and drain into the nasal cavity through an opening superior to each superior nasal concha.

ETHMOIDAL SINUSES

The ethmoidal sinuses or *ethmoid air cells* are a variable number of small cavities located deep within each lateral mass of the ethmoid bone that are partly completed by the surrounding articulated bones. Thus these sinuses generally cannot be palpated on a patient during an extraoral examination (see Figures 3-37 and 3-56). These paranasal sinuses are roughly divided into the anterior, middle, and posterior ethmoid air cells. The posterior ethmoid air cells open into the superior meatus of the nasal cavity, and the middle and anterior ethmoid air cells open into the middle meatus.

MAXILLARY SINUSES

The maxillary sinuses are paired paranasal sinuses located within each body of the maxillae, just posterior to the maxillary canine and premolars, if present (see Figures 3-45, 3-46, and 3-56). The sinus size varies according to individuals and their ages. However, these pyramid-shaped sinuses are usually the largest of the paranasal sinuses, and each one has an apex, three walls, a roof, and a floor.

The apex of the pyramid of the maxillary sinus points into the zygomatic arch, with the medial wall formed by the lateral wall of the nasal cavity. The anterior wall corresponds with the anterior or facial wall of the maxilla, and the posterior wall is the infratemporal surface of the maxilla that corresponds to the maxillary tuberosity. The roof

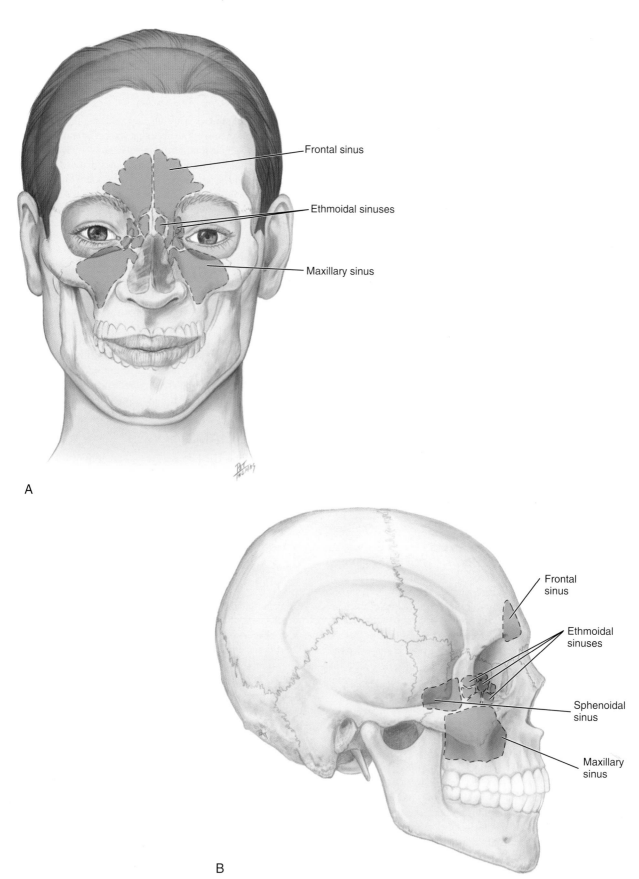

A

B

FIGURE 3-55 Anterior view of the skull with the location of the paranasal sinuses highlighted (*dashed lines*) and the superimposition of facial features and skull bones **(A),** and from a lateral view **(B).**

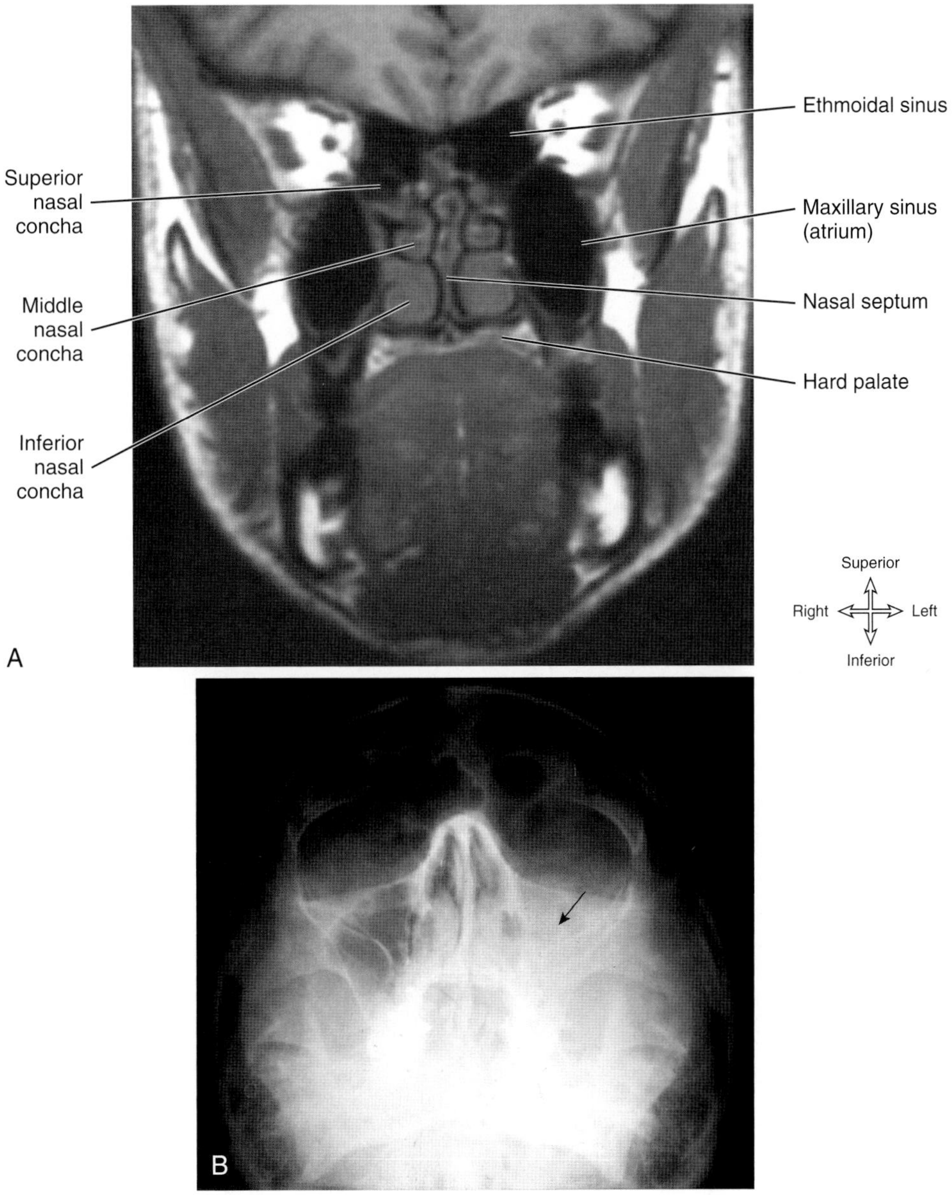

FIGURE 3-56 Coronal magnetic resonance imaging of the nasopharynx and oropharynx showing both the ethmoidal and maxillary sinuses **(A)**. From a Waters view (occipitomental sinus) radiograph showing the opacification or cloudiness of the infected left maxillary sinus *(arrow)* due to retained mucus compared with the translucent noninfected right sinus **(B)**. *(From Reynolds PA, Abrahams PH: McMinn's interactive clinical anatomy: head and neck, ed 2, London, 2010, Elsevier.)*

of the maxillary sinus is the orbital floor, and the floor is the alveolar process of each maxilla. Each maxillary sinus is further divided into communicating compartments by bony walls or septa.

The maxillary sinus drains into the middle meatus on each side by way of the ostium. Drainage of the maxillary sinus is complicated and may promote a prolonged or chronic sinusitis because the draining ostium of each sinus is higher than the floor of the sinus cavity when in anatomic position (see next discussion). Surgery to allow drainage may be required in the case of chronic maxillary sinusitis.

During an extraoral examination, visually inspect and bilaterally palpate on a patient the maxillary sinuses (Figure 3-58). A part of the sinuses can be noted on various radiographs of the maxillary posterior teeth. Due to the proximity of the maxillary sinus to the alveolar process containing the roots of the maxillary posterior teeth, the

periodontium of these teeth may be in direct contact with the mucosa of the maxillary sinus (see Figure 3-46). Additionally, the discomfort associated with a primary maxillary sinus infection can also mimic the discomfort of endodontic or periodontal infection of the maxillary posterior teeth.

With age, the enlarging maxillary sinus may even begin to surround the roots of the maxillary posterior teeth and extend its margins into the body of the zygomatic bone. If the maxillary posterior teeth are extracted and the alveolar process is resorbed, the maxillary sinus may expand even more, thinning the bony floor of the alveolar process so that only a thin shell of bone is present. These instances of proximity can cause serious clinical problems such as secondary sinusitis and perforation during infection (see Chapter 12), extraction, or trauma related to the maxillary posterior teeth.

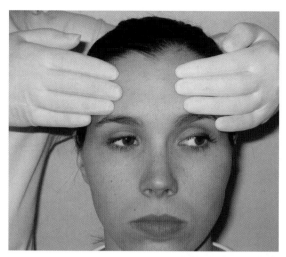

FIGURE 3-57 Demonstration of palpation of the frontal sinuses on a patient during an extraoral examination. *(Courtesy Margaret J. Fehrenbach, RDH, MS.)*

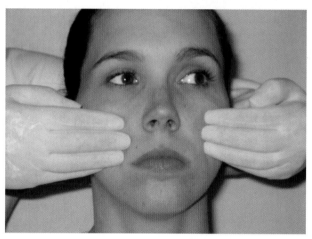

FIGURE 3-58 Demonstration of palpation of the maxillary sinuses on a patient during an extraoral examination. *(Courtesy Margaret J. Fehrenbach, RDH, MS.)*

SKULL FOSSAE

Three large deeper depressions or fossae are present on the external surface of the skull: the temporal, infratemporal, and pterygopalatine fossae. The bony borders for these paired fossae should be located on both the skull and skull figures as well as on peers and patients (Table 3-6). This is because these fossae are prominent landmarks of the skull that can be used for locating associated muscles as well as the nerves and blood vessels that travel within the fossae (Table 3-7).

TEMPORAL FOSSA

The temporal fossa is a flat fan-shaped paired depression on the lateral surface of the skull (Figure 3-59 and see Figures 3-12 and 3-13). The temporal fossa is formed by parts of five different bones: the zygomatic bone, frontal bone, sphenoid bone (its greater wing), temporal bone, and parietal bone.

The borders of the temporal fossa include: superiorly and posteriorly, the inferior temporal line; anteriorly, the frontal process of the zygomatic bone; medially, the surface of the temporal bone;

Clinical Considerations With Paranasal Sinus Pathology

The mucous membranes of the sinuses can become inflamed and congested with mucus with the presence of **primary sinusitis**, which can involve allergies or an infection occurring in the sinus. The symptoms of sinusitis are headache, usually near the involved sinus, and foul-smelling nasal or pharyngeal discharge, possibly with systemic signs of infection such as fever and weakness. The skin over the involved sinus can be tender, hot, and even reddened due to the inflammatory process in the region. On radiographs, there is opacification (or cloudiness) of the usually translucent sinus due to retained mucus (see Figure 3-56).

Recent studies have found that the cause of chronic sinus infections lies in the nasal mucus, not in the nasal and sinus tissue targeted by standard treatment. This suggests a beneficial effect of treatments that target primarily the underlying and presumably damage-inflicting nasal and sinus membrane inflammation, instead of the secondary bacterial infection that has been the primary target of past treatments for the disease. Also, surgical procedures with chronic sinus infections are now changing with the direct removal of the mucus, which is loaded with toxins from the inflammatory cells, rather than removal of the inflamed tissue during surgery. Leaving the mucus behind might predispose early recurrence of the chronic sinus infection. If any surgery is performed, it is usually to enlarge the ostia in the lateral walls of the nasal cavity to create adequate drainage.

An infection in one sinus can travel through the nasal cavity to other sinuses, leading to serious complications. Because the maxillary posterior teeth are close to the maxillary sinus, this can also cause clinical problems if any dental disease processes are present, such as an infection in any of these teeth (see **Chapter 12**). These clinical problems can include **secondary sinusitis**, the inflammation of the sinuses from another source such as an infection of the adjacent teeth. A **perforation**, an abnormal hole formed in the wall of the sinus due to the inflammatory process, also can occur with infection.

and laterally, the zygomatic arch. Inferiorly, the border between the temporal fossa and the infratemporal fossa is the infratemporal crest on the greater wing of the sphenoid bone.

The temporal fossa includes: a narrow strip of the parietal bone, the squamous part of the temporal bone, the temporal surface of the frontal bone, and the temporal surface of the greater wing of the sphenoid bone. The temporal fossa contains the body of the temporalis muscle and regional nerves and blood vessels that travel through it (see Figure 4-22).

INFRATEMPORAL FOSSA

The infratemporal fossa is a paired depression that is inferior to the anterior part of the temporal fossa (see Figure 3-59). The infratemporal crest on the greater wing of the sphenoid bone contributes to both the adjoining temporal fossa and infratemporal fossa. The infratemporal fossa can also be viewed in its entirety from the inferior aspect of the skull after removing the mandible (Figure 3-60).

The borders of the infratemporal fossa include: superiorly, the greater wing of the sphenoid bone; anteriorly, the maxillary tuberosity of the maxilla; medially, the lateral pterygoid plate of the sphenoid bone; and laterally, the mandibular ramus and zygomatic arch. No bony inferior or posterior border exists, only soft tissue.

Some structures pass from the infratemporal fossa into the orbit through the inferior orbital fissure, which is located at the anterior

TABLE 3-6	Skull Fossae Borders		
BORDERS OF EACH FOSSA	**TEMPORAL FOSSA**	**INFRATEMPORAL FOSSA**	**PTERYGOPALATINE FOSSA**
Superior	Inferior temporal line	Greater wing of the sphenoid bone	Inferior surface of body of sphenoid bone
Anterior	Frontal process of the zygomatic bone	Maxillary tuberosity of the maxilla	Maxillary tuberosity of the maxilla
Medial	Surface of the temporal bone	Lateral pterygoid plate of the sphenoid bone	Vertical plate of the palatine bone pierced by sphenopalatine foramen
Lateral	Zygomatic arch	Mandibular ramus and zygomatic arch	Pterygomaxillary fissure
Inferior	Infratemporal crest of the sphenoid bone	No bony border	Pterygopalatine canal
Posterior	Inferior temporal line	No bony border	Pterygoid process of the sphenoid bone

TABLE 3-7	Skull Fossae Contents		
STRUCTURES	**TEMPORAL FOSSA**	**INFRATEMPORAL FOSSA**	**PTERYGOPALATINE FOSSA**
Muscles	Temporalis muscle	Pterygoid muscles	
Blood vessels	Regional blood vessels	Maxillary artery and its second part branches including middle meningeal artery, inferior alveolar artery, and posterior superior alveolar artery as well as pterygoid plexus of veins	Maxillary artery and its third part branches including infraorbital and sphenopalatine arteries
Nerves	Regional nerves	Mandibular nerve (or third division) of fifth cranial or trigeminal nerve including inferior alveolar and lingual nerves	Maxillary nerve (or second division) of fifth cranial or trigeminal nerve and its branches as well as pterygopalatine ganglion

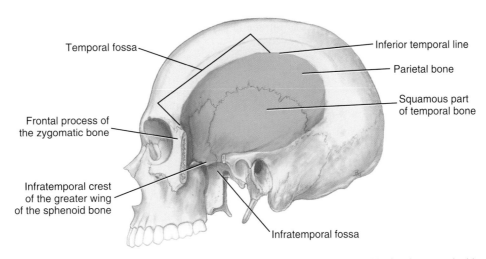

FIGURE 3-59 Lateral view of the skull and the temporal fossa highlighted and its borders noted with parts of the zygomatic and temporal bones removed.

and superior end of the fossa. Other structures pass into the infratemporal fossa from the cranial cavity (see Figures 9-3 and 9-31).

The infratemporal fossa contains a part of the maxillary artery and its second part branches that arise here, including the middle meningeal artery, which goes into the cranial cavity through the foramen spinosum; the inferior alveolar artery, which enters the mandible through the mandibular foramen; and the posterior alveolar artery, which enters the maxilla through the posterior superior alveolar foramina on the infratemporal surface of the maxilla (see Table 3-3). The fossa also contains the pterygoid plexus of veins and the pterygoid muscles (see Figure 6-12).

The infratemporal fossa also contains a part of the mandibular nerve (or third division) of the fifth cranial or trigeminal nerve including the inferior alveolar and lingual nerves. The mandibular

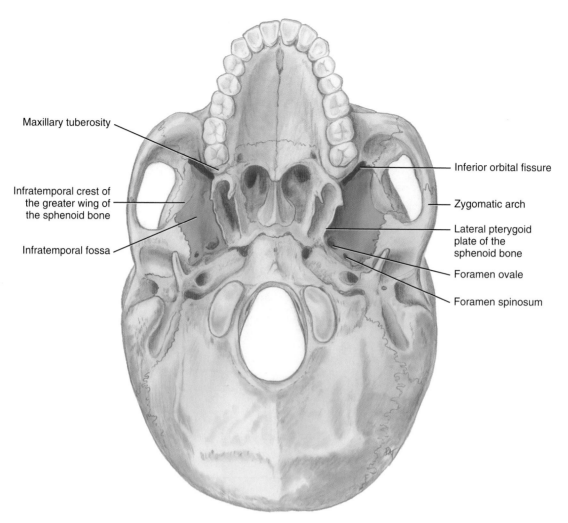

Maxillary tuberosity

Infratemporal crest of
the greater wing of
the sphenoid bone

Infratemporal fossa

Inferior orbital fissure

Zygomatic arch

Lateral pterygoid
plate of the
sphenoid bone

Foramen ovale

Foramen spinosum

FIGURE 3-60 Inferior view of the skull with the mandible removed and the infratemporal fossae highlighted with its borders and features noted.

nerve enters by way of the foramen ovale, passing between the cranial cavity and oral cavity (see Table 3-3).

PTERYGOPALATINE FOSSA

The pterygopalatine fossa is a cone-shaped paired depression deep to the infratemporal fossa and posterior to the maxilla on each side of the skull (Figure 3-61). This smaller fossa is located between the pterygoid process and the maxillary tuberosity, close to the apex of the orbit. The pterygopalatine fossa communicates via fissures and foramina in its walls with the following: the cranial cavity, infratemporal fossa, orbit, nasal cavity, and oral cavity.

The borders of the pterygopalatine fossa include: superiorly, the inferior surface of the body of the sphenoid bone; anteriorly, the maxillary tuberosity of the maxilla; medially, the vertical plate of the palatine bone; laterally, the pterygomaxillary fissure; inferiorly, the pterygopalatine canal; and posteriorly, the pterygoid process of the sphenoid bone.

The pterygopalatine fossa contains a part of the maxillary artery and its third part branches that arise here, including the infraorbital and sphenopalatine arteries, and part of the maxillary nerve (or second division) of the fifth cranial or trigeminal nerve and its branches, as well as the pterygopalatine ganglion (see Table 3-3). The

foramen rotundum is the entrance route for the maxillary nerve; a second foramen in the pterygoid process, the pterygoid canal, transmits autonomic fibers to the pterygopalatine ganglion. The pterygopalatine canal also connects with the greater and lesser palatine foramina of the palatine bones of the posterior hard palate.

CERVICAL BONES
CERVICAL VERTEBRAE

Each **cervical vertebra** (plural, **vertebrae**) (ver-tuh-bruh, ver-tuh-bree) of the spine is located in the neck between the base of the skull and the thoracic vertebrae in the trunk. All seven cervical vertebrae are bony rings with a central **vertebral foramen** (ver-tuh-bruhl) for the spinal cord and associated tissue. However, in contrast to most other vertebrae, the cervical vertebrae are characterized by the presence of a **transverse foramen** in the **transverse process** on each side of the vertebral foramen. The vertebral artery runs through these transverse foramina.

Only the first two cervical vertebrae are described in this chapter because their anatomy is unusual and they are located near the skull; the other cervical vertebrae can be studied from reference materials (see Appendix A). Importantly, damage to any vertebrae can affect dental treatment because the patient may experience a range of

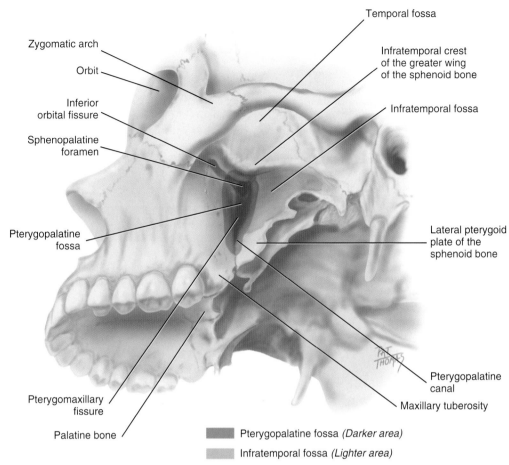

Temporal fossa

Zygomatic arch

Infratemporal crest
of the greater wing
of the sphenoid bone

Orbit

Inferior
orbital fissure

Infratemporal fossa

Sphenopalatine
foramen

Pterygopalatine
fossa

Lateral pterygoid
plate of the
sphenoid bone

Pterygomaxillary
fissure

Pterygopalatine
canal

Palatine bone

Maxillary tuberosity

▮ Pterygopalatine fossa *(Darker area)*

▮ Infratemporal fossa *(Lighter area)*

FIGURE 3-61 Oblique lateral view of the base of the skull and the roof of the infratemporal fossa (*lighter area*) and pterygopalatine fossa (*darker area*) highlighted with their borders and features noted.

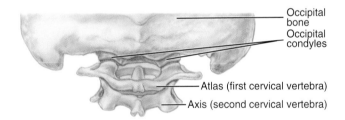

Occipital
bone
Occipital
condyles

Atlas (first cervical vertebra)

Axis (second cervical vertebra)

FIGURE 3-62 Posterior view of the skull and the first and second cervical vertebrae.

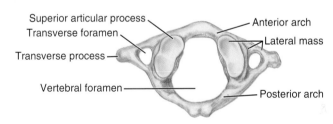

Superior articular process

Transverse foramen

Anterior arch

Transverse process

Lateral mass

Vertebral foramen

Posterior arch

FIGURE 3-63 Superior view of the disarticulated first cervical vertebra, the atlas.

complications that can affect dental care, from difficulty in movement to paralysis.

First Cervical Vertebra. The first cervical vertebra or **atlas** (at-luhs) articulates with the skull at the occipital condyles of the occipital bone (Figure 3-62). The atlas has the form of an irregular ring consisting of two **lateral masses of the atlas** connected by a short **anterior arch** and a longer **posterior arch** (Figures 3-63 and 3-66). This cervical bone lacks a body and a spine.

The lateral masses of the atlas can be effectively bilaterally palpated on a patient by placing fingers between both the mastoid processes and the angles of the mandible. More medially, the lateral masses present large, concave **superior articular processes** for the corresponding occipital condyles of the skull. The lateral masses also have circular **inferior articular processes** for articulation with the second cervical vertebra.

Second Cervical Vertebra. The second cervical vertebra or **axis** (ak-sis) is characterized by having a **dens** (denz) (Figure 3-64). The dens or *odontoid process* articulates anteriorly with the anterior arch of the first cervical vertebra (Figures 3-65 and 3-66). The body of the axis is inferior to the dens and the spine of the axis is located posterior to the body. The body and the adjoining transverse process present superior articular processes for additional articulation with the inferior articulating surfaces of the atlas. In addition, the inferior aspect of the axis presents inferior articular processes for articulating with the articular processes of the third cervical vertebra.

HYOID BONE

The hyoid bone is suspended in the neck from the styloid process of the temporal bone by the paired stylohyoid ligaments. With its orientation within a horizontal plane, the bone forms the base of both the tongue and larynx. Thus the hyoid bone does not articulate with any other bones, giving it its characteristic mobility, which is necessary for mastication, swallowing, and speech. Instead of bony articulation, regional muscles attach to the hyoid bone (see Chapter 4).

The hyoid bone is inferior to and medial to both angles of the mandible. The hyoid bone can be effectively palpated on a patient during an extraoral examination by feeling inferior and medial to the angles of the mandible; the bone can also be moved slightly side to side. It is important to not confuse the hyoid bone with the inferiorly placed thyroid cartilage (the "Adam's apple") when palpating the neck (see Figure 2-24). The hyoid bone is superior and anterior to the thyroid cartilage of the larynx; it is usually at the level of the third cervical vertebra but rises during swallowing and other activities. The hyoid bone is lowered after swallowing by the broad thyrohyoid membrane, a fibrous layer that connects the bone to the thyroid cartilage.

The "U"-shaped hyoid bone consists of five parts as noted from an anterior view (see Figures 3-65 and 3-66). The anterior part is the midline **body of the hyoid bone**. There is also a pair of projections on both sides of the hyoid bone, the **greater cornu** and **lesser cornu**. These projecting horns serve as attachments for muscles and ligaments (see Figure 4-24).

INTERNAL SKULL FROM SAGITTAL VIEW

Now that the external and internal parts of the skull have been viewed and discussed as well as the individual bones of the skull, it is also useful to consider an internal view of the skull on a sagittal section to understand the overall placement of bony structures as well as associated soft tissue as shown in Figure 3-66. For further identification of structures within a similar sagittal section, see Figure 8-4, *B*. For other sections involving the head and neck, see Chapter 11.

> ### Clinical Considerations With Skeletal System Pathology
>
> Bone fracture can occur with severe blows to the face. Fractures of the facial skeleton tend to occur at its points of buttress with the cranium. These buttress points include: the medial aspect of the orbit, the articulation of the zygomatic bone with both the frontal bone and temporal bones, the articulation of the pterygoid plates of the sphenoid bone, the palatine bones, and each maxilla. When the skull is fractured, reconstructive surgeons also rely upon these buttresses as anchor points for plates, screws, and other devices.
>
> The fracture of the bone may be detected by gentle palpation of the patient during an extraoral examination after radiographic analysis. If the fracture is bilateral, the entire facial skeleton can be pushed posteriorly, resulting in upper respiratory tract obstruction. These fractures may also heal poorly, resulting in abnormal bony contours.
>
> Abnormal bony contours can lead to facial asymmetry and nodular-appearing intraoral areas (Figures 3-67 and 3-68). The growth related to palatal or mandibular tori are considered oral variations, but others can be due to endocrine diseases causing abnormal bone growth. Bone can also enlarge with neoplastic growth of bone or other tissue, such as hard dental tissue (enamel) as in the case of the benign tumor of ameloblastoma. The dental professional needs to record any abnormal areas of bone noted and make any appropriate referrals. Pathology associated with the temporomandibular joint is discussed in Chapter 5.

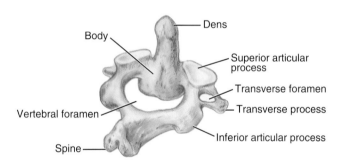

FIGURE 3-64 Posterosuperior view of the disarticulated second cervical vertebra, the axis.

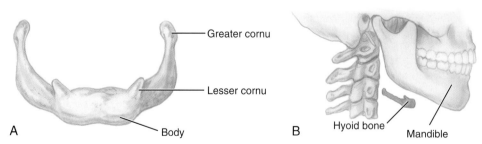

FIGURE 3-65 Anterior view of the hyoid bone **(A)** and with its location highlighted on a lateral view of the lower skull and the nearby cervical vertebrae **(B)**.

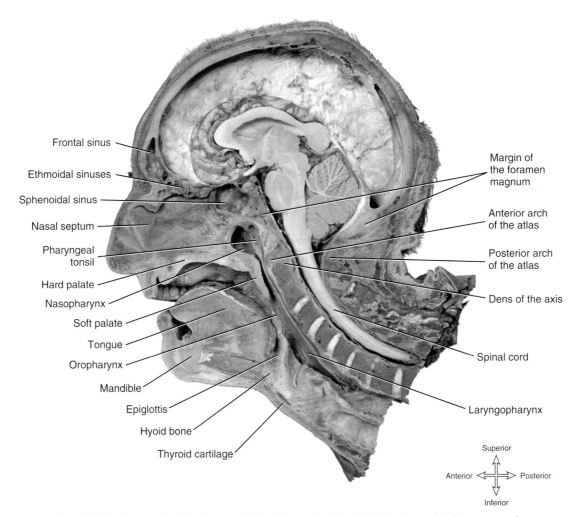

FIGURE 3-66 Dissection showing a sagittal section of the internal skull and associated bony and soft tissue structures. For further identification of the section, see Figure 8-4, *B*. *(From Reynolds PA, Abrahams PH: McMinn's interactive clinical anatomy: head and neck, ed 2, London, 2010, Elsevier.)*

Labels (left side, top to bottom): Frontal sinus, Ethmoidal sinuses, Sphenoidal sinus, Nasal septum, Pharyngeal tonsil, Hard palate, Nasopharynx, Soft palate, Tongue, Oropharynx, Mandible, Epiglottis, Hyoid bone, Thyroid cartilage

Labels (right side, top to bottom): Margin of the foramen magnum, Anterior arch of the atlas, Posterior arch of the atlas, Dens of the axis, Spinal cord, Laryngopharynx

Orientation: Superior, Anterior, Posterior, Inferior

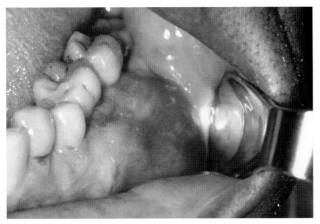

FIGURE 3-67 Nodular bony enlargement of ameloblastoma, a benign neoplasm of hard dental tissue (enamel) in the mandible that may result in facial asymmetry. *(Courtesy Margaret J. Fehrenbach, RDH, MS.)*

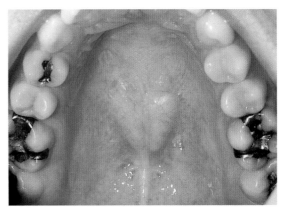

FIGURE 3-68 Nodular bony enlargement of a palatal torus noted on the hard palate, a benign growth of bone that may interfere with dental treatment. *(Courtesy Margaret J. Fehrenbach, RDH, MS.)*

REVIEW QUESTIONS

1. Which of the following features is located on the temporal bone?
   A. Superior temporal line
   B. Foramen rotundum
   C. External acoustic meatus
   D. Cribriform plate
   E. Orbital plate

2. Which area is immediately posterior to the MOST distal tooth in the upper arch of the dentition?
   A. Retromolar triangle
   B. Postglenoid process
   C. Cribriform plate
   D. Maxillary tuberosity
   E. Hamular process

3. In addition to the zygomatic bone, which of the following bones has a process that forms the other part of the zygomatic arch?
   A. Temporal
   B. Maxillae
   C. Sphenoid
   D. Palatine

4. Which of the following is the location of the articulation of the parietal bones and the occipital bone?
   A. Coronal suture
   B. Squamosal suture
   C. Sagittal suture
   D. Lambdoidal suture

5. Which of the following bony landmarks form an articulation with each other?
   A. Occipital condyles with atlas
   B. Occipital condyles with axis
   C. Mandibular fossa with coronoid notch
   D. Mandibular fossa with coronoid process

6. Which of the following features is located on the lateral surface of the mandible?
   A. Lingula
   B. Submandibular fossa
   C. Genial tubercles
   D. External oblique line
   E. Mandibular foramen

7. The orbital apex is composed of the lesser wing of the sphenoid bone and the
   A. ethmoid bone.
   B. frontal bone.
   C. maxillae.
   D. palatine bone.
   E. lacrimal bone.

8. Which of the following landmarks is formed by the maxillae?
   A. Mental spine
   B. Median palatine suture
   C. Retromolar triangle
   D. Hamulus
   E. Inferior orbital fissure

9. Which of the following structures is located or travels within the infratemporal fossa?
   A. Masseter muscle
   B. Pterygopalatine ganglion
   C. Posterior superior alveolar artery
   D. Maxillary division of the fifth cranial nerve

10. The concavity noted on the anterior border of the coronoid process of the mandibular ramus is the
    A. mandibular notch.
    B. coronoid notch.
    C. temporal fossa.
    D. infratemporal fossa.

11. Which of the following landmarks serves to locate the hyoid bone during an extraoral examination on a patient?
    A. Level of the first cervical vertebra
    B. Superior and anterior to the thyroid cartilage
    C. Articulation with the cartilage of the larynx
    D. Inferior and posterior to the "Adam's apple"

12. Which of the following structures forms the floor of each maxillary sinus?
    A. Alveolar process of the maxilla
    B. Facial wall of the maxilla
    C. Infratemporal surface of the maxilla
    D. Lateral wall of the nasal cavity

13. Which of the following processes is located just inferior and medial to the external acoustic meatus?
    A. Pterygoid process
    B. Styloid process
    C. Mastoid process
    D. Hamulus

14. The spaces located under the three conchae of the lateral walls of the nasal cavity are the nasal
    A. ostia.
    B. ducts.
    C. meatuses.
    D. inferior nasal conchae.
    E. vestibules.

15. Which of the following bones and their processes form the hard palate?
    A. Maxillary processes of the maxillae and horizontal plates of the palatine bones
    B. Palatal processes of the maxillae and maxillary plates of the palatine bones
    C. Horizontal plates of the palatine bones and palatine processes of the maxillae
    D. Maxillary plates of the palatine bones and horizontal processes of the maxillae

16. Which of the following cranial nerves is associated with the stylomastoid foramen?
    A. Fifth cranial nerve
    B. Seventh cranial nerve
    C. Ninth cranial nerve
    D. Tenth cranial nerve
    E. Eleventh cranial nerve

17. Which of the following bones of the skull is paired?
    A. Sphenoid
    B. Ethmoid
    C. Occipital
    D. Vomer
    E. Parietal

18. Which of the following bony plates is perforated to allow the passage of the olfactory nerves for the sense of smell?
    A. Medial plate of sphenoid bone
    B. Lateral plate of sphenoid bone
    C. Perpendicular plate of ethmoid bone
    D. Cribriform plate of ethmoid bone

19. Which of the following bones of the skull is considered a cranial bone?
    A. Vomer
    B. Maxilla
    C. Sphenoid
    D. Zygomatic
    E. Mandible
20. Which part of the temporal bone is involved in the temporomandibular joint?
    A. Squamous
    B. Tympanic
    C. Petrous
    D. Mastoid
21. Which is a single bone located at the midline of the skull?
    A. Temporal
    B. Zygomatic
    C. Sphenoid
    D. Inferior nasal conchae
22. Which of the following structures is a short windowlike opening found in healthy bone?
    A. Fossa
    B. Foramen
    C. Fissure
    D. Perforation
23. Which of the following bones forms the jugular foramen along with the jugular notch of the temporal bone?
    A. Occipital
    B. Mandible
    C. Parietal
    D. Sphenoid
24. Which of the following is a faint ridge noted where the right and left mandibular processes fused together in early childhood?
    A. Mylohyoid line
    B. Mental protuberance
    C. Mandibular symphysis
    D. External oblique line
25. In which bone are BOTH the infraorbital foramen and infraorbital canal located?
    A. Frontal
    B. Maxillae
    C. Sphenoid
    D. Zygomatic
26. Which of the following structures is a large, roughened projection related to the petrous part of the temporal bone?
    A. Notch
    B. Process
    C. Air cells
    D. Sinus
27. Which of the following landmarks is an anterior process located on the sphenoid bone?
    A. Wing
    B. Notch
    C. Body
    D. Angle
28. The lacrimal gland is located just inside the lateral part of the
    A. glabella.
    B. supraorbital rim.
    C. supraorbital notch.
    D. nasion.
29. The occipital condyles are located _____ and _____ to the foramen magnum.
    A. Medial, anterior
    B. Lateral, anterior
    C. Medial, posterior
    D. Lateral, posterior
30. Which bone forms BOTH the superior and middle nasal conchae?
    A. Occipital
    B. Mandible
    C. Maxilla
    D. Frontal
    E. Ethmoid

Identification Exercises

Identify the structures on the following diagrams by filling in each blank with the correct anatomic term. You can check your answers by looking back at the figure indicated in parentheses for each identification diagram.

1. (Figure 3-4)

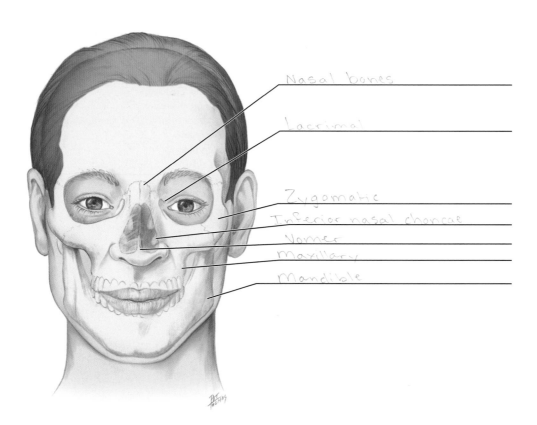

Nasal bones

Lacrimal

Zygomatic

Inferior nasal choncae

Vomer

Maxillary

Mandible

2. (Figures 3-5, 3-6, and 3-7)

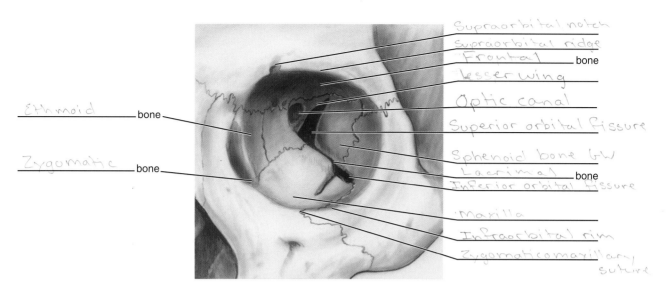

Supraorbital notch
Supraorbital ridge
Frontal _____ bone
Lesser wing
Optic canal
Superior orbital fissure
Sphenoid bone GW
Lacrimal _____ bone
Inferior orbital fissure
Maxilla
Infraorbital rim
Zygomaticomaxillary suture

Ethmoid _____ bone

Zygomatic _____ bone

3. (Figures 3-20, 3-23, and 3-27)

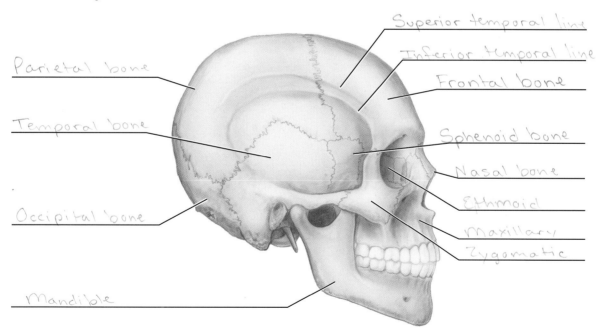

Superior temporal line
Inferior temporal line
Frontal bone
Sphenoid bone
Nasal bone
Ethmoid
Maxillary
Zygomatic

Parietal bone

Temporal bone

Occipital bone

Mandible

4. (Figure 3-22, *A*)

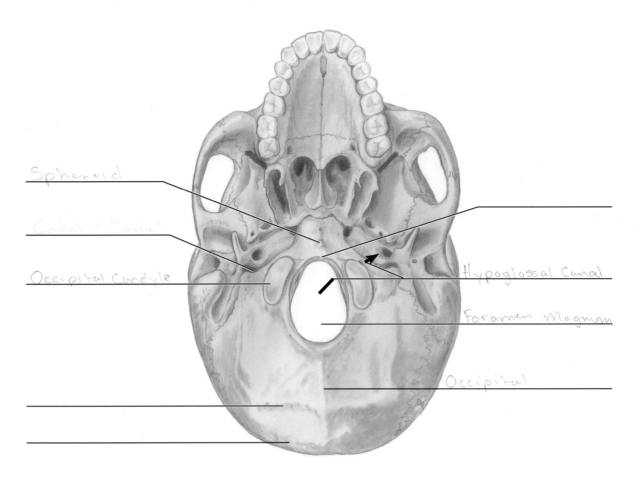

Sphenoid

Carotid Canal

Occipital Condyle

Hypoglossal Canal

Foramen Magnum

Occipital

5. (Figures 3-28, 3-29, and 3-30)

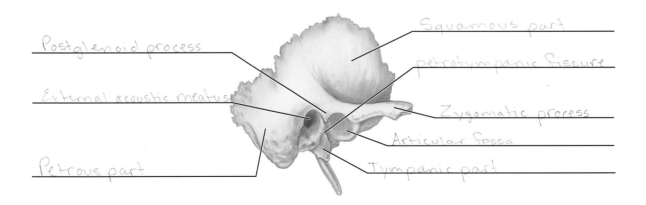

Postglenoid process

External acoustic meatus

Petrous part

Squamous part

petrotympanic fissure

Zygomatic process

Articular fossa

Tympanic part

6. (Figures 3-31 and 3-32, *A*)

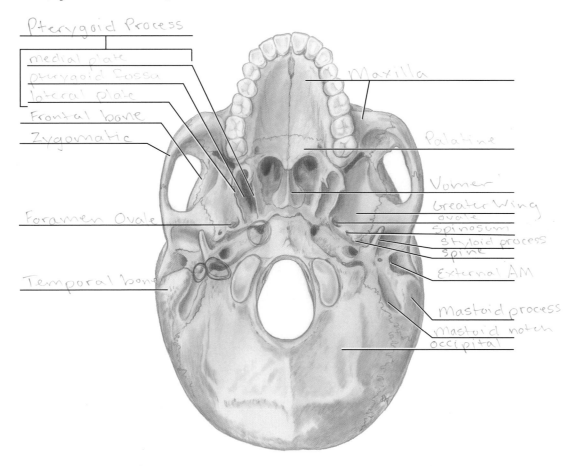

Pterygoid Process
medial plate
pterygoid fossa
lateral plate
Frontal bone
Zygomatic
Foramen Ovale
Temporal bone

Maxilla
Palatine
Vomer
Greater Wing
ovale
spinosum
Styloid process
spine
External AM
Mastoid process
Mastoid notch
occipital

7. (Figure 3-33, *A*)

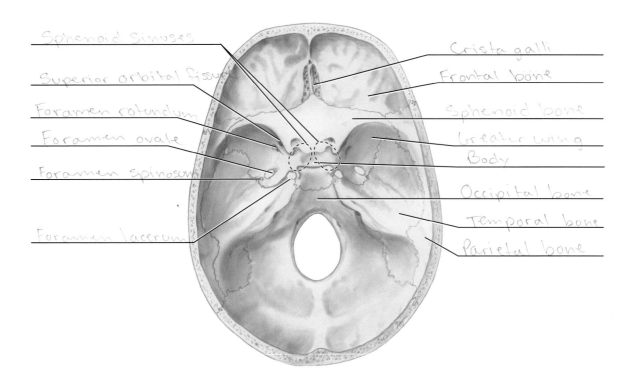

Sphenoid Sinuses
Superior orbital fissure
Foramen rotundum
Foramen ovale
Foramen spinosum
Foramen lacerum

Crista galli
Frontal bone
Sphenoid bone
Greater wing
Body
Occipital bone
Temporal bone
Parietal bone

8. (Figure 3-35, *A*)

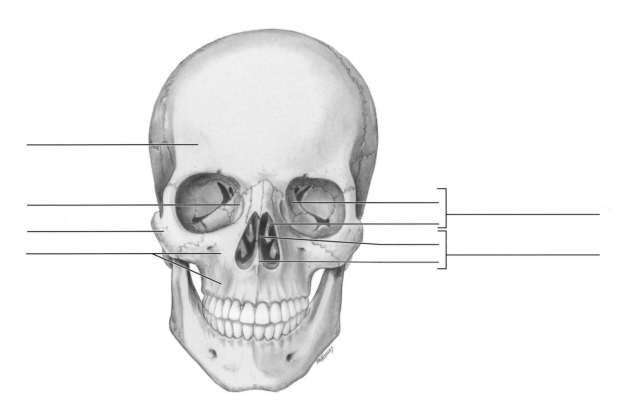

9. (Figure 3-38)

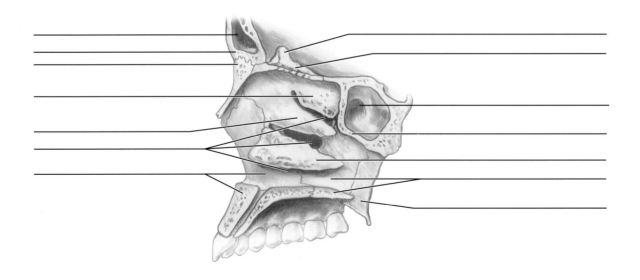

10. (Figures 3-40 and 3-41)

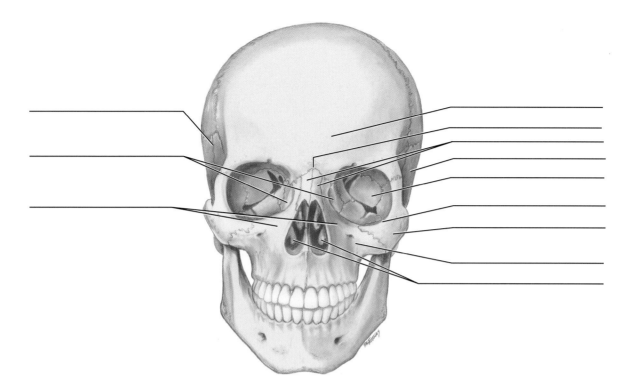

11. (Figure 3-42)

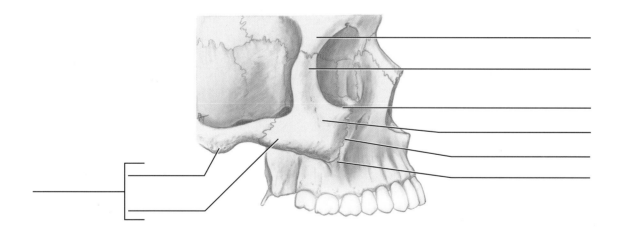

12. (Figure 3-44)

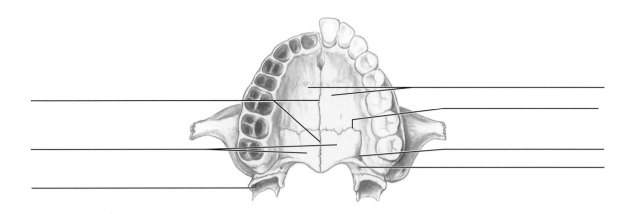

13. (Figure 3-45)

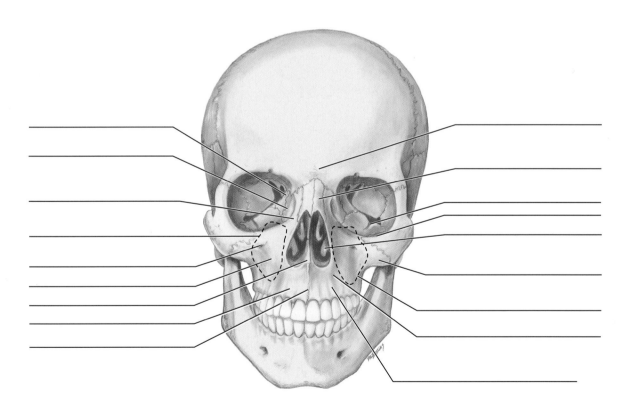

14. (Figure 3-47, *A*)

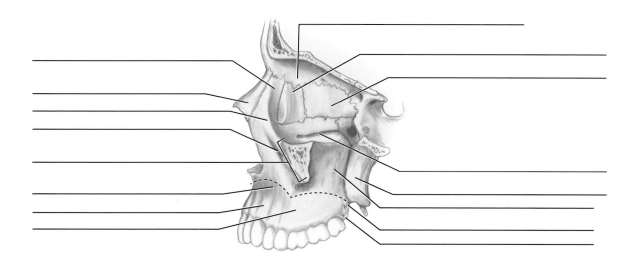

15. (Figures 3-52, *A* and 3-55, *B*)

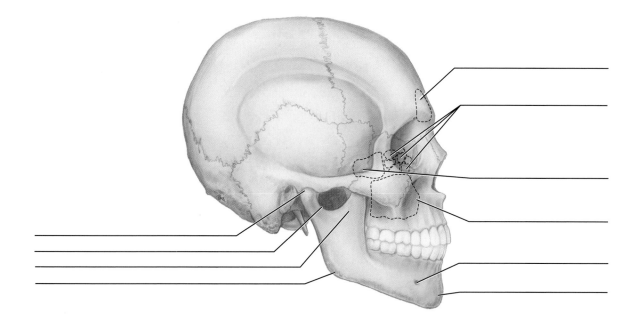

16. (Figure 3-60)

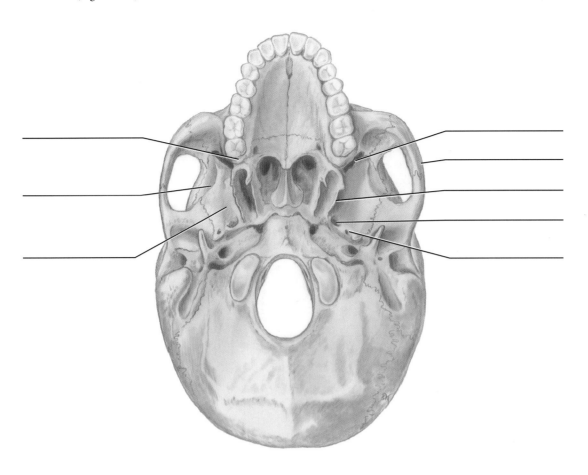

17. (Figure 3-61)

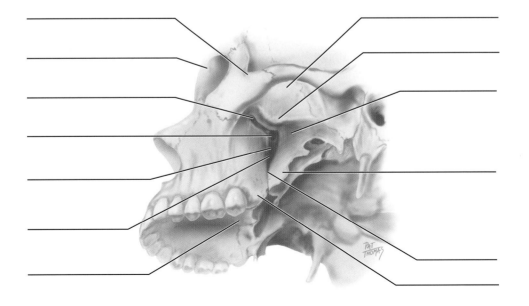

18. (Figure 3-62)

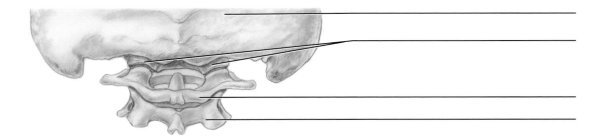

19. (Figure 3-65, *A*)

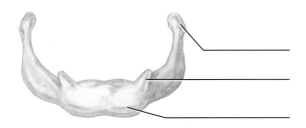

20. (Figure 3-65, *B*)

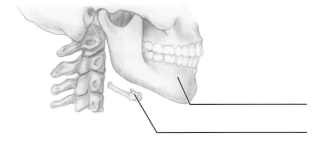

CHAPTER 4

Muscular System

1. Define and pronounce the **key terms** and **anatomic terms** in this chapter.
2. Locate and identify the muscles of the head and neck on a diagram, skull, and patient.
3. Describe the origin, insertion, action, and innervation of each muscle of the head and neck.
4. Discuss the processes of mastication, speech, and swallowing with regard to anatomic

considerations involving the muscles of the head and neck.
5. Discuss the pathology associated with the muscles of the head and neck.
6. Correctly complete the review questions and activities for this chapter.
7. Integrate an understanding of the muscles of the head and neck into the clinical dental practice.

●●● KEY TERMS

Action Movement accomplished by a muscle when muscle fibers contract.
Facial paralysis (puh-**ral**-i-sis) Loss of the action of facial muscles.

Insertion End of the muscle attached to more movable structure.
Muscle Body tissue that shortens under neural control, causing soft tissue and bony structures to move.

Muscular system System that includes skeletal muscle tissue.
Origin End of muscle attached to least movable structure.

MUSCULAR SYSTEM OVERVIEW

The muscular system includes skeletal muscle tissue. A muscle within the muscular system shortens under neural control, causing soft tissue and bony structures of the body to move. Each muscle is attached at both ends of these moving structures, with each end categorized according to its role in movement. The origin is the end of the muscle that is attached to the least movable structure. The insertion is the other end of the muscle and is attached to the more movable structure.

Generally, the insertion of the muscle moves toward the origin where the muscle arises when the muscle is contracted. The movement that is accomplished when the muscle fibers contract is the action of the muscle. The muscles have specific innervation that is discussed in this chapter, but a more thorough explanation of the nervous system can be found in Chapter 8. The blood supply to the muscular area is further discussed in Chapter 6. However, it is important to remember that unlike innervation to the muscles, which is a one-to-one relationship, blood supply is regional. Arteries supply the muscles in their vicinity, and veins receive blood from the nearby muscles.

HEAD AND NECK MUSCLES

The dental professional needs to determine the location and action of the skeletal muscles of the head and neck in order to perform a

thorough patient examination (see Appendix B). This information is important because the placement of other structures such as bones, nerves, blood vessels, and lymph nodes is related to the location of these skeletal muscles. These muscles may also malfunction and be involved in temporomandibular joint disorders (see Chapter 5), occlusal trauma, and certain nervous system diseases (discussed later). Muscles of the head and neck and their attachments define many of the spaces in the face and neck and are also a consideration in the spread of dental infections (see Chapters 11 and 12, respectively).

The muscles of the head and neck are divided according to function into six main groups: the cervical muscles, muscles of facial expression, muscles of mastication, hyoid muscles, muscles of the tongue, and muscles of the pharynx. Muscle groups of the ears, eyes, and nose are not included in this chapter but can be studied from reference materials (see Appendix A).

CERVICAL MUSCLES

There are two **cervical muscles** considered in this chapter. Both are superficially located on the neck and serve to hold and stabilize the head as well as position the head in relation to the rest of the body. The two cervical muscles include: the sternocleidomastoid muscle and trapezius muscle.

STERNOCLEIDOMASTOID MUSCLE

One of the largest and most superficial cervical muscles is the paired sternocleidomastoid (SCM) muscle (Figure 4-1). As a thick muscle of the neck, it serves as a primary muscular landmark of the neck during an extraoral examination of a patient since it divides the neck region into anterior and posterior cervical triangles. This helps define the location of structures, such as the lymph nodes of the head and neck (see Figures 2-23, 2-25, and 2-26 and see discussion in Chapters 2 and 10).

Origin and Insertion. The muscle originates from the medial part of the clavicle and the sternum's superior and lateral surfaces and passes posteriorly and superiorly to insert on the mastoid process of the temporal bone as well as by a thin aponeurosis or layer of flat broad tendons into the lateral half of the superior nuchal line of the occipital bone (see Figures 3-22 and 3-31). This insertion is just posterior and inferior to the external acoustic meatus of each ear.

Action. If one of the muscles contracts, the head and neck bend to the ipsilateral side, and the face and anterior part of the neck rotate to the contralateral side. If both muscles contract at the same time, the head will flex at the neck and extend at the junction between the neck and skull. The SCM muscle is effectively palpated on each side of the neck during an extraoral examination when the patient moves the head to the contralateral side (Figure 4-2). This makes the important landmark of the muscle more prominent and increases accessibility for effective palpation of the nearby cervical nodes as discussed.

Innervation. The muscle is innervated by the eleventh cranial or accessory nerve.

TRAPEZIUS MUSCLE

The other important superficial cervical muscle is the paired **trapezius muscle** (truh-**pee**-zee-us), which is superficial to both the lateral and posterior surfaces of the neck (Figure 4-3). It is a broad flat triangular muscle.

Origin and Insertion. The muscle originates from the external surface of the occipital bone at the superior nuchal line (see Figure 3-22) and the posterior midline of the cervical and thoracic regions. It then inserts on the lateral third of the clavicle and parts of the scapula.

Action. The cervical fibers of the muscle act to lift the clavicle and scapula, as when the shoulders are shrugged. With this action, the muscle is then used as a base for palpation of structures such as the cervical lymph nodes during an extraoral examination.

Innervation. The muscle is innervated by the eleventh cranial or accessory nerve, as well as the third and fourth cervical nerves.

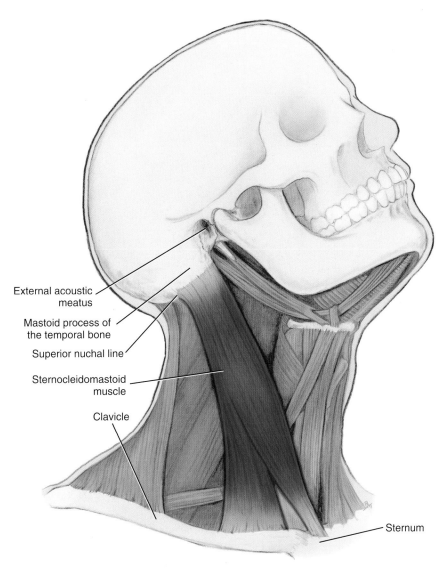

External acoustic meatus

Mastoid process of the temporal bone

Superior nuchal line

Sternocleidomastoid muscle

Clavicle

Sternum

FIGURE 4-1 Origin and insertion of the highlighted right sternocleidomastoid muscle.

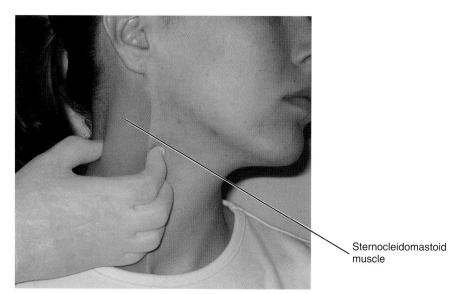

FIGURE 4-2 Demonstration of palpation of the highlighted sternocleidomastoid muscle of a patient during an extraoral examination with the patient turning the head to the contralateral side, which makes the muscle more prominent. *(Courtesy of Margaret J. Fehrenbach, RDH, MS.)*

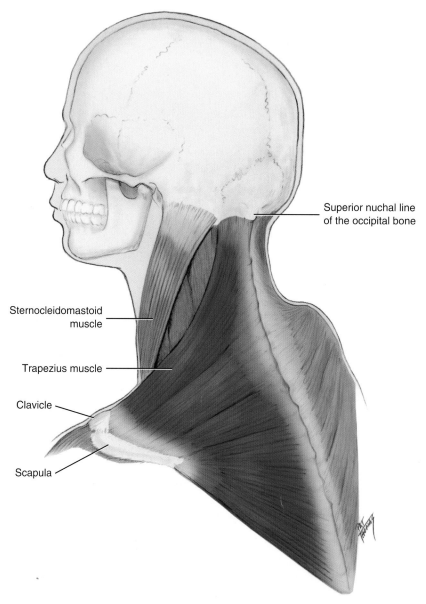

FIGURE 4-3 Origin and insertion of the highlighted left trapezius muscle.

MUSCLES OF FACIAL EXPRESSION

The **muscles of facial expression** are paired muscles within the superficial fascia of the facial tissue (Figures 4-4 and 4-5). Use of these muscles is noted during an extraoral examination, assuring function of the nerves to these muscles. The use of a mirror when performing various facial expressions is helpful in learning about the location and function of each of these muscles.

Origin and Insertion. The origins and insertions of the muscles of facial expression vary; however, these muscles may be further grouped according to whether they are situated in the scalp, orbital region, or oral region (Table 4-1). All the muscles of facial expression originate from the surface of the skull bone (rarely the fascia) and insert on the dermis of skin.

Action. When the muscles of facial expression contract, the skin moves. These muscles also cause wrinkles at right angles to the muscles' action line. During facial expression, the muscles of facial expression act in various combinations to show varying expressions to change the appearance of the face; this group involvement is similar to the muscles of mastication discussed later (Table 4-2).

Innervation. All the muscles of facial expression are innervated by the seventh cranial or facial nerve, with each nerve serving the muscles on one side of the face (see Figure 8-22). Branches have been designated according to location across the face.

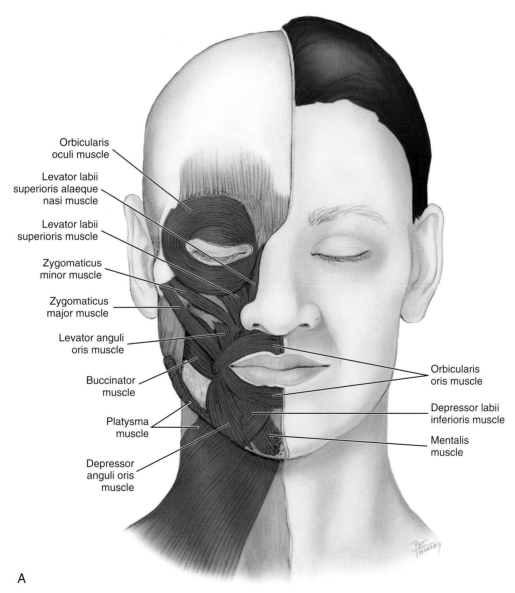

A

FIGURE 4-4 Muscles of facial expression are highlighted from an anterior view (**A**). See next page for part **B**.

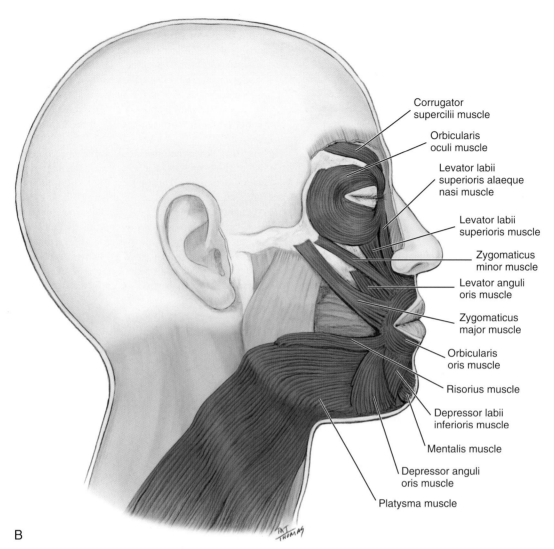

B

FIGURE 4-4, cont'd B, Muscles of facial expression are highlighted from a lateral view.

TABLE 4-1	**Muscles of Facial Expression**	
MUSCLE	**ORIGIN**	**INSERTION**
Epicranial	Frontal belly or frontalis muscle: epicranial aponeurosis Occipital belly or occipitalis muscle: occipital and temporal bones	Frontal belly or frontalis muscle: eyebrow and root of nose Occipital belly or occipitalis muscle: epicranial aponeurosis
Orbicularis oculi	Orbital rim, frontal bone, and maxilla	Lateral canthus area, some encircle eye
Orbicularis oris	Vermilion zone fibers: encircles mouth Non-vermilion zone fibers: cross the midline	Labial commissure Diffusely in the lip or nose
Buccinator	Maxilla, mandible, and pterygomandibular raphe	Labial commissure
Risorius	Fascia superficial to masseter muscle	Labial commissure
Levator labii superioris	Maxilla	Upper lip
Levator labii superioris alaeque nasi	Maxilla	Ala of nose and upper lip
Zygomaticus major	Zygomatic bone	Labial commissure
Zygomaticus minor	Zygomatic bone	Upper lip
Levator anguli oris	Maxilla	Labial commissure
Depressor anguli oris	Mandible	Labial commissure
Depressor labii inferioris	Mandible	Lower lip
Mentalis	Mandible	Chin
Platysma	Clavicle and shoulder	Mandible and muscles of the mouth

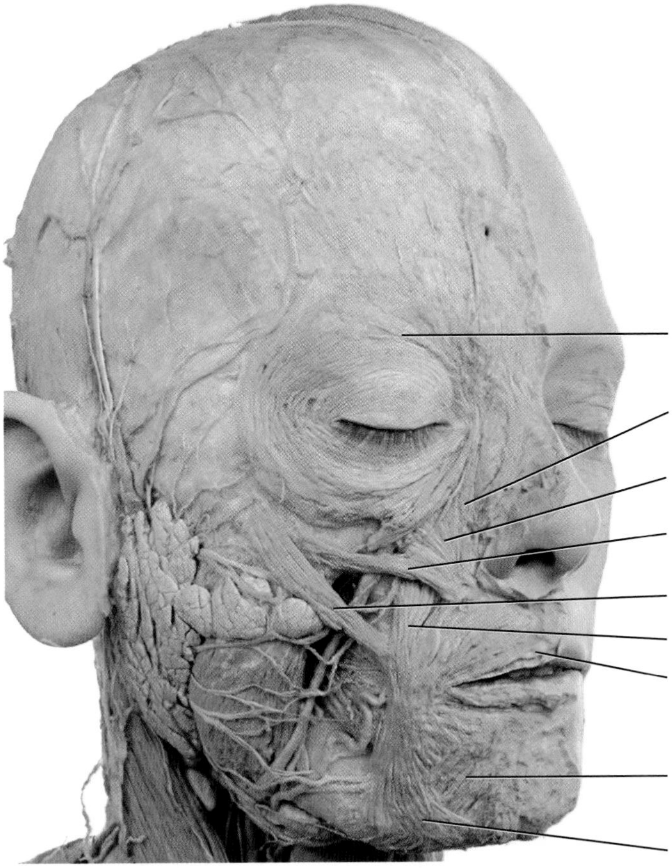

Orbicularis oculi
muscle

Levator labii superioris
alaeque nasi muscle

Levator labii
superioris muscle

Zygomaticus
minor muscle

Zygomaticus
major muscle

Levator anguli oris muscle

Orbicularis oris muscle

Depressor labii
inferioris muscle

Depressor anguli
oris muscle

FIGURE 4-5 Superficial dissection of the face showing most of the muscles of facial expression. *(From Reynolds PA, Abrahams PH:* McMinn's interactive clinical anatomy: head and neck, *ed 2, London, 2001, Elsevier.)*

TABLE 4-2	Muscles of Facial Expression and Associated Facial Expressions
MUSCLE	**FACIAL EXPRESSION(S)**
Epicranial	Surprise
Orbicularis oculi	Closing eyelid and squinting
Corrugator supercilii	Frowning
Orbicularis oris	Closing and pursing lips as well as pouting and grimacing
Buccinator	Compresses the cheeks during chewing
Risorius	Stretching lips
Levator labii superioris	Raising upper lip
Levator labii superioris alaeque nasi	Raising upper lip and dilating nares with sneer
Zygomaticus major	Smiling
Zygomaticus minor	Raising upper lip to assist in smiling
Levator anguli oris	Smiling
Depressor anguli oris	Frowning
Depressor labii inferioris	Lowering lower lip
Mentalis	Raising chin and protruding lower lip
Platysma	Raising neck skin and grimacing

Clinical Considerations With Muscles of Facial Expression Pathology

An inability to form facial expressions on one side of the face may be the first sign of damage to the seventh cranial or facial nerve that innervates the muscles of facial expression. The nerve damage results in **facial paralysis** of the muscles of facial expression on the involved side (Figure 4-6). Paralysis is the loss of voluntary muscle action that can be on either a temporary or permanent basis. Facial paralysis can occur with a stroke (or cerebrovascular accident), Bell palsy, or possibly with parotid salivary gland cancer because the seventh cranial or facial nerve travels through the gland (see Figure 8-22). Twitching, spasms, and weakness can also be evident along with excessive drooling and altered taste sensations. These cases of facial paralysis may resolve over time or with specific treatment.

The facial nerve within the parotid salivary gland can also become anesthetized with an incorrectly administered inferior alveolar or Vazirani-Akinosi mandibular blocks leading to transient facial paralysis (see Figure 9-37 and 9-56) or permanently damaged by oral surgery in the region.

MUSCLES OF FACIAL EXPRESSION IN SCALP REGION

Epicranial Muscle. The **epicranial muscle** (ep-ee-**kray**-nee-uhl) or *epicranius* is a muscle of facial expression in the scalp region (Figure 4-7). This muscle and its tendon are one of the layers that form the scalp. This muscle has two bellies: the frontal and occipital bellies.

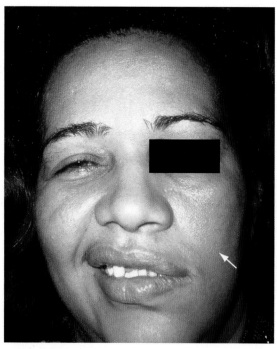

FIGURE 4-6 Unilateral paralysis of the facial muscles due to muscle damage from Bell palsy *(arrow)*. The patient is trying to smile during an extraoral examination; however, she is unable to show any facial expression on her involved left side. *(Courtesy of Margaret J. Fehrenbach, RDH, MS.)*

The bellies are separated by a large, spread-out scalpal tendon, the **epicranial aponeurosis** (ap-o-noo-**row**-sis) or *galea aponeurotica*.

Origin and Insertion. The frontal belly of the epicranial muscle arises from the epicranial aponeurosis, having no bony attachment. The epicranial aponeurosis is at the most superior part of the skull (see Figure 3-22). The frontal belly or **frontalis muscle** (**frun**-tal-is) then inserts into the skin of the eyebrow and root of the nose (see Figure 2-7). The occipital belly or **occipitalis muscle** (ok-sip-i-**ta**-lis) originates from both the superior nuchal line of the occipital bone and the mastoid process of the temporal bone and then inserts in the epicranial aponeurosis (see Figure 3-31).

Action. Both bellies of the muscle raise the eyebrows and scalp, as when a person shows surprise (Figure 4-8). However, the two bellies of the muscle can also act independently of each other during certain facial expressions.

MUSCLES OF FACIAL EXPRESSION IN ORBITAL REGION

Orbicularis Oculi Muscle. The **orbicularis oculi muscle** (or-bik-u-**lare**-is ok-yule-eye) is a muscle of facial expression that encircles the orbit (Figure 4-9). This muscle has important functions in protecting and moistening the eye, as well as in facial expression. Thus loss of its use can possibly damage the eye(s) due to the subsequent dryness.

Origin and Insertion. The muscle originates on the orbital rim, the nasal process of the frontal bone, and the frontal process of the maxilla (see Figure 3-7). Most of the fibers insert into the skin at the lateral canthus, although some inner fibers completely encircle the orbit.

Action. The muscle closes the eyelid. If all fibers are active, the eye can be squinted, and wrinkles or "crow's feet" form at the lateral canthus; these lines become especially defined with aging.

Corrugator Supercilii Muscle. The **corrugator supercilii muscle** (kor-uh-**gay**-tuhr soo-per-**sil**-ee-eye) is a muscle of facial expression in the orbital region, deep to the superior part of the orbicularis oculi muscle (see Figure 4-9).

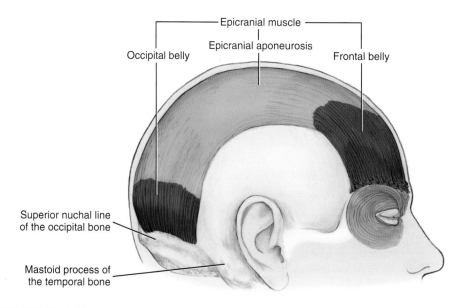

FIGURE 4-7 Origin and insertion of the highlighted frontal and occipital bellies of the right epicranial muscle.

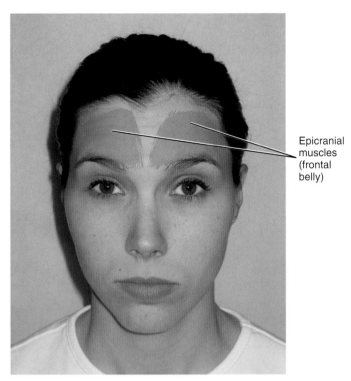

FIGURE 4-8 Use of the highlighted epicranial muscle to raise the eyebrows and scalp to show surprise.

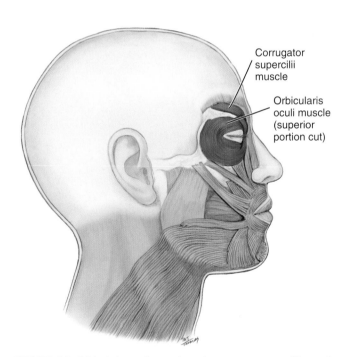

FIGURE 4-9 Orbicularis oculi muscle and corrugator supercilii muscle are highlighted.

Origin and Insertion. This muscle originates on the frontal bone in the supraorbital region. It then passes superiorly and laterally to insert into the skin of the eyebrow.

Action. The muscle draws the skin of the eyebrow medially and inferiorly toward the nose, which causes vertical wrinkles in the glabella area of the forehead and horizontal wrinkles at the bridge of the

nose, as when a person frowns (see Figure 4-14, *B*). It works in concert with the muscles of the nasal region.

MUSCLES OF FACIAL EXPRESSION IN ORAL REGION

Orbicularis Oris Muscle. The **orbicularis oris muscle (or**-is) is an important muscle of facial expression in the oral region since it acts to shape and control the size of the mouth opening and is important for creating the lip positions and movements during speech (Figure 4-10).

Origin and Insertion. The vermilion zone fibers of the muscle encircle the mouth between the skin and labial mucosa of the lips, with no bony attachment. These fibers then insert into the skin of the lips at both labial commissures. Within the upper lip, these fibers also insert on the ridges of the philtrum. The non-vermilion zone fibers cross the midline, diffusely ending by inserting into the other muscles of the lip or nose.

Action. The muscle has four relatively distinct lip-related movements: the pressing together (with closing lips), tightening and thinning (with pursing lips), rolling inward between the teeth (with grimacing), and thrusting outward (with pouting and kissing). This muscle can show more defined wrinkling with cigarette use or other prolonged oral habits.

Buccinator Muscle. The **buccinator muscle (buk**-sin-nay-tuhr) is a thin quadrilateral muscle of facial expression that forms the anterior part of the cheek or the lateral wall within the buccal region of the oral cavity (Figure 4-11 and see Figure 2-9).

Origin and Insertion. The muscle originates from three areas: the alveolar processes of the maxilla and of the mandible, as well as the fibrous structure, the **pterygomandibular raphe (ter**-i-go-man-**dib**-u-luhr **ray**-fee). The pterygomandibular raphe is a tendinous band located posterior to the most distal mandibular molar as it spans the area between the mandible and the point at which the hard and soft palates meet; it is noted on a patient in the oral cavity as the pterygomandibular fold (see Figures 2-21, 3-34 and 4-31). The pterygomandibular fold is a landmark for the administration of the inferior alveolar block (see Figures 9-35 and 9-37).

The buccinator and superior pharyngeal constrictor muscles of the pharynx (discussed later) are attached to each other at the pterygomandibular raphe. The buccinator muscle fibers from the alveolar process of the maxilla and the superior part of the pterygomandibular raphe travel obliquely downward toward the lower lip, while fibers from the alveolar process of the mandible and inferior part of the pterygomandibular raphe travel obliquely upward toward the upper lip, creating an intersecting pattern at the ipsilateral labial commissure. Between the origin and insertion, the fibers from the buccinator muscle intersect and take on an overall "braided" effect.

Action. The muscle pulls each labial commissure laterally and shortens the cheek both vertically and horizontally. This action when both muscles are activated causes the muscle to keep food pushed back on the occlusal or masticatory surface of the posterior teeth, as when a person chews. By keeping the food in the correct position when chewing, the buccinator muscles assist the muscles of mastication. In infants, the muscles provide suction for nursing. In addition, because of its importance in expelling air through wind instruments, it has also been called the "trumpet muscle."

Risorius Muscle. The **risorius muscle** (ri-**sore**-ee-us) is a thin muscle of facial expression in the oral region (Figure 4-12).

Origin and Insertion. The muscle originates from fascia superficial to the masseter muscle and then passes anteriorly to insert into the skin at the ipsilateral labial commissure.

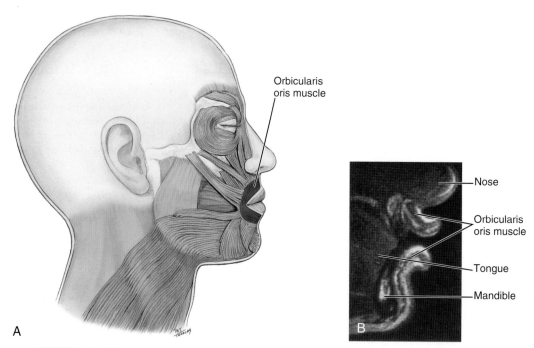

FIGURE 4-10 Orbicularis oris muscle highlighted **(A)**, and sagittal magnetic resonance imaging of a kiss **(B)**. (*B from Reynolds PA, Abrahams PH: McMinn's interactive clinical anatomy: head and neck, ed 2, London, 2001, Elsevier.*)

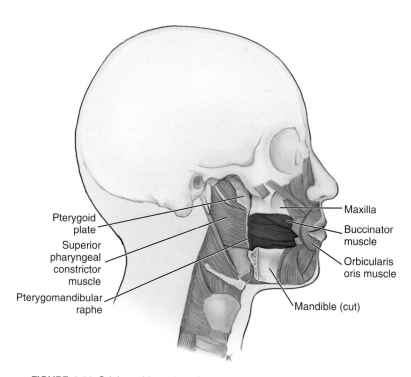

FIGURE 4-11 Origin and insertion of the buccinator muscle are highlighted.

Action. The muscle acts to stretch the lips laterally to retract the labial commissure, and thus widen the mouth (see Figure 4-14, *A*). The muscle has been thought (erroneously) to produce "grinning" or "smiling" but really produces more of a grimace. The risorius has a connection with the platysma muscle in that it often contracts with it (see Figure 4-18).

Levator Labii Superioris Muscle. The **levator labii superioris muscle** (le-**vay**-tuhr **lay**-be-eye **soo**-per-ee-**or**-is) is a broad flat muscle of facial expression in the oral region (Figure 4-13).

Origin and Insertion. The muscle originates from the infraorbital rim of the maxilla (see Figure 3-7). It then passes inferiorly to insert into the skin of the upper lip.

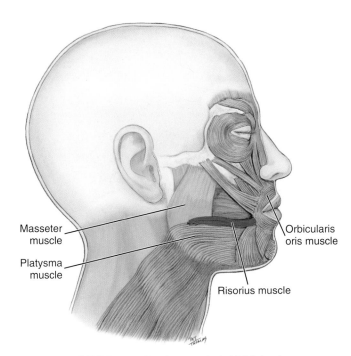

FIGURE 4-12 Risorius muscle is highlighted.

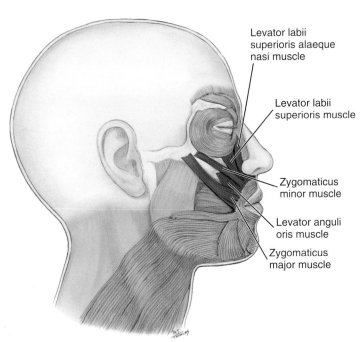

FIGURE 4-13 Levator labii superioris alaeque nasi, levator labii superioris, zygomaticus minor, levator anguli oris, and zygomaticus major muscles are highlighted.

Action. The muscle elevates the upper lip (Figure 4-14, *A*).

Levator Labii Superioris Alaeque Nasi Muscle. The **levator labii superioris alaeque nasi muscle** (a-luh-kwee **nay**-zy) is a muscle of facial expression in the oral region (see Figure 4-13).

Origin and Insertion. The muscle originates from the frontal process of the maxilla (see Figure 3-45). It then passes inferiorly to insert into two areas: the skin of the ala of the nose and upper lip.

Action. The muscle elevates the upper lip and ala of the nose, thus also dilating each naris, as in a sneering expression (Figure 4-14, *B*).

Zygomaticus Major Muscle. The **zygomaticus major muscle** (zy-go-**mat**-i-kus) is a muscle of facial expression in the oral region that is located lateral to the zygomaticus minor muscle (see Figure 4-13).

Origin and Insertion. The muscle originates from the zygomatic bone, lateral to the zygomaticus minor (see Figure 3-42). It then passes anteriorly and inferiorly to insert into the skin at the ipsilateral labial commissure, in and around the orbicularis oris.

Action. The muscle elevates the ipsilateral labial commissure of the upper lip and pulls it laterally, as when a person smiles (see Figure 4-14, *A*). Some research suggests that the difference between a genuine smile and a perfunctory (or faux) smile is that when a person truly feels happy, the zygomatic major muscle contracts together with the orbicularis oculi muscle of the orbit.

Zygomaticus Minor Muscle. The **zygomaticus minor muscle** is a small variable muscle of facial expression in the oral region, medial to the zygomaticus major muscle (see Figure 4-13).

Origin and Insertion. The muscle originates on the body of the zygomatic bone (see Figure 3-42). It then inserts in the skin of the upper lip adjacent to the insertion of the levator labii superioris.

Action. The muscle elevates the upper lip, assisting in smiling (see Figure 4-14, *A*).

Levator Anguli Oris Muscle. Deep to both the zygomaticus major and zygomaticus minor muscles of facial expression in the oral region is the **levator anguli oris muscle** (**an**-gu-ly) (see Figure 4-13).

Origin and Insertion. The muscle originates in the canine fossa of the maxilla, usually superior to the root of the maxillary canine (see Figure 3-47). It then passes inferiorly to insert into the skin at the ipsilateral labial commissure, intermingling with fibers of the zygomaticus major, depressor anguli oris, and orbicularis oris muscles.

Action. The muscle elevates the ipsilateral labial commissure, as when a person smiles (see Figure 4-14, *A*).

Depressor Anguli Oris Muscle. The **depressor anguli oris muscle** (de-**pres**-uhr) is a triangular muscle of facial expression in the oral region (Figure 4-15).

Origin and Insertion. The muscle originates on the inferior border of the mandible (see Figure 3-51). It then passes superiorly to insert into the skin at the ipsilateral labial commissure.

Action. The muscle depresses the ipsilateral labial commissure, as when a person frowns (see Figure 4-14, *B*).

Depressor Labii Inferioris Muscle. Deep to the depressor anguli oris muscle is the **depressor labii inferioris muscle** (in-**fere**-ee-o-ris), a small quadrilateral muscle of facial expression in the oral region (see Figure 4-15).

Origin and Insertion. The muscle originates from the inferior border of the mandible (see Figure 3-51). It then passes superiorly to insert into the skin of the lower lip.

Action. The muscle depresses the lower lip, exposing the mandibular incisor teeth.

Mentalis Muscle. The **mentalis muscle** (men-**ta**-lis) is a short thick muscle of facial expression superior and medial to the mental nerve in the oral region (Figure 4-16).

Origin and Insertion. The muscle originates on the mandible near the midline (see Figure 3-51). It then inserts in the skin of the chin.

Action. The muscle raises the chin, wrinkling its skin, causing the displaced lower lip to protrude, narrowing the oral vestibule. Thus when active, these fibers may dislodge a complete denture in an edentulous patient who has lost alveolar process height.

Platysma Muscle. The **platysma muscle** (pluh-**tiz**-muh) is a muscle of facial expression that runs from the neck all the way to the mouth superficial to the anterior cervical triangle and external jugular vein (Figure 4-17 and see Figure 2-23).

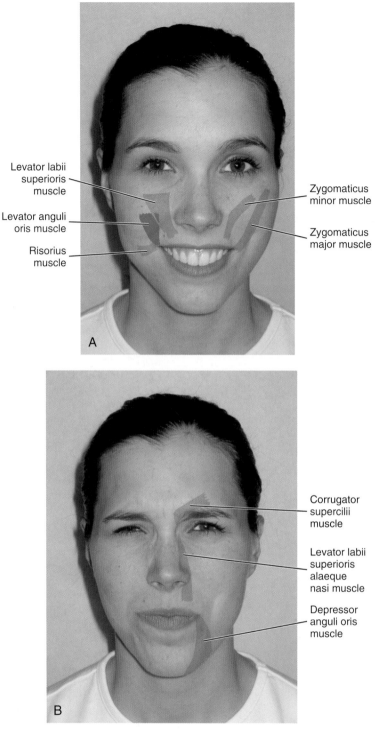

Levator labii
superioris
muscle

Levator anguli
oris muscle

Risorius
muscle

Zygomaticus
minor muscle

Zygomaticus
major muscle

A

Corrugator
supercilii
muscle

Levator labii
superioris
alaeque
nasi muscle

Depressor
anguli oris
muscle

B

FIGURE 4-14 Use of highlighted muscles of facial expression when smiling **(A)**, and when disgusted **(B)**.

Origin and Insertion. The muscle originates in the skin superficial to the clavicle and shoulder. It then passes anteriorly to insert on the inferior border of the mandible and into the other muscles surrounding the mouth (see earlier discussion).

Action. The muscle raises the skin of the neck to form noticeable vertical and horizontal ridges and depressions. It can also pull the ipsilateral labial commissures down, as when a person grimaces (Figure 4-18).

MUSCLES OF MASTICATION

The **muscles of mastication** (mass-ti-**kay**-shuhn) are four paired muscles that are located deeper within the face than the muscles of facial expression. These muscles are all attached in some manner to the mandible and include: the masseter, temporalis, medial pterygoid, and lateral pterygoid muscles. These muscles may be involved in pathology associated with the temporomandibular joint (see also

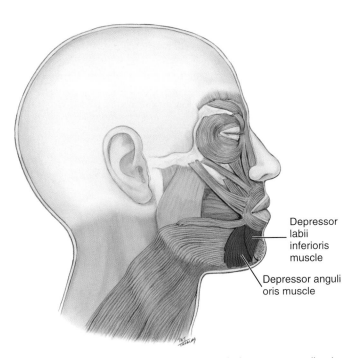

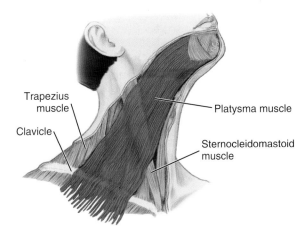

FIGURE 4-17 Origin and insertion of the right platysma muscle are highlighted.

FIGURE 4-15 Depressor labii inferioris and depressor anguli oris muscles are highlighted.

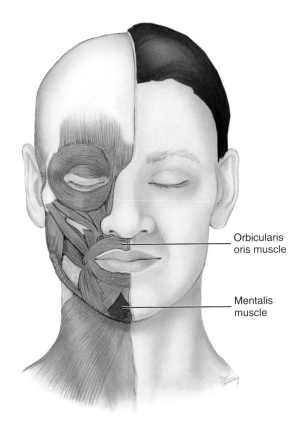

FIGURE 4-16 Mentalis muscle is highlighted.

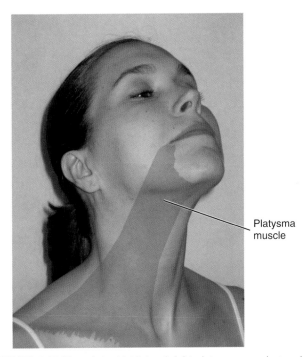

FIGURE 4-18 Use of the highlighted right platysma muscle to raise the skin of the neck.

Chapter 5). All the muscles of mastication are embryologic derivatives of the first branchial arch or mandibular arch.

Origin and Insertion. The origin and insertion of each muscle of mastication varies; however, all the muscles of mastication generally originate on the cranium and insert on the mandible (Table 4-3).

Action. The muscles of mastication work with the temporomandibular joint to accomplish movements of the mandible so as to allow mastication. Similar to the muscles of facial expression, these muscles can work in combination. Mastication is the process of chewing food in preparation for swallowing and digestion (see Figure 5-6 and further discussion in Chapter 5). Thus the muscles of mastication are responsible for closing the jaws, moving the lower jaw forward or backward, and shifting the lower jaw to one side.

These jaw movements involve the movement of the mandible, while the rest of the skull remains relatively stable. The movements of the mandible include: depression, elevation, protrusion, retraction, and lateral deviation. The dental professional needs to understand the association of the muscles of mastication with the movements of the mandible (Table 4-4).

Innervation. All muscles of mastication are innervated by branches of the mandibular nerve (or third division) of the fifth cranial or trigeminal nerve, with each nerve serving one side of the face.

TABLE 4-3	Muscles of Mastication	
MUSCLE	**ORIGIN**	**INSERTION**
Masseter	Superficial head: zygomatic process of maxilla and anterior two-thirds of inferior border of zygomatic arch Deep head: posterior one-third and medial surface of the zygomatic arch	Superficial head: angle of mandible Deep head: mandibular ramus
Temporalis	Inferior temporal line superiorly and inferiorly by the infratemporal crest of the sphenoid bone within temporal fossa	Coronoid process of the mandibular ramus
Medial pterygoid	Deep head: pterygoid fossa on lateral pterygoid plate of the sphenoid bone Superficial head: lateral surfaces of the pyramidal process of the palatine bone and maxillary tuberosity of the maxilla	Both heads: medial surface of the mandibular ramus and angle of the mandible
Lateral pterygoid	Superior head: infratemporal surface and infratemporal crest of the greater wing of the sphenoid bone Inferior head: lateral pterygoid plate of the sphenoid bone	Superior head: on the anterior surface of the neck of the mandibular condyle at pterygoid fovea of the mandible as well as temporomandibular joint disc and capsule Inferior head: on the anterior surface of the neck of the mandibular condyle at pterygoid fovea of the mandible

TABLE 4-4	Muscles of Mastication and Associated Mandibular Movements
MUSCLE	**MANDIBULAR MOVEMENT(S)**
Masseter	Bilateral contraction: elevation of mandible during closing of jaws
Temporalis	Bilateral contraction of entire muscle: elevation of mandible during closing of jaws Bilateral contraction of only posterior part: retraction of mandible, mandible backward
Medial pterygoid	Bilateral contraction: elevation of mandible during closing of jaws
Lateral pterygoid	Unilateral contraction: lateral deviation of mandible, shift mandible to contralateral side Bilateral contraction: mainly protrusion of mandible with mandible forward, slight depression of mandible during opening of jaws

MASSETER MUSCLE

The most obvious muscle of mastication is the masseter muscle since it is the most superficial and one of the strongest (Figure 4-19 and see Figure 2-9). The muscle is a broad, thick, flat rectangular muscle (almost quadrilateral) on each side of the face that is anterior to the parotid salivary gland. The masseter muscle has two heads that differ in depth: the superficial and deep heads.

Origin and Insertion. Both heads of the muscle originate from the zygomatic arch but from differing locations (see Figure 3-14). The superficial head originates from the zygomatic process of the maxilla, and from the anterior two-thirds of the inferior border of the zygomatic arch. The deep head originates from the posterior one-third and the entire medial surface of the zygomatic arch. The deep head is partly concealed by the superficial head of the muscle.

Both heads then pass inferiorly to insert on different parts of the external surface of the mandible: the superficial head on the lateral surface of the angle of the mandible and the deep head on the mandibular ramus superior to the angle of the mandible (see Figure 3-52).

Action. The action of the muscle during bilateral contraction of the entire muscle is to elevate the mandible, raising the lower jaw. Elevation of the mandible occurs during the closing of the jaws. The masseter parallels the nearby medial pterygoid muscle in action, but the effect is stronger overall. During an extraoral examination, visually inspect and bilaterally palpate both masseter muscles. Place the fingers of each hand over each muscle as the patient clenches the teeth together several times (Figure 4-20).

Innervation. The muscle is innervated by the masseteric nerve, a branch of the mandibular nerve (or third division) of the fifth cranial or trigeminal nerve.

Clinical Considerations With Masseter Muscle Pathology

The masseter muscle can become enlarged in patients who habitually clench or grind their teeth (as with bruxism) and even in those who constantly chew gum. This masseteric hypertrophy is asymptomatic and only slightly firm; it is usually bilateral but can be unilateral. Even if the hypertrophy is bilateral, there still may be asymmetry of the face due to unequal enlargement of the muscles (Figure 4-21).

This extraoral enlargement may be confused with dental infections, parotid salivary gland disease, and maxillofacial neoplasms. However, only those intraoral signs involved with changes in occlusion are present such as attrition and abfraction. The enlargement corresponds with the outline of the muscle and there are no symptoms of tenderness or pain as with other etiologies for muscle enlargement. Most patients seek medical attention because of comments about facial appearance. It is important to note that this situation may be associated with further pathology of the temporomandibular joint (see **Chapter 5**).

TEMPORALIS MUSCLE

The **temporalis muscle** (tem-puh-**ral**-is) is a broad fan-shaped muscle of mastication on each side of the head that fills the temporal fossa, and is located superior to the zygomatic arch (Figure 4-22).

Origin and Insertion. The muscle originates from the entire temporal fossa on the temporal bone that is bordered superiorly by the inferior temporal line and inferiorly by the infratemporal crest (see Figure 3-59). It then passes inferiorly to insert onto the medial

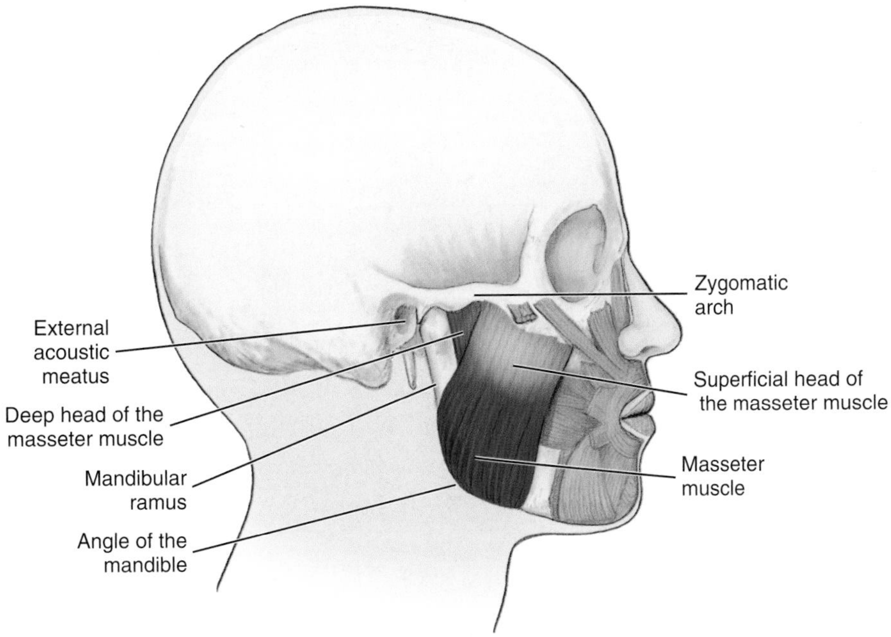

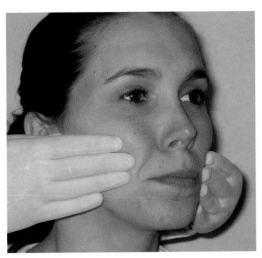

External
acoustic
meatus

Zygomatic
arch

Superficial head of
the masseter muscle

Deep head of the
masseter muscle

Masseter
muscle

Mandibular
ramus

Angle of the
mandible

FIGURE 4-19 Origin and insertion of the masseter muscle with both its superficial head and its deep head highlighted.

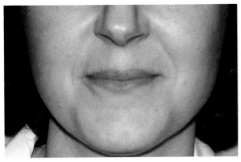

FIGURE 4-20 Demonstration of palpation of the masseter muscles during an extraoral examination while the patient clenches the teeth together several times. *(Courtesy of Margaret J. Fehrenbach, RDH, MS.)*

FIGURE 4-21 Bilateral enlargement of the masseter muscle due to bruxism, or grinding of the teeth, which alters the facial dimensions.

surface, apex, and anterior border of the coronoid process of the mandible at the anteromedial border of the mandibular ramus (see Figure 3-52).

Action. If the entire muscle contracts, the main action is to elevate the mandible, raising the mandible. Elevation of the mandible occurs during the closing of the jaws. If only the posterior part contracts, the muscle moves the lower jaw backward, which occurs with retraction of the mandible. Retraction of the jaw often accompanies the closing of the jaws. This muscle also maintains the mandible in its physiologic rest position, allowing for freeway space.

Innervation. The muscle is innervated by the deep temporal nerves, branches of the mandibular nerve (or third division) of the fifth cranial or trigeminal nerve.

MEDIAL PTERYGOID MUSCLE

Deeper, yet similar in its rectangular form to the more superficial masseter, is another muscle of mastication, the **medial pterygoid muscle (ter**-i-goid) or *internal pterygoid muscle* (Figure 4-23). The medial pterygoid muscle also has two heads due to their differing depth, again similar to the masseter muscle: the deep and superficial heads. However, even with these two differing heads, this is the deepest muscle of mastication.

Origin and Insertion. The larger deep head of the muscle originates from the pterygoid fossa on the medial surface of the lateral pterygoid plate of the sphenoid bone (see Figures 3-32). The smaller superficial head of the muscle originates from the lateral surfaces of both the pyramidal process of the palatine bone and maxillary tuberosity of the maxilla (see Figures 3-43 and 3-47). Both heads then pass inferiorly, posteriorly, and laterally to insert on the medial surface of the mandibular ramus and angle of the mandible, as far superior as the mandibular foramen (see Figure 3-52).

Action. The muscle elevates the mandible, raising the lower jaw. Elevation of the mandible occurs during the closing of the jaws. The medial pterygoid muscle parallels the action of masseter muscle, but the effect is smaller overall.

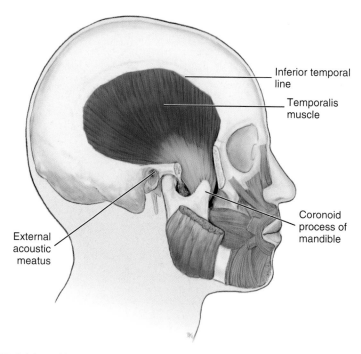

FIGURE 4-22 Origin and insertion of the temporalis muscle with both the zygomatic arch and superior part of the masseter muscle removed.

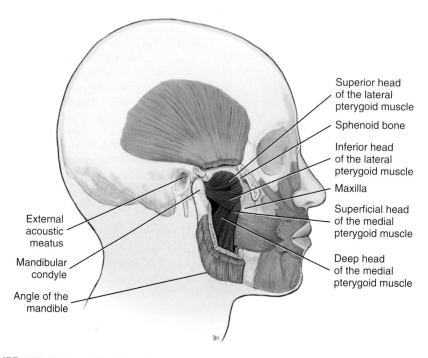

FIGURE 4-23 Origin and insertion of both the medial pterygoid muscle and lateral pterygoid muscle with both heads of each muscle highlighted. Note that the inferior part of the temporalis muscle, zygomatic arch, and most of the mandibular ramus have been removed.

Innervation. The muscle is innervated by the medial pterygoid nerve, a branch of the mandibular nerve (or third division) of the fifth cranial or trigeminal nerve.

LATERAL PTERYGOID MUSCLE

The **lateral pterygoid muscle** or *external pterygoid muscle* is a short, thick, almost conical muscle of mastication superior to the medial pterygoid muscle (see Figures 4-23). The lateral pterygoid muscle has two separate heads of origin: the superior and inferior heads. The two heads are separated anteriorly by a slight interval but fuse together posteriorly. The entire muscle lies within the infratemporal fossa, deep to the temporalis muscle, with the muscle surrounded by the pterygoid plexus of veins (see Figures 3-60 and 6-13).

Origin and Insertion. The superior head of the muscle originates from the infratemporal surface and infratemporal crest of the greater wing of the sphenoid bone and passes inferiorly to insert on the anterior surface of the neck of the mandibular condyle at the pterygoid fovea of the mandible as well as the anterior margin of the temporomandibular joint disc and capsule (see Figures 3-32, 3-52 and 5-4). The inferior head of the muscle originates from the lateral surface of the lateral pterygoid plate of the sphenoid bone and also inserts on the anterior surface of the neck of the mandibular condyle at the pterygoid fovea.

Action. Unlike the other three muscles of mastication, the lateral pterygoid is the only muscle of mastication that assists in depressing the mandible, lowering the mandible, as it moves forward or protrudes. Depression of the mandible occurs during the opening of the jaws. However, the main action when both muscles contract is to bring the mandible forward, thus causing the protrusion of the mandible. Protrusion of the mandible occurs during opening of the jaws. If only one muscle is contracted, the mandible shifts to the contralateral side, causing lateral deviation of the mandible.

Innervation. The muscle is innervated by the lateral pterygoid nerve, a branch of the mandibular nerve (or third division) of the fifth cranial or trigeminal nerve.

HYOID MUSCLES

The hyoid bone is a horseshoe-shaped bone suspended inferior to the mandible; it does not articulate with any other bone and has only muscular and ligamental attachments through the **hyoid muscles** (**hi**-oid) (see Figure 3-65). These muscles can be further grouped based on their vertical position in relationship to the hyoid bone: the suprahyoid or infrahyoid muscles (Box 4-1).

Action. The muscles assist in the actions of mastication and swallowing through their attachment to the hyoid bone.

Origin and Insertion. Most of these muscles are in a superficial position in the neck tissue. Both groups of the hyoid muscles are mainly attached to the hyoid bone, except for the sternothyroid muscle (Figure 4-24 and Table 4-5).

SUPRAHYOID MUSCLES

The **suprahyoid muscles** (**soo**-pruh-**hi**-oid) are superior to the hyoid bone (Figures 4-25 and 4-26 and see Figure 4-24). These superiorly located muscles may be further divided according to their horizontal position in relationship to the hyoid bone, being in either the anterior or posterior suprahyoid muscle groups. The **anterior suprahyoid muscle group** includes: the anterior belly of the digastric, mylohyoid, and geniohyoid muscles. The **posterior suprahyoid muscle group** includes: the posterior belly of the digastric and stylohyoid muscles.

Action. Two actions associated with mastication result from muscle contraction of the suprahyoid muscles. One action of both the anterior and posterior suprahyoid muscles is to cause the elevation of the hyoid bone and larynx if the mandible is stabilized by contraction of the muscles of mastication. This action occurs during swallowing.

BOX 4-1	Hyoid Muscles and Relationship to Hyoid Bone

Suprahyoid Muscles	Infrahyoid Muscles
Digastric	Omohyoid
Mylohyoid	Sternohyoid
Stylohyoid	Sternothyroid
Geniohyoid	Thyrohyoid

The other action associated with mastication results from the contraction of the anterior suprahyoid muscles, which causes the mandible to depress and the jaws to open. Thus jaw opening involves the lateral pterygoid muscles, which protrude the mandible, and the anterior suprahyoid muscles, which lower the mandible. Some of the suprahyoid muscles have additional specific actions that are also discussed.

Digastric Muscle. The **digastric muscle** (di-**gas**-trik) is a suprahyoid muscle that has two separate bellies: the anterior and posterior bellies (see Figure 4-25). The anterior belly of the muscle is a part of the anterior suprahyoid muscle group, and the posterior belly is a part of the posterior suprahyoid muscle group. Each digastric muscle demarcates the superior part of the anterior cervical triangle, forming (with the mandible) a submandibular triangle on each side of the neck; the right and left anterior bellies of the muscle also form a single midline submental triangle (see Figure 2-25).

Origin and Insertion. The anterior belly of the muscle originates on the **intermediate tendon of the digastric muscle**, which is loosely attached to the body and the greater cornu of the hyoid bone, and then passes superiorly and anteriorly to insert onto the digastric fossa on the medial surface of the mandible (see Figure 3-54). The posterior belly of the muscle arises from the mastoid notch, medial to the mastoid process of the temporal bone, and then passes anteriorly and inferiorly to insert on the intermediate tendon (see Figure 3-31).

Action. The muscle either elevates the hyoid bone or depresses the mandible.

Innervation. The anterior belly of the muscle is innervated by the mylohyoid nerve, which is a branch of the mandibular nerve (or third division) of the fifth cranial or trigeminal nerve. In contrast, the posterior belly of the muscle is innervated by the posterior digastric nerve, which is a branch of the seventh cranial or facial nerve.

Mylohyoid Muscle. The **mylohyoid muscle** (my-lo-**hi**-oid) is an anterior suprahyoid muscle deep to the digastric muscle with fibers running transversely between the two mandibular rami (see Figures 4-25, 4-26, and 4-28).

Origin and Insertion. The muscle originates from the mylohyoid line from the medial surface of the mandible (see Figure 3-54). The right and left muscles then pass inferiorly to unite medially at the **mylohyoid raphe**, forming the floor of the mouth. The most posterior fibers of the muscle then insert on the body of the hyoid bone.

Action. In addition to either elevating the hyoid bone or depressing the mandible, this muscle also forms the floor of the mouth and helps elevate the tongue.

Innervation. The muscle is innervated by the mylohyoid nerve, which is a branch of the mandibular nerve (or third division) of the fifth cranial or trigeminal nerve.

Stylohyoid Muscle. The **stylohyoid muscle** (sty-lo-**hi**-oid) is a thin posterior suprahyoid muscle that has two slips: superficial and deep slips, which are located on either side of the intermediate tendon of the digastric muscle discussed earlier (see Figure 4-25).

Origin and Insertion. This muscle originates from the styloid process of the temporal bone, then passes anteriorly and inferiorly to insert on the body of the hyoid bone (see Figure 3-31).

Action. The muscle either elevates the hyoid bone or depresses the mandible.

Innervation. The muscle is innervated by the stylohyoid nerve, which is a branch of the seventh cranial or facial nerve.

Geniohyoid Muscle. The **geniohyoid muscle** (ji-nee-o-**hi**-oid) is an anterior suprahyoid muscle superior to the medial border of the mylohyoid muscle (see Figures 4-26 and 4-28).

Origin and Insertion. The muscle originates from the medial surface of the mandible, at the genial tubercles near the mandibular symphysis, with both the right and left muscles in contact with each

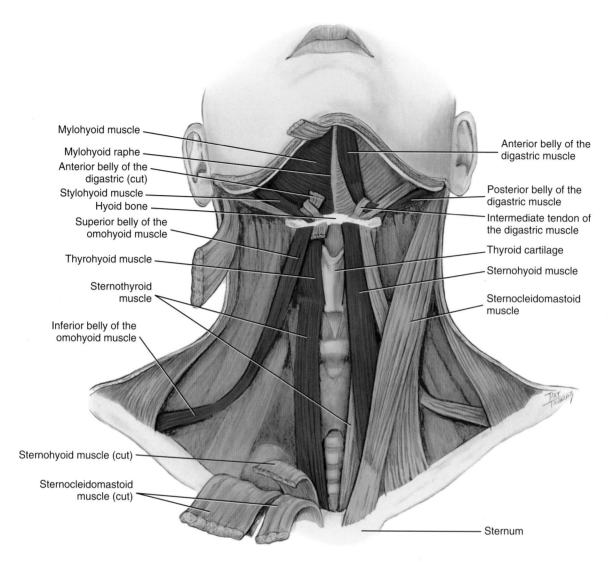

Mylohyoid muscle

Mylohyoid raphe

Anterior belly of the digastric (cut)

Stylohyoid muscle

Hyoid bone

Superior belly of the omohyoid muscle

Thyrohyoid muscle

Sternothyroid muscle

Inferior belly of the omohyoid muscle

Sternohyoid muscle (cut)

Sternocleidomastoid muscle (cut)

Anterior belly of the digastric muscle

Posterior belly of the digastric muscle

Intermediate tendon of the digastric muscle

Thyroid cartilage

Sternohyoid muscle

Sternocleidomastoid muscle

Sternum

FIGURE 4-24 Anterior view of the head and neck as well as the hyoid bone with the hyoid muscles highlighted and with their origins and insertions noted. Note that many overlying muscles have been cut and the geniohyoid muscle is not included.

other. It then passes posteriorly and inferiorly to insert on the body of the hyoid bone.

Action. The muscle either elevates the hyoid bone or depresses the mandible.

Innervation. The muscle is innervated by the first cervical nerve, which is conducted by way of the twelfth cranial or hypoglossal nerve.

INFRAHYOID MUSCLES

The **infrahyoid muscles** (in-fruh-**hi**-oid) are four pairs of hyoid muscles inferior to the hyoid bone (Figure 4-27 and see Figure 4-24). The infrahyoid muscles include: the omohyoid, sternohyoid, sternothyroid, and thyrohyoid muscles.

Action. Most of the infrahyoid muscles depress the hyoid bone; some have additional specific actions that are also discussed.

Innervation. All the infrahyoid muscles are innervated by the first, second, and third cervical nerves.

Omohyoid Muscle. The **omohyoid muscle** (o-moh-**hi**-oid) is an infrahyoid muscle lateral to both the sternothyroid and thyrohyoid muscles. The omohyoid muscle has two separate bellies: the superior

and inferior bellies. The superior belly divides the inferior part of the anterior cervical triangle into the carotid and muscular triangles. In the posterior cervical triangle, the inferior belly serves to demarcate the subclavian triangle inferiorly from the occipital triangle superiorly (see Figures 2-25 and 2-26).

Origin and Insertion. The inferior belly of the muscle originates from the scapula. The inferior belly then passes anteriorly and superiorly, crossing the internal jugular vein deep to the SCM muscle, where it then attaches by a short tendon to the superior belly. The superior belly of the muscle originates from the short tendon attached to the inferior belly and then inserts on the lateral border of the body of the hyoid bone.

Action. The muscle depresses the hyoid bone.

Sternohyoid Muscle. The **sternohyoid muscle** (ster-no-**hi**-oid) is an infrahyoid muscle superficial to the sternothyroid as well as the thyroid cartilage and thyroid gland.

Origin and Insertion. The muscle originates from the posterior and superior surfaces of the sternum, near to where the sternum joins each clavicle. The muscle then passes superiorly to insert on the body of the hyoid bone.

TABLE 4-5	**Hyoid Muscles**	
	ACTIONS	
Suprahyoid Muscles	Elevation of hyoid bone and larynx if mandible is stabilized by muscles of mastication	
Anterior Suprahyoid Muscles	Depress mandible and open jaws; mylohyoid forms floor of mouth and helps elevate tongue	
	ORIGIN	**INSERTION**
Digastric	Anterior belly: intermediate tendon	Anterior belly: digastric fossa on medial surface of mandible
Mylohyoid	Mylohyoid line of medial surface of mandible	Mylohyoid raphe and body of hyoid bone
Geniohyoid	Genial tubercles of mandible	Body of hyoid bone
Posterior Suprahyoid Muscles	**ORIGIN**	**INSERTION**
Digastric	Posterior belly: mastoid notch of temporal bone	Posterior belly: intermediate tendon
Stylohyoid	Styloid process of temporal bone	Body of hyoid bone
	ACTIONS	
Infrahyoid Muscles	Most depress hyoid bone, except sternothyroid, which depresses only thyroid cartilage and larynx; thyrohyoid also raises thyroid cartilage and larynx	
	ORIGIN	**INSERTION**
Omohyoid	Inferior belly: scapula Superior belly: inferior belly via intermediate tendon	Inferior belly: superior belly via intermediate tendon Superior belly: body of hyoid bone
Sternohyoid	Posterior and superior surfaces of sternum	Body of hyoid bone
Sternothyroid	Posterior surface of sternum	Thyroid cartilage
Thyrohyoid	Thyroid cartilage	Body and greater cornu of hyoid bone

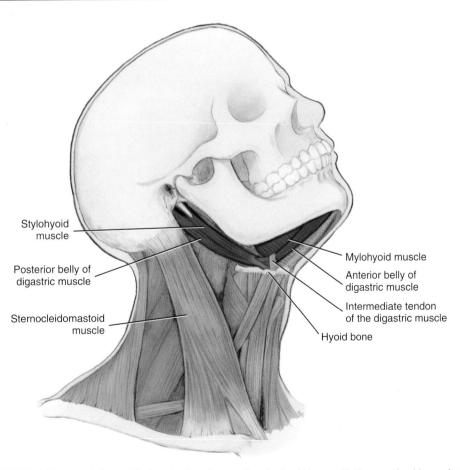

FIGURE 4-25 Lateral view of the head and neck as well as the hyoid bone with the suprahyoid muscles highlighted and with their origins and insertions noted. Note that the geniohyoid muscle is not included.

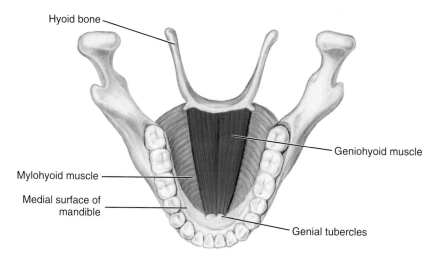

FIGURE 4-26 Superior view of the floor of the oral cavity as well as the mandible and hyoid bone showing the origin and insertion of the highlighted geniohyoid muscle.

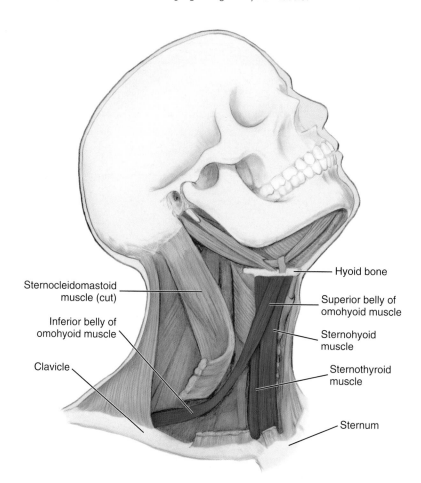

FIGURE 4-27 Lateral view of the head and neck as well as the hyoid bone and the highlighted infrahyoid muscles with their origins and insertions noted; see Figure 4-24 for the thyrohyoid muscle.

Action. The muscle depresses the hyoid bone.

Sternothyroid Muscle. The **sternothyroid muscle** (ster-no-**thy**-roid) is an infrahyoid muscle superficial to the thyroid gland.

Origin and Insertion. The muscle originates from the posterior surface of the sternum, deep and medial to the sternohyoid muscle, at the level of the first rib. It then passes superiorly to insert on the thyroid cartilage (see Figure 2-24).

Action. The muscle depresses the thyroid cartilage and larynx, yet does not directly depress the hyoid bone.

Thyrohyoid Muscle. The **thyrohyoid muscle** (thy-roh-**hi**-oid) is deep to both the omohyoid and sternohyoid muscles.

Origin and Insertion. The muscle originates on the thyroid cartilage and inserts on the body and greater cornu of the hyoid bone; it appears as a continuation of the sternothyroid (see Figures 4-24 and 2-24).

Action. In addition to depressing the hyoid bone, the muscle raises the thyroid cartilage and larynx.

MUSCLES OF TONGUE

The tongue is a thick vascular mass of voluntary muscle surrounded by a mucous membrane that is anchored to the floor of the mouth by the lingual frenum. The tongue has complex movements during mastication, speaking, and swallowing; these movements are a result of the combined action of **muscles of the tongue**. The tongue consists of symmetric halves divided from each other by the **median septum**

(**me**-dee-uhn **sep**-tuhm), which is a deep tendinous band located within the midline. The median septum corresponds with the median lingual sulcus, a midline depression on the tongue's dorsal surface (see Figure 2-17). The tongue is further divided into a base at the posterior and a body at the anterior, both having multiple surfaces (dorsal, lateral, ventral), as well as an apex.

The muscles of the tongue can be grouped according to their location: the intrinsic and extrinsic groups, with the intrinsic and extrinsic tongue muscles of both groups intertwining within the structure of the tongue (Figure 4-28). Each half of the tongue has muscular groups within these two main groups, separated by the median septum.

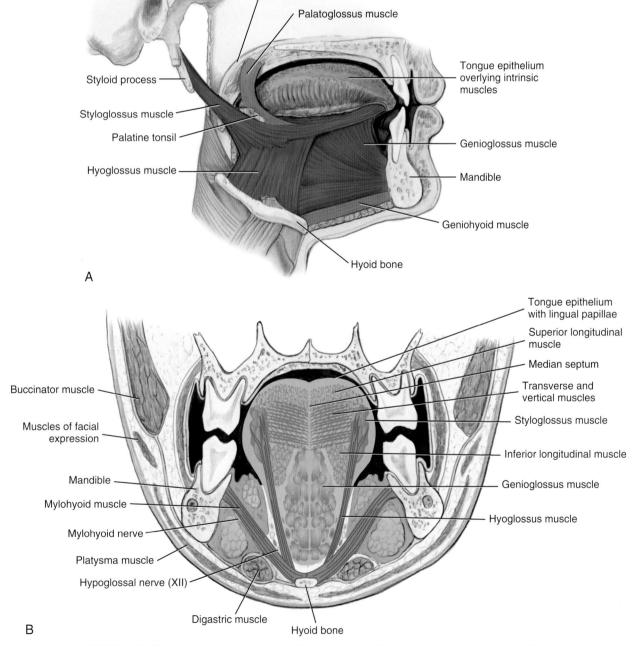

FIGURE 4-28 Tongue with intrinsic and extrinsic muscles as well as associated structures noted. Parasagittal section with extrinsic muscles highlighted and intrinsic muscles noted **(A)**. Frontal section just distal to the mandibular first molar with both extrinsic and intrinsic muscles of the tongue noted **(B)**.

Origin and Insertion. Intrinsic muscles are located entirely inside the tongue. Extrinsic muscles have their origin outside the tongue yet have their insertion inside the tongue.

Action. The intrinsic muscles change the shape of the tongue, while the extrinsic muscles also move the tongue while suspending and anchoring the tongue to bony structures of the mandible, the styloid process, and the hyoid bone.

Innervation. All of the muscles of the tongue are innervated by the twelfth cranial or hypoglossal nerve.

INTRINSIC TONGUE MUSCLES

The four pairs of **intrinsic tongue muscles** (in-**trin**-sik) are located entirely inside the tongue (see Figure 4-28). These muscles are grouped by their orientation to the tongue surface: the superior longitudinal, transverse, vertical, and inferior longitudinal muscles.

Origin and Insertion. The **superior longitudinal muscle** is the most superficial of the intrinsic muscles and runs in an oblique and longitudinal direction close to the dorsal surface from the base to the apex. Deep to the superior longitudinal muscle is the **transverse muscle** (tranz-**vurs**), which runs in a transverse direction from the median septum to pass outward toward the lateral surface. The **vertical muscle** runs in a vertical direction from the dorsal surface to the ventral surface in the body. The **inferior longitudinal muscle** is close to the ventral surface of the tongue and runs in a longitudinal direction from the base to the apex.

Action. The superior and inferior longitudinal muscles both act together to change the shape of the tongue by shortening and thickening it and act singly to help it curl in various directions. The transverse and vertical muscles both act together to make the tongue long and narrow.

Innervation. Intrinsic tongue muscles are innervated by the twelfth cranial or hypoglossal nerve.

EXTRINSIC TONGUE MUSCLES

There are three pairs of **extrinsic tongue muscles** (eks-**trin**-sik). Each of these muscles first takes on a name indicating its location and then ends in "glossus," the Greek word for *tongue*. The extrinsic tongue muscles include: the styloglossus, genioglossus, and hyoglossus muscles. Anatomists sometimes include the palatoglossus muscle in this category because it is involved in tongue movement; however, it is discussed with the muscles of the soft palate in this chapter due to its involvement with that structure.

Origin and Insertion. The extrinsic tongue muscles all have differing origins outside the tongue but all their insertions are inside the tongue (Table 4-6 and see Figure 4-28).

TABLE 4-6	Extrinsic Tongue Muscles*		
MUSCLES	**ORIGIN**	**INSERTION**	**ACTION**
Styloglossus	Styloid process of temporal bone	Tongue	Retracts tongue
Genioglossus	Genial tubercles on medial surface of mandible	Hyoid bone and tongue	Protrudes tongue and depresses parts
Hyoglossus	Greater cornu and body of hyoid bone	Tongue	Depresses tongue

*The palatoglossus muscle is noted under the muscles of the soft palate.

Innervation. All the extrinsic tongue muscles are innervated by the twelfth cranial or hypoglossal nerve.

Styloglossus Muscle. The **styloglossus muscle** (sty-lo-**gloss**-us) is an extrinsic tongue muscle.

Origin and Insertion. The muscle originates from the styloid process of the temporal bone (see Figure 3-31). It then passes inferiorly and anteriorly to insert into two parts on the lateral surface of the tongue, at the apex and also at the border between the body and base.

Action. The muscle retracts the tongue, moving it superiorly and posteriorly.

Genioglossus Muscle. The **genioglossus muscle** (ji-nee-o-**gloss**-us) is a fan-shaped extrinsic tongue muscle superior to the geniohyoid.

Origin and Insertion. The muscle arises from the genial tubercles on the medial surface of the mandible (see Figure 3-54). A few of its most inferior fibers insert on the hyoid bone, but most of its fibers insert into the tongue from its base almost to the apex. The right and left muscles are separated by the tongue's median septum, which was discussed earlier.

Action. Different parts of the muscle can protrude or "stick" the tongue out of the oral cavity or depress parts of the tongue surface. The protrusive activity of the muscle helps to prevent the tongue from sinking back and obstructing respiration; therefore, during general anesthesia the mandible is sometimes pulled forward to achieve the same effect to ensure unobstructed respiration. In addition, the genioglossus is often used to test the function of the twelfth cranial or hypoglossal nerve by asking a patient to "stick out" the tongue.

Hyoglossus Muscle. The **hyoglossus muscle** (hi-o-**gloss**-us) is an extrinsic tongue muscle.

Origin and Insertion. The muscle originates on both the greater cornu and a part of the body of the hyoid bone. It then inserts into the lateral surface of the body of the tongue.

Action. The muscle depresses the tongue.

MUSCLES OF PHARYNX

The **muscles of the pharynx** or *pharyngeal muscles* are involved in speaking, swallowing, and middle ear function (Figure 4-29). These muscles are specifically responsible for initiating the swallowing process. The pharynx is part of both the respiratory and digestive tracts and is also connected to both the nasal and oral cavities. The pharynx consists of three parts: the nasopharynx, oropharynx, and laryngopharynx (see Figure 2-20). The muscles of the pharynx include: the stylopharyngeus muscle, pharyngeal constrictors, and muscles of the soft palate.

Stylopharyngeus Muscle. The **stylopharyngeus muscle** (sty-lo-fuh-**rin**-je-us) is a paired longitudinal muscle of the pharynx.

Origin and Insertion. The muscle originates from the styloid process of the temporal bone (see Figure 3-31). It then inserts into the lateral and posterior pharyngeal walls.

Action. The muscle elevates and simultaneously widens the pharynx.

Innervation. The muscle is innervated by the ninth cranial or glossopharyngeal nerve.

Pharyngeal Constrictor Muscles. The **pharyngeal constrictor muscles** (fuh-**rin**-je-uhl kuhn-**strik**-tor) form the lateral and posterior walls of the pharynx. They consist of three paired muscles based on their vertical placement within the pharynx: the superior, middle, and inferior pharyngeal constrictor muscles.

Origin and Insertion. The origin of each muscle is different, although the muscles overlap each other and have similar insertions. The superior pharyngeal constrictor originates from the hamulus of

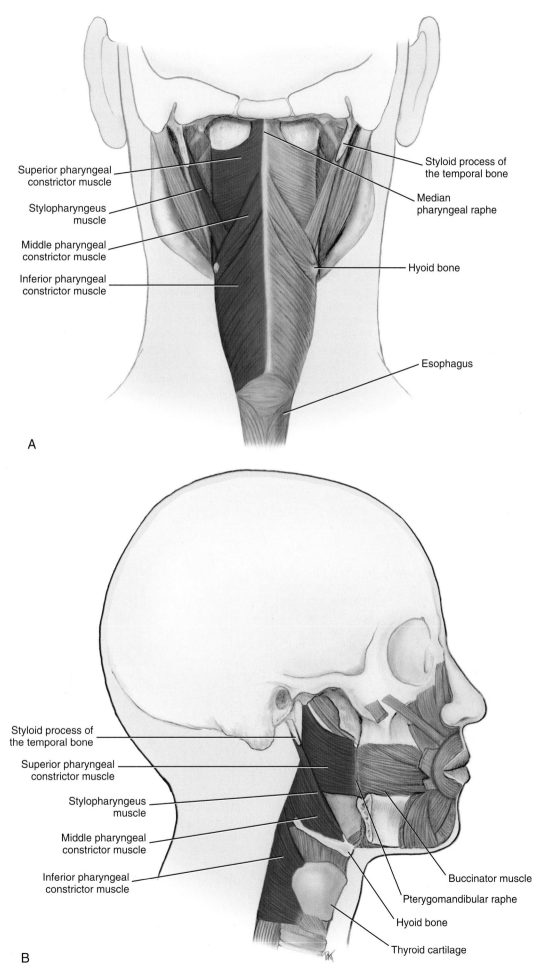

Superior pharyngeal
constrictor muscle

Stylopharyngeus
muscle

Middle pharyngeal
constrictor muscle

Inferior pharyngeal
constrictor muscle

Styloid process of
the temporal bone

Median
pharyngeal raphe

Hyoid bone

Esophagus

A

Styloid process of
the temporal bone

Superior pharyngeal
constrictor muscle

Stylopharyngeus
muscle

Middle pharyngeal
constrictor muscle

Inferior pharyngeal
constrictor muscle

Buccinator muscle

Pterygomandibular raphe

Hyoid bone

Thyroid cartilage

B

FIGURE 4-29 Muscles of the pharynx are highlighted and their origins and insertions noted from a
posterior view of the head and neck **(A)** and from a lateral view of the head and neck **(B)**.

the medial pterygoid plate, mandible, and pterygomandibular raphe (see Figures 3-34 and 3-52). The superior pharyngeal constrictor muscles of the pharynx and buccinator muscles are attached to each other at the pterygomandibular raphe.

The middle pharyngeal constrictor originates on the hyoid bone and stylohyoid ligament. The stylohyoid ligament runs from the tip of the styloid process of the temporal bone to the lesser cornu of the hyoid bone.

The inferior pharyngeal constrictor originates from both the thyroid and cricoid cartilage of the larynx. When these three muscles overlap, the inferior is most superficial. These muscles then all insert into the **median pharyngeal raphe**, which is a midline tendinous band of the posterior wall of the pharynx that is itself attached to the base of the skull.

Action. These muscles raise the pharynx and larynx and help drive food inferiorly into the esophagus during swallowing.

Innervation. The pharyngeal constrictor muscles are all innervated by the tenth cranial or vagus nerve through the pharyngeal plexus.

Muscles of the Soft Palate. There are five paired **muscles of the soft palate** (**pal**-uht) (see Figures 4-30 and 4-31). The soft palate forms the nonbony posterior part of the roof of the mouth or the oropharynx and connects laterally with the tongue (see Figure 2-20). The muscles of the soft palate include: the palatoglossus, palatopharyngeus, levator veli palatini, and tensor veli palatini muscles, and muscle of the uvula (Table 4-7). Anatomists sometimes consider the palatoglossus muscle to be an extrinsic muscle of the tongue because

it is involved in tongue movement, but it is considered under the muscles of the soft palate in this chapter since it is involved with that structure and shares the same innervation as most of the rest of the muscles nearby.

Action. The muscles of the soft palate are all involved in speaking and swallowing. When the muscles of the soft palate are relaxed, the soft palate extends posteriorly to define the anterior oropharynx. The combined actions of several muscles of the soft palate move the soft palate superiorly and posteriorly to contact the posterior pharyngeal wall that is being moved anteriorly. This movement of both the soft palate and pharyngeal wall brings a separation between the nasopharynx and oral cavity during swallowing to prevent food from entering the nasal cavity while eating. Specific actions of each muscle of the soft palate will also be discussed.

Innervation. All of the muscles of the soft palate, except the tensor veli palatini muscle, are innervated by the tenth cranial or vagus nerve through the pharyngeal plexus; the tensor veli palatini muscle is supplied by the medial pterygoid nerve, a branch of the mandibular nerve (or third division) of the fifth cranial or trigeminal nerve.

Palatoglossus Muscle. The **palatoglossus muscle** (pal-uh-toh-**gloss**-us) forms the anterior faucial pillar in the oral cavity, a vertical fold anterior to each palatine tonsil (see Figures 2-2 and 10-19).

Origin and Insertion. The muscle originates from the posterior part of the median palatine raphe, which is a midline tendinous band of the palate. The median palatine raphe is a surface feature demarcating the deeper median palatine suture between the palatine processes

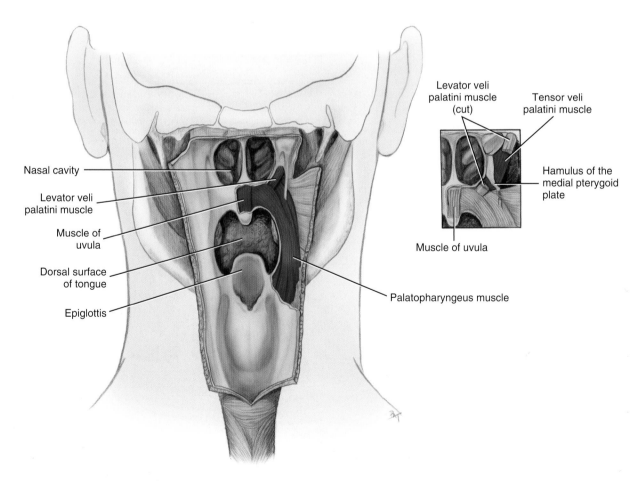

FIGURE 4-30 Posterior view of the head and neck as well as the muscles of the soft palate highlighted with their origins and insertions noted. Note that the pharyngeal constrictor muscles have been cut and mucous membranes partially removed (see inset).

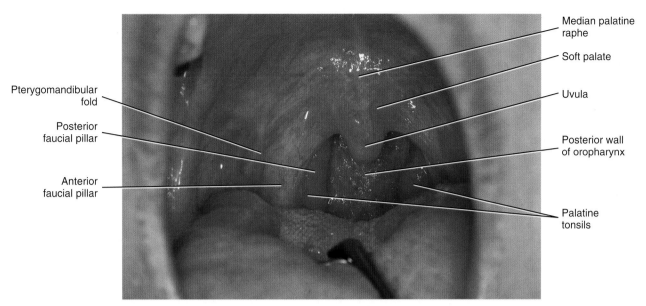

Median palatine raphe

Soft palate

Uvula

Posterior wall of oropharynx

Palatine tonsils

Pterygomandibular fold

Posterior faucial pillar

Anterior faucial pillar

FIGURE 4-31 Intraoral view of the oral cavity noting the soft palate, pterygomandibular fold, median palatine raphe, uvula, and anterior and posterior faucial pillars with palatine tonsils between the vertical folds. These oral cavity structures noted are all related to underlying muscles or other structures. See Figure 2-21 for a more detailed view.

TABLE 4-7	Muscles of Soft Palate		
MUSCLES	**ORIGIN**	**INSERTION**	**ACTION**
Palatoglossus (forming anterior faucial pillar)	Median palatine raphe	Lateral surface of tongue	Elevates and arches tongue to soft palate, depressing soft palate toward tongue; forms sphincter, separating oral cavity from pharynx
Palatopharyngeus (forming posterior faucial pillar)	Soft palate	Laryngopharynx and thyroid cartilage	Moves palate posteroinferiorly and posterior pharyngeal wall anterosuperiorly to help close off nasopharynx; elevates pharynx
Levator veli palatini	Temporal bone	Median palatine raphe	Raises soft palate to contact the posterior pharyngeal wall to help close off nasopharynx
Tensor veli palatini	Auditory (pharyngotympanic) tube and inferior surface of sphenoid bone	Becomes tendon near hamulus of medial pterygoid plate; tendon forms palatine aponeurosis and inserts at median palatine raphe	Tenses and slightly lowers soft palate
Muscle of the uvula	Tissue projection that hangs inferiorly from posterior soft palate in uvula		Soft palate closely adapts to posterior pharyngeal wall to help close off nasopharynx

of the maxillae anteriorly and the horizontal plates of the palatine bones posteriorly. It spans the palate from the incisive papilla to the uvula. Posteriorly, it is the locus for the origin of this muscle as well as other muscles of the soft palate. The muscle inserts into the lateral surface of the tongue.

Action. The muscle elevates the base of the tongue, arching the tongue against the soft palate, and depresses the soft palate toward the tongue. The muscles on both sides also form a sphincter, separating the oral cavity from the pharynx.

Palatopharyngeus Muscle. The **palatopharyngeus muscle** (pal-uh-toh-fuh-**rin**-je-us) forms the posterior faucial pillar in the oral cavity, a vertical fold posterior to each palatine tonsil (see Figures 2-21 and 10-19).

Origin and Insertion. The muscle originates in the soft palate and then inserts in the walls of the laryngopharynx and on the thyroid cartilage.

Action. The muscle moves the palate posteroinferiorly and the posterior pharyngeal wall anterosuperiorly to help close off the nasopharynx during swallowing.

Levator Veli Palatini Muscle. The **levator veli palatini muscle** (vee-ly pal-uh-**ti**-ni) is mainly located superior to the soft palate (see Figure 4-30).

Origin and Insertion. The muscle originates from the inferior surface of the temporal bone (see Figure 3-31). It then inserts into the median palatine raphe, which is a midline tendinous band of the palate discussed earlier (see Figures 2-15).

Action. The muscle raises the soft palate and helps bring it into contact with the posterior pharyngeal wall to close off the nasopharynx during speech and swallowing.

Tensor Veli Palatini Muscle. The **tensor veli palatini muscle** (tensor vee-ly) is a special muscle that stiffens the soft palate. This muscle is usually active during all palatal movements; some of its fibers are also responsible for opening the auditory (pharyngotympanic) tube to allow air to flow between the pharynx and middle ear cavity.

Origin and Insertion. The muscle originates from the auditory (pharyngotympanic) tube area and the inferior surface of the sphenoid bone (see Figure 3-34). It then passes inferiorly between the medial pterygoid muscle and medial pterygoid plate, forming a tendon near the hamulus of the medial pterygoid plate. The tendon winds around the hamulus, using it as a pulley and then spreads out to insert into the median palatine raphe, which is a midline tendinous band of the palate discussed earlier (see Figures 2-15).

Action. The muscle tenses and slightly lowers the soft palate.

Muscle of the Uvula. The **muscle of the uvula** (**u**-vu-luh) is a muscle of the soft palate.

Origin and Insertion. The muscle lies entirely within the uvula of the palate, which is a midline tissue structure that hangs inferiorly from the posterior margin of the soft palate and can be noted during an intraoral examination (see Figure 2-21).

Action. The muscle shortens and broadens the uvula, changing the contour of the posterior part of the soft palate. This change in contour allows the soft palate to adapt closely to the posterior pharyngeal wall to help close off the nasopharynx during swallowing.

Clinical Considerations With Muscles Involved in Mastication, Swallowing, and Speech

Impairment of the muscles of mastication, hyoid muscles, as well as muscles of the tongue, pharynx, and soft palate can critically influence dental treatment because these muscles are involved in mastication, swallowing, and speech. The etiology of these impairments can range from systemic disease states or syndromes including stroke (or cerebrovascular accident) to a genetically determined fault in muscle function such as muscular dystrophy.

A patient with this type of impairment may have difficulty communicating with the dental staff, such as when answering questions to complete health histories, and thus would need assistance from knowledgeable caregivers. The patient may also have difficulty when asked to open the mouth or swallow (dysphagia) during the appointment. Adapting to dental procedures such as taking radiographs or impressions as well as achieving adequate homecare may also pose a concern. Conversely, mouth drop may be present unless the mandible is held shut by hand. Biomechanical machinery such as for lifesaving suctioning may need to be worked around and attended to by the caregivers. Others will need to have extra dental suctioning performed to avoid choking; rubber dam placement can be added for safety.

The tongue may become atrophied in severe cases, with the clinician needing to move it to accommodate treatment. In contrast, a more active tongue may need a mouth prop along with muscle relaxant; the increased side effects of this premedication, including saliva pooling, coughing, gagging, choking, and possibility of aspiration, may become overwhelming negative factors during treatment. However, having the patient sit slightly more upright as well as trying to turn the body to one side may help to overcome these side effects as well as any other factors related to the semi-prone dental chair position (see earlier discussion with cervical muscle pathology). Patience and adaptability are key factors when working with any challenging patient group. The dental professional will need to work in conjunction with other healthcare providers such as physical therapists and speech pathologists to be able to provide long-range comprehensive dental care.

REVIEW QUESTIONS

1. The origin of the frontal belly of the epicranial muscle and the insertion of its occipital belly are BOTH at the
   A. clavicle and sternum.
   B. mastoid process.
   C. epicranial aponeurosis.
   D. pterygomandibular raphe.

2. Which of the following muscles is considered a muscle of mastication?
   A. Buccinator
   B. Risorius
   C. Mentalis
   D. Masseter
   E. Corrugator supercilii

3. The origin of a muscle is considered to be
   A. the starting point of a muscle.
   B. where the muscle fibers join the bone tendon.
   C. the muscle end attached to the least movable structure.
   D. the muscle end attached to the most movable structure.

4. Which of the following muscle pairs is divided by a median septum?
   A. Geniohyoid
   B. Masseter
   C. Digastric
   D. Transverse
   E. Vertical

5. Which of the following paired muscles unite medially, forming the floor of the mouth?
   A. Geniohyoid
   B. Omohyoid
   C. Digastric
   D. Mylohyoid
   E. Transverse

6. Which of the following muscle groups listed below serves to depress the hyoid bone?
   A. Muscles of mastication
   B. Suprahyoid muscles
   C. Infrahyoid muscles
   D. Intrinsic tongue muscles
   E. Extrinsic tongue muscles

7. Which of the following muscles has two bellies, giving the muscle two different origins?
   A. Lateral pterygoid
   B. Geniohyoid
   C. Thyrohyoid
   D. Stylohyoid

8. Which of the following is the MOST commonly used muscle when the patient's lips close around the saliva ejector?
   A. Risorius
   B. Mentalis
   C. Mylohyoid
   D. Buccinator
   E. Orbicularis oris

9. Which of the following muscle groups is involved in BOTH elevating the hyoid bone and depressing the mandible?
   A. Muscles of mastication
   B. Suprahyoid muscles
   C. Infrahyoid muscles
   D. Intrinsic tongue muscles
   E. Extrinsic tongue muscles

10. Which of the following muscle groups listed below is innervated by the cervical nerves?
    A. Muscles of mastication
    B. Muscles of facial expression
    C. Suprahyoid muscles
    D. Infrahyoid muscles
    E. Intrinsic tongue muscles

11. Which muscle can make the patient's oral vestibule shallower, thereby making dental work sometimes difficult?
    A. Mentalis
    B. Zygomaticus major
    C. Depressor anguli oris
    D. Levator anguli oris

12. Which of the following muscle groups is innervated by the facial nerve?
    A. Intrinsic tongue muscles
    B. Extrinsic tongue muscles
    C. Muscles of facial expression
    D. Muscles of mastication

13. Which of the following muscle groups inserts DIRECTLY on the hyoid bone?
    A. Geniohyoid, stylohyoid, and omohyoid muscles
    B. Masseter, stylohyoid, and digastric muscles
    C. Masseter, buccinator, and omohyoid muscles
    D. Palatopharyngeus and palatoglossus muscles and muscle of the uvula

14. Which of the following muscles is used when a patient grimaces?
    A. Epicranial
    B. Corrugator supercilii
    C. Risorius
    D. Mentalis

15. Which of the following muscles is an extrinsic muscle of the tongue?
    A. Geniohyoid muscle
    B. Hyoglossus muscle
    C. Mylohyoid muscle
    D. Transverse muscle
    E. Vertical muscle

16. Which muscle of facial expression compresses the cheeks during chewing assisting the muscles of mastication?
    A. Risorius
    B. Buccinator
    C. Mentalis
    D. Orbicularis oris
    E. Masseter

17. The superior pharyngeal constrictor muscle is noted to
    A. originate from the larynx.
    B. insert on the median pharyngeal raphe.
    C. overlap the stylopharyngeus muscle.
    D. be a longitudinal muscle of the pharynx.

18. Which of the following descriptions concerning the masseter muscle is CORRECT?
    A. Most superficial muscle of facial expression
    B. Originates from the zygomatic arch
    C. Inserts on the medial surface of the mandible's angle
    D. Depresses the mandible during jaw movement

19. Which of the following muscles forms the anterior faucial pillar in the oral cavity?
    A. Palatoglossus
    B. Palatopharyngeus
    C. Stylopharyngeus
    D. Tensor veli palatini

20. Which of the following situations occurs when BOTH sternocleidomastoid muscles are used at the same time by the patient?
    A. Neck is drawn laterally
    B. Head flexes at the neck
    C. Chin moves superiorly to the contralateral side
    D. Head rotates and is drawn to the shoulders

21. Which muscle does NOT aid in smiling with the lips when it contracts?
    A. Zygomatic major muscle
    B. Levator anguli oris muscle
    C. Zygomaticus minor muscle
    D. Epicranial muscle

22. Which muscle is located just deep to the skin of the neck?
    A. Platysma
    B. Buccinator
    C. Risorius
    D. Mentalis

23. Which muscle listed is considered MOST superiorly located on the head and neck?
    A. Corrugator supercilii muscle
    B. Zygomatic major muscle
    C. Superior pharyngeal constrictor muscle
    D. Superior belly of the omohyoid muscle

24. Which muscle listed below when contracted causes a frown?
    A. Zygomaticus minor muscle
    B. Levator anguli oris muscle
    C. Depressor anguli oris muscle
    D. Risorius muscle

25. Which muscle listed below is MOST superficial in regard to location?
    A. Masseter muscle
    B. Medial pterygoid muscle
    C. Lateral pterygoid muscle
    D. Superior pharyngeal constrictor muscle

26. Which of the following muscle pairs are considered to be intrinsic tongue muscles?
    A. Superior longitudinal
    B. Genioglossus
    C. Styloglossus
    D. Hyoglossus

27. All the muscles of the pharynx are known to be involved in
    A. closing the jaws.
    B. facial expression.
    C. middle ear function.
    D. stabilization of the mandible.

28. The posterior belly of the digastric muscle is also considered a(n)
    A. muscle of facial expression.
    B. posterior suprahyoid muscle.
    C. intrinsic muscle of the tongue.
    D. extrinsic muscle of the tongue.

29. Which of the following nerves innervates the temporalis muscle?
    A. First cervical nerve by way of the hypoglossal nerve
    B. Ninth cranial nerve or glossopharyngeal nerve
    C. Maxillary branch of the trigeminal nerve
    D. Mandibular branch of the trigeminal nerve
    E. Seventh cranial nerve or facial nerve

30. Which muscle's activity helps to prevent the tongue from sinking back and obstructing respiration?
    A. Genioglossus muscle
    B. Stylopharyngeus muscle
    C. Inferior longitudinal muscle
    D. Palatoglossus muscle

Identification Exercises

Identify the structures on the following diagrams by filling in each blank with the correct anatomic term. You can check your answers by looking back at the figure indicated in parentheses for each identification diagram.

1. (Figure 4-4, *A*)

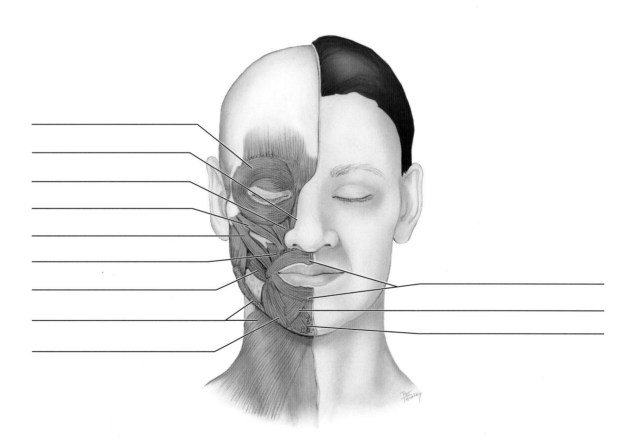

2. (Figure 4-4, *B*)

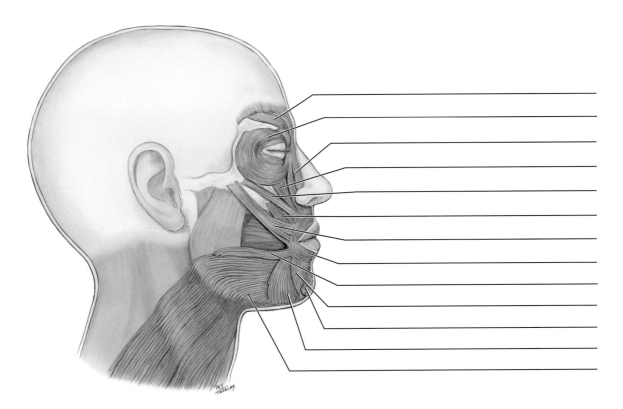

3. (Figures 4-22 and 4-23)

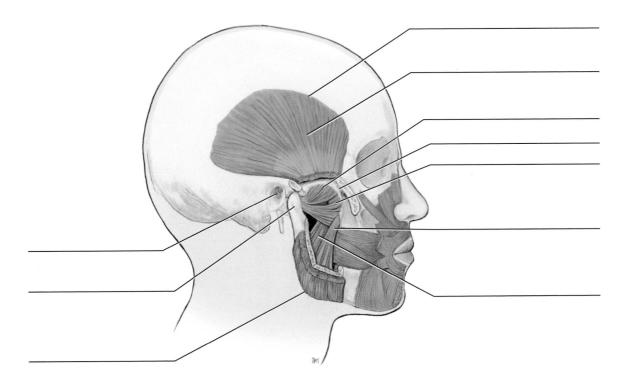

4. (Figure 4-24)

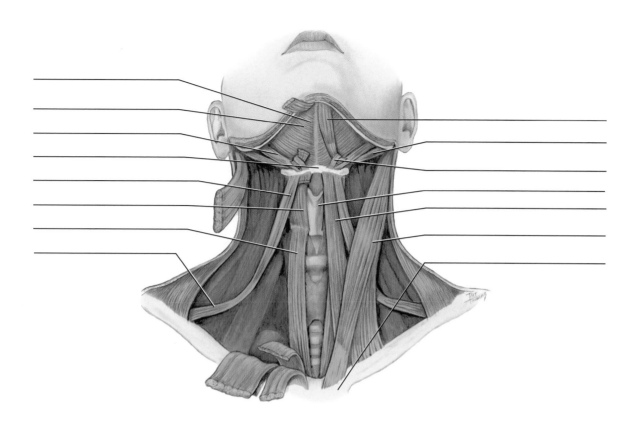

5. (Figures 4-25 and 4-27)

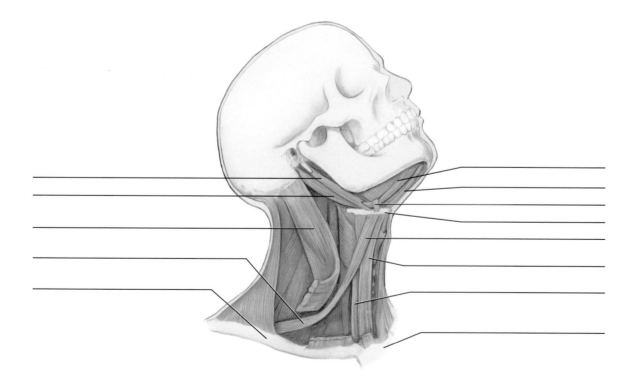

6. (Figure 4-28, *A*)

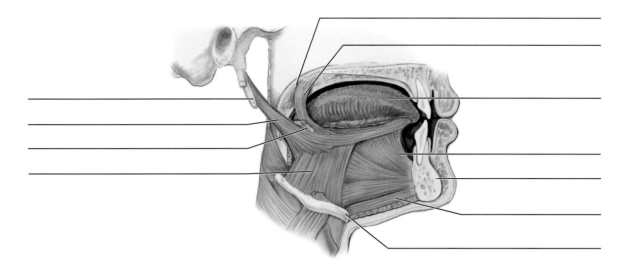

7. (Figure 4-29, *B*)

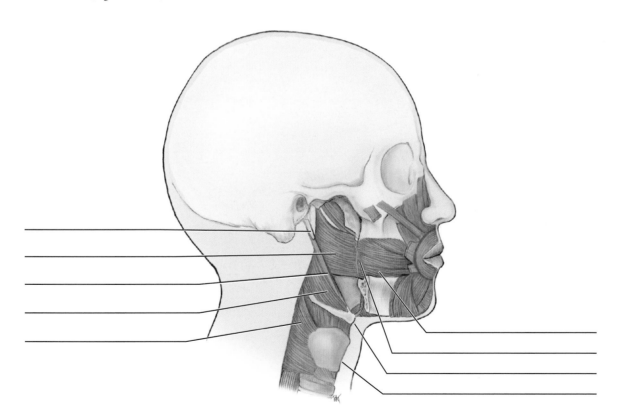

8. (Figure 4-30)

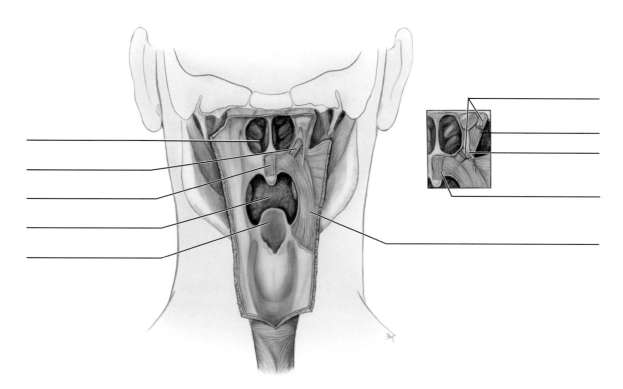

Temporomandibular Joint

●●● LEARNING OBJECTIVES

1. Define and pronounce the **key terms** and **anatomic terms** in this chapter.
2. Locate and identify the landmarks of the temporomandibular joint on a diagram, skull, and patient.
3. Describe the movements of the temporomandibular joints and their relationship with the muscles in the head and neck region.
4. Discuss temporomandibular joint pathology and related patient care.
5. Correctly complete the review questions and activities for this chapter.
6. Integrate an understanding of the anatomy of the temporomandibular joint into clinical dental practice.

●●● KEY TERMS

Depression of the mandible (de-presh-uhn) (man-di-buhl) Lowering of lower jaw.
Elevation of the mandible (el-uh-vay-shuhn) Raising of lower jaw.
Joint Site of a junction or union between two or more bones.
Lateral deviation of the mandible (dee-vee-ay-shuhn) Shifting of lower jaw to one side.

Ligament (lig-uh-muhnt) Band of fibrous tissue connecting bones.
Protrusion of the mandible (pro-troo-zhuhn) Bringing forward of lower jaw.
Retraction of the mandible (re-trak-shuhn) Bringing backward of lower jaw.
Subluxation (sub-luhk-say-shuhn) Acute episode in which both joints become dislocated.

Temporomandibular disorder (TMD) (tem-puh-roh-man-dib-u-luhr) Disorder involving one or both temporomandibular joints.
Trismus (triz-muhs) Reduced opening of the jaws.

TEMPOROMANDIBULAR JOINT OVERVIEW

The temporomandibular joint (TMJ) is a joint on each side of the head that allows for movement of the mandible for mastication, speech, and respirations (see Figure 2-9 and Chapter 4). A **joint** is a site of junction or union between two or more bones (see Chapter 3). The TMJ is classified as a ginglymoarthrodial joint, which denotes a joint having the form of both ginglymus and arthrodia joints, or hinge and sliding joints (discussed later).

Since a patient may have a disorder associated with one or both TMJs, the dental professional must understand its anatomy and its movements and be able to perform an extraoral examination of it, noting any pathology (see Appendix B).

The TMJ has its sensory innervation by the auriculotemporal and masseteric branches of the mandibular nerve (or third division) of the fifth cranial or trigeminal nerve; motor function is by the muscles of mastication (discussed later). The blood supply to the joint is from branches of the external carotid artery, predominantly the superficial temporal branch. The venous return is by the superficial temporal, maxillary, and pterygoid plexus of veins. The lymph from the TMJ is drained deeply into the superior deep cervical nodes.

JOINT BONES

The TMJ is the articulation of the temporal bone and the mandible on each side of the head, the bones of which give the joint its name (Figure 5-1). An articulation is an area where the bones are joined to each other. Both articulating bony surfaces of the joint are covered by fibrocartilage. For more specific information on both of these bones of the joint, see Chapter 3.

TEMPORAL BONE

The temporal bone is a cranial bone that articulates with the facial bone of the mandible at the TMJ by way of the joint disc (Figure 5-2). The articulating area on the temporal bone of the joint is located on

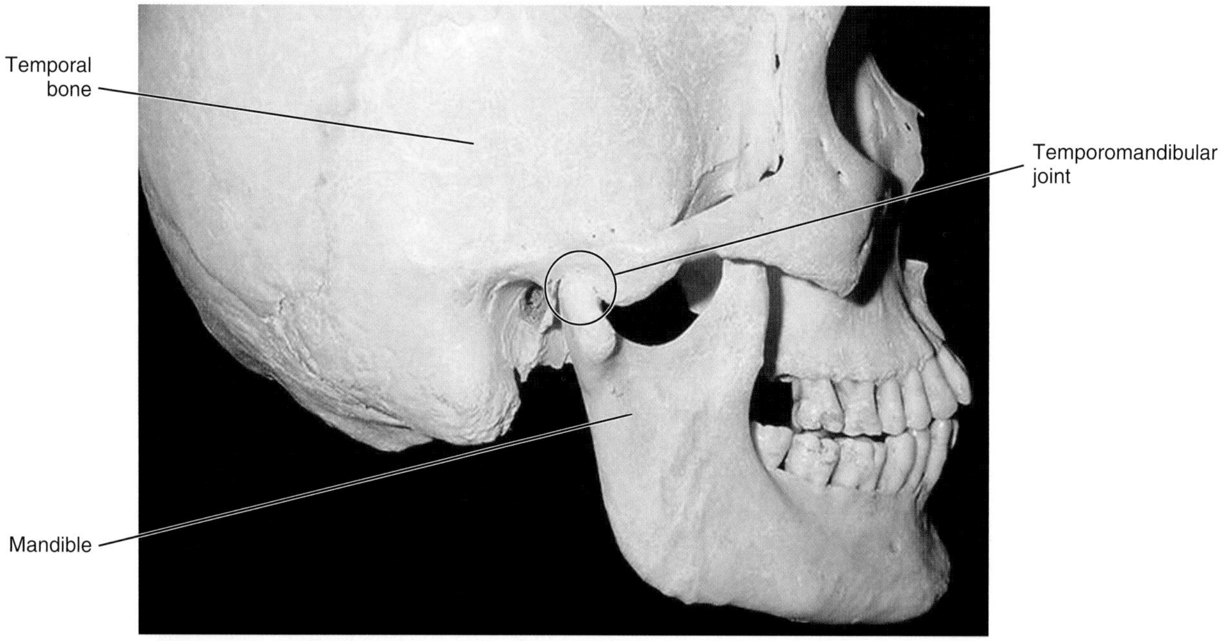

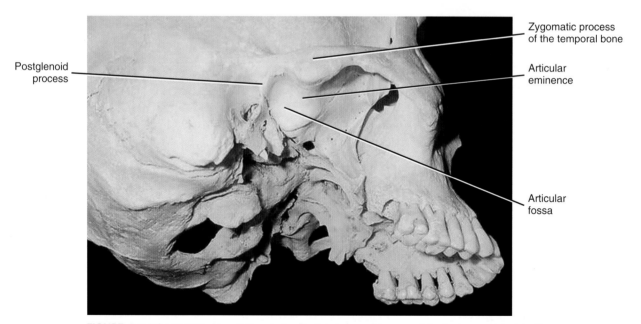

FIGURE 5-1 Lateral view of the skull noting the temporomandibular joint (*circle*), which is an articulation between the temporal bone and the mandible.

FIGURE 5-2 Inferolateral view of the skull with the temporal bone and its features related to the temporomandibular joint noted.

the bone's inferior aspect, involving its squamous part (see Figure 3-29). This articulating area includes the temporal bone's articular eminence and articular fossa. The articular eminence consists of a rounded protuberance on the inferior aspect of the zygomatic process.

The articular fossa, which is also known as the *mandibular fossa* or *glenoid fossa,* is posterior to the articular eminence. This fossa consists of an oval-shaped depression on the temporal bone, which is posterior and medial to the zygomatic process of the temporal bone. Posterior to the articular fossa is a sharper ridge, the postglenoid process.

MANDIBLE

The mandible is a facial bone that articulates with the temporal bone of the cranium. This articulation is accomplished by way of the joint disc working with the knuckle-shaped posterosuperior process of the mandibular ramus. The head of this process is the mandibular condyle, and its superior surface is the articulating surface of the condyle (Figure 5-3 and see Figures 3-49 to 3-54). The articulating surface of the condyle is strongly convex in the anteroposterior direction and only slightly convex mediolaterally.

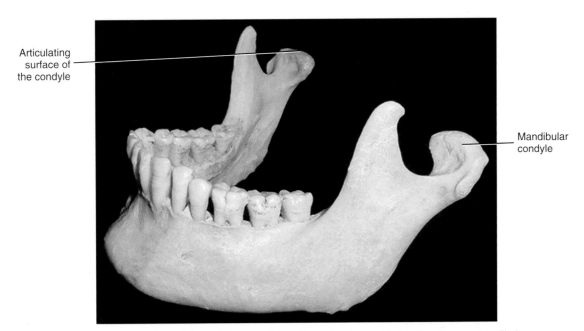

FIGURE 5-3 Anterolateral view of the mandible with its features related to the temporomandibular joint noted.

JOINT CAPSULE

A fibrous **joint capsule** completely encloses the TMJ (Figure 5-4). Superiorly, the capsule wraps around the margin of the temporal bone's articular eminence and articular fossa. Inferiorly, the capsule wraps around the level posteriorly and laterally at the neck, but anteriorly and medially it attaches just to the margin of the articular surface of the condyle.

JOINT DISC

The fibrous **joint disc** or *meniscus* is located between the temporal bone and mandibular condyle on each side, allowing articulation between the two bones (see Figures 5-4 and 9-3). The margins of the joint disc are continuous with the joint capsule or attach into the joint capsule. On section, the disc appears caplike on the mandibular condyle, with its superior aspect concavoconvex from anterior to posterior and its inferior aspect concave (see Figure 5-9). This shape of the disc conforms to the shape of both the adjacent articulating bones of the TMJ and is related to joint movements.

The disc completely divides the TMJ into two compartments or **synovial cavities** (sy-**no**-vee-uhl): the upper and lower synovial cavities. The membranes lining the inside of the joint capsule secrete synovial fluid that helps lubricate the joint and fills the synovial cavities. **Synovial fluid** is a clear viscous liquid, rather like egg white.

The disc is attached to the lateral and medial poles of the mandibular condyle. The disc is not attached to the temporal bone anteriorly, except indirectly through the capsule. Posteriorly, the disc is divided into two areas or divisions: the upper and lower divisions. The upper division of the posterior part of the disc is attached to the temporal bone's postglenoid process, and the lower division attaches to the neck of the condyle. The disc blends with the capsule at these points. This posterior area of attachment of the disc to the capsule is one of the locations where nerves and blood vessels enter the joint; the periphery is innervated and vascularized. However, the disc is both aneural (having no nervous tissue) and avascular (having no blood vessels) in its thinner middle or force-bearing intermediate zone.

With aging or trauma to the area, the joint disc can become thinner or even perforated. Recent studies suggest this disc degeneration may also cause calcifications within the disc, changes that may lead to impaired movement of the joint. At any age, the disc may become dislocated by injury to its attachments. Both perforation and displacement can lead to clinical problems noted during dental treatment (discussed later).

LIGAMENTS ASSOCIATED WITH JOINT

The mandible is joined to the cranium by ligaments of the TMJ. A ligament is a band of fibrous tissue that connects bones. Three paired ligaments are associated with the TMJ: the temporomandibular, stylomandibular, and sphenomandibular ligaments (Figure 5-5). The temporomandibular ligament is considered the major ligament for the joint since it provides strength to the joint. The other two are minor ligaments even though they still connect the mandible to the cranium as does the temporomandibular ligament; however, neither minor ligament provides much strength to the joint itself.

TEMPOROMANDIBULAR JOINT LIGAMENT

The **temporomandibular ligament** (tem-puh-roh-man-**dib**-u-luhr) is located on the lateral side of each joint forming a reinforcement of the lateral part of the joint capsule of the TMJ. Thus it amounts to a thickening of the capsule in this area to create the ligament itself. The base of this triangular ligament is attached to the zygomatic process of the temporal bone lateral to the articular eminence; its apex is fixed to the lateral side of the neck of the mandible. This ligament prevents the excessive retraction or moving backward of the mandible, a situation that might lead to difficulties with the movement of the TMJ.

STYLOMANDIBULAR LIGAMENT

The **stylomandibular ligament** (sty-lo-man-**dib**-u-luhr) is a variable ligament formed from thickened cervical fascia in the area.

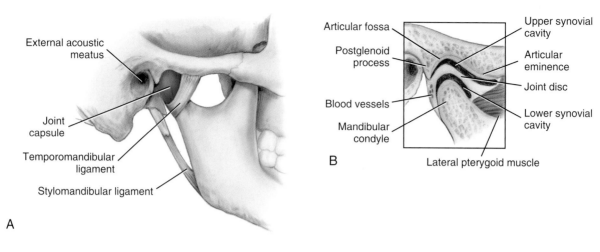

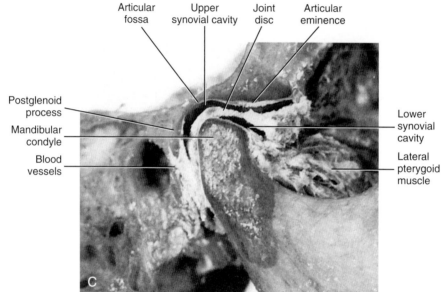

FIGURE 5-4 Joint capsule of the temporomandibular joint from a lateral view **(A)**, and with the capsule removed to show the upper and lower synovial cavities and their relationship to the joint disc **(B)**, and with a block dissection **(C)**. **(B** *from Fehrenbach MJ, Topowics T:* Illustrated dental embryology, histology, and anatomy, *ed 4, St Louis, 2016, Elsevier; **C** from Liebgott WB: The anatomical basis of dentistry, St. Louis, 1986, Mosby.)*

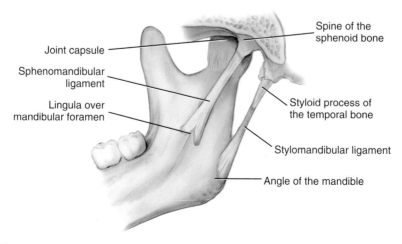

FIGURE 5-5 Medial view of the temporomandibular joint with its joint capsule and associated ligaments noted.

This ligament runs from the styloid process of the temporal bone to the angle of the mandible, which separates the parotid and submandibular salivary glands. It also becomes taut when the mandible is protruded.

SPHENOMANDIBULAR LIGAMENT

The **sphenomandibular ligament** (sfe-no-man-**dib**-u-luhr) is not strictly considered part of the TMJ but is located on the medial side of the mandible, at some distance from the joint. This long membranous band runs from the angular spine of the sphenoid bone to the lingula over the mandibular foramen on the medial aspect of the mandible. The inferior alveolar nerve descends between the sphenomandibular ligament and the mandibular ramus to gain access to the mandibular foramen. The sphenomandibular ligament, because of its attachment to the lingula, overlaps the opening of the foramen. It is a vestige of Meckel cartilage, which is part of the embryonic lower jaw.

Although it is not part of the TMJ, the ligament becomes accentuated and taut when the mandible is protruded. The sphenomandibular ligament is involved in troubleshooting the inferior alveolar block due to its location (see Figure 9-37). The ligament may actually act as an outer barrier to the diffusion of the local anesthetic agent if the medial surface of the mandible is not contacted with the needle at the deeper mandibular foramen with the inferior alveolar nerve.

JAW MOVEMENTS WITH MUSCLE RELATIONSHIPS

The TMJ allows for the movement of the mandible during speech and mastication by way of each muscle attached to the cranium and the mandible (Figure 5-6). There are two basic types of movement performed by the joint and its associated muscles: gliding (or sliding) and rotational (or hinge) movements.

The gliding movement of the TMJ occurs mainly between the disc and the articular eminence of the temporal bone in the upper synovial cavity, with the disc plus the condyle moving forward or backward, and down and up the articular eminence. The gliding movement allows the lower jaw to move forward or backward. Bringing the lower jaw forward involves protrusion of the mandible. Bringing the lower jaw backward involves retraction of the mandible. Protrusion involves the bilateral contraction of both of the lateral pterygoid muscles. The contraction of the posterior parts of both temporalis muscles is involved during retraction of the mandible.

The rotational movement of the TMJ occurs mainly between the disc and the mandibular condyle in the lower synovial cavity. The axis of rotation of the disc plus the condyle is approximately transverse, and the movements accomplished are depression or elevation of the mandible. Depression of the mandible is the lowering

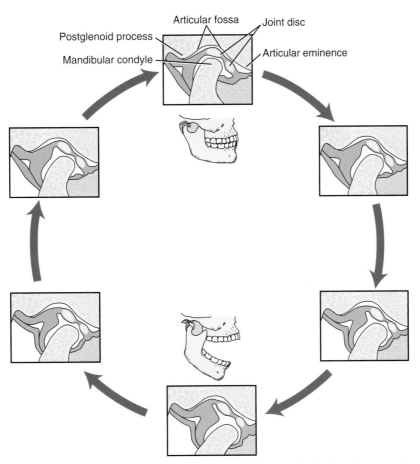

Articular fossa
Joint disc
Postglenoid process
Mandibular condyle
Articular eminence

FIGURE 5-6 Movements of the mandible related to the temporomandibular joint demonstrating what occurs during the opening and closing of the mouth. *(From Fehrenbach MJ, Popowics T:* Illustrated dental embryology, histology, and anatomy, *ed 4, St Louis, 2016, Elsevier.)*

of the lower jaw. **Elevation of the mandible** is the raising of the lower jaw.

With these two types of movement, gliding and rotational and with the right and left TMJs working together, the finer movements of the jaw can be accomplished. These include opening and closing the jaws and shifting the lower jaw to one side.

Opening the jaws involves both depression and protrusion of the mandible. Closing the jaws involves both elevation and retraction of the mandible. Thus opening and closing the jaws involves a combination of gliding and rotational movements of the TMJs in their respective joint cavities. The disc plus the condyle glide on the articular fossa in the upper synovial cavity, moving forward or backward on the articular eminence. Roughly at the same time, the mandibular condyle rotates on the disc in the lower synovial cavity.

Muscles are involved in mandibular movements as already noted (see **Chapter 4** for related figures with specific origins and insertions). The muscles of mastication involved in elevating the mandible during closing of the jaws include the bilateral contractions of the masseter, temporalis, and medial pterygoid muscles. The anterior suprahyoid muscles are involved in depressing the mandible when they bilaterally contract during opening of the jaws with the hyoid bone stabilized by the other hyoid muscles. The lateral pterygoid muscles are primarily involved in the protrusion that accompanies opening. Because the protruded condyle articulates with the articular eminence rather than the articular fossa, a slight depression is associated with protrusion.

Lateral deviation of the mandible or *lateral excursion* involves shifting the lower jaw to one side. Lateral deviation involves both the gliding and rotational movements of the contralateral TMJs in their respective joint cavities. During lateral deviation, the contralateral disc plus the condyle glide forward and medially on the articular eminence in the upper synovial cavity while the contralateral condyle and disc remain relatively stable in the articular fossa. This produces a rotation around the more stable condyle.

Contraction of the contralateral lateral pterygoid muscles, the one on the protruding side, is involved during lateral deviation. When the mandible laterally deviates to the left, the right lateral pterygoid muscle contracts, moving the right condyle forward while the left condyle stays in position, thus causing the mandible to move to the left. The reverse situation occurs when the mandible laterally deviates to the right.

During mastication, the power stroke, when the teeth crunch the food, involves a movement from a laterally deviated position back to the midline. If the food is on the right, the mandible will be deviated to the right by the left lateral pterygoid muscle. The power stroke will return the mandible to the center, so the movement is to the left and involves a retraction of the left side. This is accomplished by the left posterior part of the temporalis muscle. At the same time, all the closing jaw muscles on the right side contract to crush the food. The reverse situation occurs if the food is on the left.

The resting position of the TMJ is not with the teeth biting together. Instead, the muscular balance and proprioceptive feedback allow a physiologic rest for the mandible, an interocclusal clearance or *freeway space*, which is approximately 2 to 4 mm between the opposing teeth of each dental arch. When a large number of teeth become lost over time, the jaw may overclose, which is often uncomfortable for the patient and may cause trauma to the teeth and surrounding oral region. Likewise, replacement dentures that "jack" the jaw open are intolerable for a patient.

To palpate the joint and its associated muscles effectively during an extraoral examination, have the patient go through all the movements of the mandible while bilaterally palpating the joint just anterior to the external acoustic meatus of each ear (Figure 5-7 and Table 5-1). Thus the TMJ is palpated laterally at a depression inferior to the zygomatic arch and approximately 1 to 2 cm anterior to the tragus. This includes asking the patient to open and close the mouth several times and then to move the opened lower jaw to the left, then to the right, and then forward. To further assess the mandible moving at the TMJ, use digital palpation by gently placing a finger into the outer part of the external acoustic meatus (Figure 5-8).

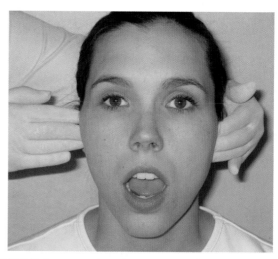

FIGURE 5-7 Demonstration of palpation of the temporomandibular joint during an extraoral examination while the patient undergoes movement involving both joints. *(Courtesy of Margaret J. Fehrenbach, RDH, MS.)*

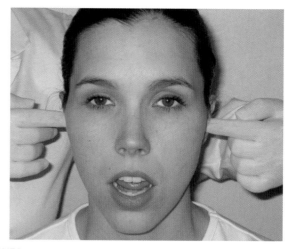

FIGURE 5-8 Demonstration of further palpation of the temporomandibular joint by gently placing a finger into the outer part of the external acoustic meatus of the patient during an extraoral examination. *(Courtesy of Margaret J. Fehrenbach, RDH, MS.)*

TABLE 5-1	Mandibular Movements of Temporomandibular Joint and Muscles	
MANDIBULAR MOVEMENT(S)	**TEMPOROMANDIBULAR JOINT MOVEMENT(S)**	**ASSOCIATED MUSCLES**
Protrusion of mandible, moving mandible forward	Gliding in both upper synovial cavities	Lateral pterygoid with bilateral contraction
Retraction of mandible, moving mandible backward	Gliding in both upper synovial cavities	Posterior part of temporalis and suprahyoid with bilateral contraction
Elevation and retraction of mandible, closing jaws	Gliding in both upper synovial cavities and rotation in both lower synovial cavities	Masseter, temporalis, medial pterygoid with bilateral contraction
Depression and protrusion of mandible, opening jaws	Gliding in both upper synovial cavities and rotation in both lower synovial cavities	Suprahyoid and lateral pterygoid with bilateral contraction
Lateral deviation of mandible to shift mandible to contralateral side	Gliding in one upper synovial cavity and while the condyle and disc of other side spin around an approximately vertical axis within upper synovial cavity	Lateral pterygoid with unilateral contraction

Clinical Considerations With Temporomandibular Joint Pathology

A patient may have pathology associated with one or both of the TMJs or a **temporomandibular disorder (TMD)**. The patient may experience chronic joint tenderness, swelling, and painful muscle spasms. Also present may be difficulties of joint movement such as a limited or deviated mandibular opening. The dental professional plays an important role in the recognition, treatment, and maintenance of patients with this disorder.

Recognition of TMD includes palpation of the joint as the patient performs all the movements of the joint as well as palpation of the related muscles of mastication during an extraoral examination as discussed earlier. All signs and symptoms related to TMD, such as the amount of mandibular opening and facial pain, as well as any parafunctional habits and related medical history, need to be recorded by the dental professional. This may mean an in-depth occlusal evaluation for the patient. The traditional skull radiograph of the joint area may be used, or magnetic resonance imaging (MRI) may be performed to aid in the diagnosis of TMD. The MRI is a noninvasive nuclear procedure for imaging soft tissue with high fat and water content. This imaging makes it possible to distinguish any abnormalities in the joint (Figure 5-9).

Not all patients with TMD have abnormalities in the joint disc or the joint itself. Most symptoms seem to originate from the muscles supporting the joint. In addition, recent studies do not support the role of TMD in directly causing headaches, or neck or back pain or instability; headaches are usually caused by muscle tension or vascular changes. Cyclic episodes of TMD and other incidents of chronic body pain are commonly encountered in the TMD population, with smoking now shown to increase pain levels.

Joint sounds occur because of disc derangement. The posterior part of the joint disc gets caught between the condyle head and the articular eminence. However, joint sounds are not a reliable indicator of TMD because they can change over time in a patient. Thus the clicking, grinding, and popping of the joint during movement present with TMD is also found in 40% to 60% of persons without TMD.

Many controversies surround the etiology and thus treatment of TMD, and fewer than half of TMD patients seek treatment for their disorder. Most recent studies have determined that malocclusion and occlusal discrepancies are not involved in most cases, but lack of overbite may be an additive factor. Accordingly, occlusal adjustment, jaw repositioning, and orthodontic therapy are not the treatments of choice for all patients with TMD, nor do these treatments seem to prevent this disorder.

Most cases of TMD improve over time with inexpensive and reversible conservative treatments, including patient-based or prescription pain control, relaxation therapy, stress management, habit control, moderate muscle exercises, and orofacial myology. Certain homecare steps can also work to improve any initial problems with TMD, such as by avoiding the eating of hard foods or using chewing gum as well as learning relaxation techniques to reduce overall stress and muscle tension. Maintaining good posture, especially when working at a computer such as pausing often to change position and resting hands and arms, can relieve stressed muscles. It is always important to use safety measures in certain situations to reduce the risk of fractures and dislocations of the TMJ.

A flat-plane, full-coverage oral appliance, such as a nonrepositioning stabilization splint, often is helpful to control bruxism and take stress off the TMJ, although some individuals may bite harder on it, thus worsening their condition. An anterior splint, with contact at the front teeth only, may then prove helpful if used short term. Such inexpensive and reversible treatments (i.e., ones not causing permanent jaw or dentition changes) now show the same success as more expensive and irreversible treatments such as surgery. Thus only a few patients with TMD require surgery or other extensive treatment. However, surgery of the TMJ can now make use of arthroscopy with an endoscope and lasers. Replacement of the jaw joint(s) or disc(s) with TMJ implants is still considered a treatment of last resort.

An acute episode of TMD can occur when a patient opens the mouth too wide, causing maximal depression and protrusion of the mandible, as when yawning or receiving prolonged dental care. This causes **subluxation** or dislocation of both joints (Figure 5-10). Subluxation happens when the head of each condyle moves too far anteriorly on the articular eminence. When the patient tries to close and elevate the mandible, the condylar heads cannot move posteriorly because the muscles of mastication have become spastic. The patient now has **trismus**, which refers to reduced opening of the jaws. Trismus can also occur with odontogenic infections (see **Chapters 11** and **12**).

Treatment of subluxation consists of relaxing these muscles and having the clinician carefully shift the mandible downward and back gently with the finger and thumbs of both hands, equally on both sides. The condylar heads will then be able to assume their posterior position in relationship to the articular eminence by the muscular action of the elevating muscles of mastication. Future care of these patients involves avoidance of extreme depression of the mandible such as with prolonged dental treatment.

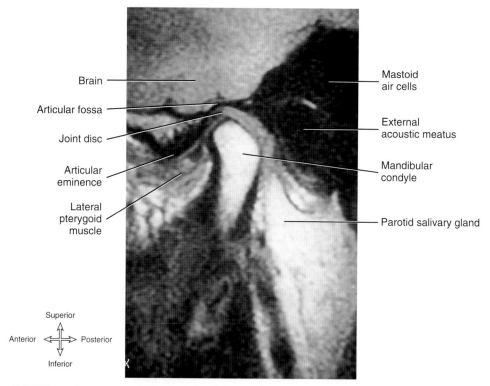

Brain

Articular fossa

Joint disc

Articular eminence

Lateral pterygoid muscle

Mastoid air cells

External acoustic meatus

Mandibular condyle

Parotid salivary gland

Superior

Anterior ⟷ Posterior

Inferior

FIGURE 5-9 Coronal magnetic resonance imaging in an asymptomatic individual with a closed temporomandibular joint. Note that this has been reconstructed as a parasagittal section. *(From Quinn PD: Color atlas of temporomandibular joint surgery, St Louis, 1998, Elsevier.)*

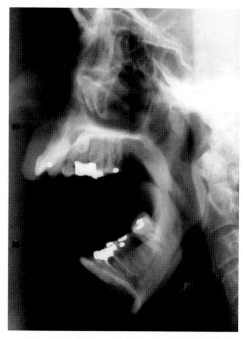

FIGURE 5-10 Lateral radiographic view of an individual with a dislocation or subluxation of both of the temporomandibular joints. *(From Reynolds PA, Abrahams PH: McMinn's interactive clinical anatomy: head and neck, ed 2, London, 2001, Elsevier.)*

REVIEW QUESTIONS

1. Which of the following ligaments associated with the temporomandibular joint serves to reinforce the joint capsule?
   A. Styloid
   B. Stylomandibular
   C. Temporomandibular
   D. Sphenomandibular

2. Which of the following landmarks associated with the temporomandibular joint is located DIRECTLY on the mandible?
   A. Articular eminence
   B. Condyle
   C. Articular fossa
   D. Postglenoid process

3. Which of the following is an overall description of the basic movement performed by the temporomandibular joint?
   A. Gliding movement only
   B. Rotational movement only
   C. Gliding and rotational movement
   D. No movement is involved

4. Which of the following muscles is involved in the lateral deviation of the mandible?
   A. Masseter muscle
   B. Medial pterygoid muscle
   C. Lateral pterygoid muscle
   D. Temporalis muscle
   E. Digastric muscle

5. Protrusion of the mandible is an action that primarily involves
   A. opening the jaws.
   B. closing the jaws.
   C. bringing the lower jaw forward.
   D. bringing the lower jaw backward.
   E. shifting the lower jaw to one side.

6. Which of the following movements of the lower jaw is assisted through contraction by the temporalis muscle?
   A. Mandibular depression only
   B. Mandibular elevation only
   C. Mandibular retraction only
   D. Mandibular depression and elevation
   E. Mandibular elevation and retraction

7. Which of the following temporomandibular joint ligaments has the inferior alveolar nerve descending nearby in order to gain access to the mandibular foramen?
   A. Sphenomandibular ligament only
   B. Stylomandibular ligament only
   C. Temporomandibular ligament only
   D. Sphenomandibular and stylomandibular ligaments
   E. Stylomandibular and temporomandibular ligaments

8. Which of the following statements about the temporomandibular joint disc is INCORRECT?
   A. Disc separates the TMJ into synovial cavities
   B. Disc is attached anteriorly and posteriorly to the condyle
   C. Gliding movements take place between the disc and the temporal bone
   D. Inferior surface of the disc is concave

9. Which area of the mandible listed below articulates with the temporal bone at the temporomandibular joint?
   A. Lingula
   B. Mandibular notch
   C. Coronoid process
   D. Condyle

10. During both mandibular protrusion and retraction, the rotation of the articulating surface of the mandible against the joint disc in the lower synovial cavity is prevented by the
    A. facial muscles.
    B. infrahyoid muscles.
    C. muscles of mastication.
    D. ligaments of the temporomandibular joint.

11. Which structure of the temporomandibular joint secretes synovial fluid?
    A. Mandibular condyle
    B. Joint disc
    C. Inner capsule lining membranes
    D. Lateral pterygoid muscle

12. Which list is in order of location from the MOST anterior structure to the MOST posterior structure as found within the temporomandibular joint?
    A. Articular fossa, postglenoid process, articular eminence
    B. Condyle, coronoid process, mandibular notch
    C. Articular eminence, articular fossa, postglenoid process
    D. Coronoid process, condyle, mandibular notch

13. At what position does a displaced joint disc of the temporomandibular joint usually lie?
    A. Anterior to its usual position
    B. Posterior to its usual position
    C. Within the articular fossa
    D. Within the mandibular notch

14. The joint capsule of the temporomandibular joint wraps around which structure?
    A. Coronoid process
    B. Mandibular notch
    C. Mandibular condyle
    D. Zygomatic arch

15. Which of the following situations occurs when there is subluxation of the temporomandibular joint?
    A. Head of condyle moves too far anteriorly on the articular eminence.
    B. Neck of condyle moves too far posteriorly on the articular eminence.
    C. Coronoid process moves too far anteriorly on the articular eminence.
    D. Coronoid process moves too far posteriorly on the articular eminence.

16. Which of the following landmarks is located upon the temporal bone?
    A. Condyle
    B. Articular fossa
    C. Coronoid notch
    D. External oblique line

17. Which of the following provides arterial branches for the MOST direct blood supply to the temporomandibular joint?
    A. Internal carotid artery
    B. External carotid artery
    C. Common carotid artery
    D. Aorta alone

18. Which of the following is located posterior to the articular fossa within the region of the temporomandibular joint?
    A. Postglenoid process
    B. Articular eminence
    C. Bony separation of the nasal septum
    D. Zygomatic process of the temporal bone

19. Which of the following nerves innervates the temporomandibular joint?
    A. Facial nerve
    B. Hypoglossal nerve
    C. Vagus nerve
    D. Trigeminal nerve
    E. Glossopharyngeal nerve

20. Which of the following situations can possibly happen to the joint disc of the temporomandibular joint as a person ages?
    A. Increased blood supply
    B. Fewer calcifications
    C. Perforations of structure
    D. Thickening of structure

Identification Exercises

Identify the structures on the following diagrams by filling in each blank with the correct anatomic term. You can check your answers by looking back at the figure indicated in parentheses for each identification diagram.

1. (Figures 5-1, 5-2, and 5-4, *A* and *B*)

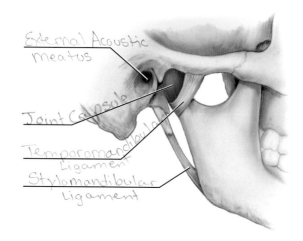

External Acoustic meatus

Joint Capsule

Temporomandibular Ligament

Stylomandibular Ligament

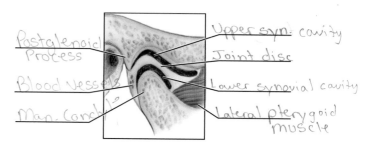

Postglenoid Process

Blood Vessels

Man. Condyle

Upper syn. cavity

Joint disc

Lower synovial cavity

lateral pterygoid muscle

2. (Figures 5-3 and 5-5)

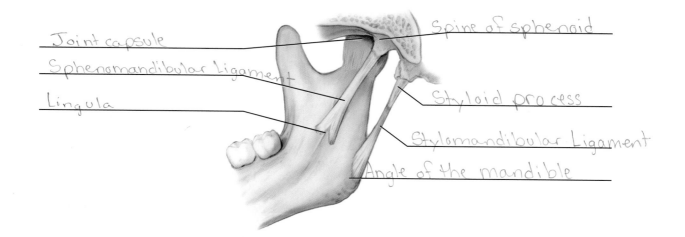

Joint capsule

Sphenomandibular Ligament

Lingula

Spine of sphenoid

Styloid process

Stylomandibular Ligament

Angle of the mandible

CHAPTER 6

Vascular System

●●● LEARNING OBJECTIVES

1. Define and pronounce the **key terms** and **anatomic terms** in this chapter.
2. Identify and trace the routes of the blood vessels of the head and neck on a diagram, skull, and patient.
3. Discuss the vascular system pathology associated with the head and neck region.
4. Correctly complete the review questions and activities for this chapter.
5. Integrate an understanding of the head and neck blood supply into clinical dental practice.

●●● KEY TERMS

Anastomosis/Anastomoses (uh-nuhs-tuh-**moh**-sis, uh-nuhs-tuh-**moh**-sees) Communication of blood vessel(s) with another blood vessel(s).

Arterial plaque Substance lining arteries consisting mainly of cholesterol.

Arteriole (ahr-**tare**-ee-ole) Smaller artery branching off artery and connecting with capillary.

Artery Blood vessel carrying blood away from the heart.

Atherosclerosis (ath-uhr-o-skluh-**roh**-sis) Narrowing and blockage of arteries by fatty arterial plaque.

Bacteremia (bak-tuhr-**ee**-me-uh) Bacteria traveling within vascular system.

Capillary (**kap**-i-lare-ee) Smaller blood vessel branching off an arteriole to supply blood directly to tissue.

Carotid pulse (kuh-**rot**-id) Reliable pulse palpated from common carotid artery.

Embolus/Emboli (**em**-bol-us, **em**-bo-lie) Foreign material(s) such as a thrombus (or thrombi) traveling in blood to block vessel.

Hematoma (he-muh-**toh**-muh) Bruise resulting when a blood vessel is injured and small amount of blood escapes into surrounding tissue and then clots.

Hemorrhage (**hem**-uh-ruhj) Large amounts of blood escaping into surrounding tissue without clotting when blood vessel is seriously injured.

Thrombus/Thrombi (**throm**-buhs, **throm**-by) Clot(s) forming on inner blood vessel wall.

Vascular plexus (**plek**-suhs) Large network of blood vessels, usually veins.

Vascular system Consists of arterial blood supply, capillary network, venous drainage.

Vein Blood vessel traveling to the heart carrying blood.

Venous sinuses (**vee**-nuhs) Blood-filled space between two layers of tissue.

Venule (**ven**-yule) Smaller vein draining capillaries and then joins larger veins.

VASCULAR SYSTEM OVERVIEW

The **vascular system** of the head and neck, as is the case in the rest of the body, consists of an arterial blood supply, a capillary network, and venous drainage. A large network of blood vessels within the system is a **vascular plexus**. The head and neck area contains certain important venous plexuses. Blood vessels also may communicate with each other within the system by an **anastomosis** (plural, **anastomoses**), a connecting channel(s) among the vessels.

An **artery** is the component of the vascular system that arises from the heart and carries blood away from it. Each artery starts as a large vessel and branches into smaller vessels, each one a smaller artery or an **arteriole**. Each arteriole branches into even smaller vessels until it becomes a network of capillaries. Each **capillary** is smaller than an arteriole and can supply blood to a larger area only because there are so many of them.

A **vein** is another component of the vascular system. A vein, unlike an artery, travels to the heart and carries blood to it. After each smaller vein or **venule** drains the capillaries of the area, the venules coalesce to become larger veins. Veins are much larger and more numerous than arteries. Veins anastomose freely and have a greater variability in location in comparison with arteries. It is a common misconception that the veins of the head do not contain one-way valves like other veins of the vascular system. In fact, most veins of the face, but not all, have valves.

There are also different kinds of venous networks found within the vascular system in the body. Superficial veins are found immediately deep to the skin. Deeper veins usually accompany larger arteries in a more protected location. **Venous sinuses** are blood-filled spaces between two layers of tissue. All these venous networks are connected by anastomoses.

Blood vessels are less numerous than lymphatic vessels. However, the pathway of venous blood vessels mainly parallels those of the lymphatic vessels (see Chapter 10). Thus these blood vessels may also spread cancer from a neoplasm to distant sites, and at a faster rate than lymphatic vessels.

The dental professional must be able to locate the larger blood vessels of the head and neck because these vessels may become compromised due to a pathologic process or during a dental procedure such as when administering a local anesthetic injection (see Chapter 9). Blood vessels may not only spread cancer but can also spread dental (or odontogenic) infection (see Chapter 12).

Initially, reviewing the pathways of the arteries and veins as they exit and enter the heart is important to understanding the origins of the blood vessels of the head and neck; the dental professional will need to review this if needed (see Appendix A). After the origins of blood supply to the head and neck are understood, diagrams of the blood vessels overlying the skull are helpful in studying this system. Correlating the structure supplied with the area's blood vessels is an additional way of understanding the location of the various blood vessels. It is important to remember that, unlike innervation to various structures, which is a one-to-one relationship, blood supply is more regional in coverage. Arteries supply the structures in their vicinity, and veins receive blood from the nearby structures.

ARTERIAL BLOOD SUPPLY TO HEAD AND NECK

The major arteries that supply the head and neck include the common carotid and subclavian arteries. The origins from the heart to the head

and neck of these two major arteries are different depending on the side of the body; in contrast, the other branching arteries of the head and neck are usually symmetric in their coverage.

ORIGINS TO HEAD AND NECK

The origins from the heart of the common carotid and subclavian arteries that supply the head and neck are different for the right and left sides of the body (Figure 6-1). For the left side of the body, the common carotid and subclavian arteries arise directly from the **aorta** (**ay**-or-tuh). For the right side of the body, the common carotid and subclavian arteries are both branches from the brachiocephalic artery. The **brachiocephalic artery** (bray-kee-o-suh-**fal**-ik) is a direct branch of the aorta.

The **common carotid artery** (kuh-**rot**-id) is branchless and travels superiorly along the neck in a lateral position to both the trachea and larynx on its way to the superior border of the thyroid cartilage (see Figure 6-1). The common carotid artery travels in the carotid sheath deep to the sternocleidomastoid (SCM) muscle; the carotid sheath also contains the internal jugular vein and the tenth cranial or vagus nerve. The carotid sheath is part of the deep cervical fasciae of the neck that is deep to the superficial cervical fasciae (see Figure 11-1). Thus the carotid sheath surrounds the vascular compartments of the neck (see Figure 11-15). The common carotid artery ends by dividing into the internal and external carotid arteries at approximately the level of the larynx; thus the carotid sheath also carries the internal carotid artery (Figure 6-2).

Just before the common carotid artery bifurcates into the internal and external carotid arteries, it exhibits a swelling, the **carotid sinus** (see Figure 6-2). When the common carotid artery is palpated against the larynx, the carotid pulse can be used for monitoring since it is the most reliable arterial pulse of the body. If the anterior border of the SCM muscle is rolled posteriorly at the level of the thyroid cartilage

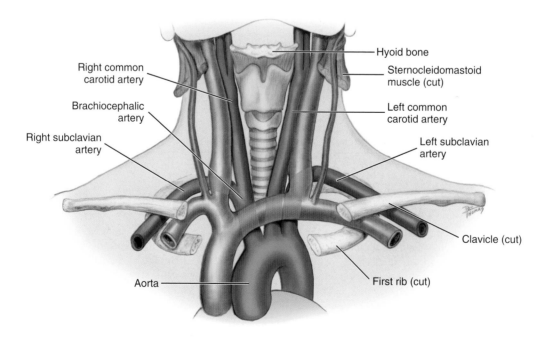

FIGURE 6-1 Origins from the heart of the arterial blood supply for the head and neck highlighting the pathways of the common carotid and subclavian arteries (*red*) contrasted with adjacent venous drainage (*blue*). Note that these pathways of these major arteries differ within either the right or left sides of the body.

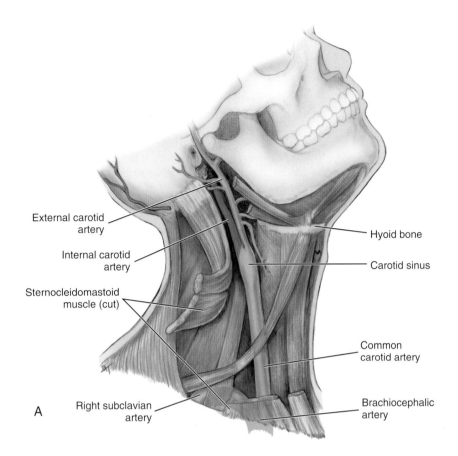

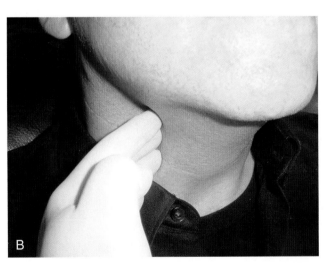

FIGURE 6-2 Pathway of the internal carotid artery after branching off from the common carotid artery is highlighted. Note the carotid sinus, which is location for obtaining the carotid pulse **(A)**. Demonstration of the palpation of the carotid sinus so as to obtain the carotid pulse; compression of the carotid sinus to obtain the carotid pulse should be avoided by dental personnel unless they have undergone specific emergency training and the situation warrants it **(B)**. *(B Courtesy of Margaret J. Fehrenbach, RDH, MS.)*

of the larynx or laryngeal eminence ("Adam's apple"), the carotid pulse can be felt in the groove of soft tissue produced (see Figure 2-24).

The carotid pulse is the most reliable on the surface of the body because the common carotid is a major artery supplying the brain. In an emergency (such as with basic life support), the common carotid remains palpable and can be monitored by qualified emergency medical service (EMS) personnel when peripheral arteries such as the radial artery are not. However, care must be taken to avoid compression of either the carotid sinus or one or both carotid arteries even by dental personnel unless it is an emergency situation and they have undergone specific training. Instead, dental personnel can continue to safely use the radial artery to record a patient's baseline pulse.

The **subclavian artery** (sub-**klay**-vee-uhn) arises lateral to the common carotid artery (see Figure 6-1). The subclavian artery gives rise to branches that supply both intracranial and extracranial structures, but its major destination is the upper extremity (at the arm).

INTERNAL CAROTID ARTERY

The **internal carotid artery** is a division that travels superiorly in a slightly lateral position in relationship to the external carotid artery after leaving the common carotid artery (see Figure 6-2). This artery is covered by the large SCM muscle on each side of the neck. The internal carotid artery has no branches located in the neck but continues adjacent to the internal jugular vein within the carotid sheath to the skull base, where it enters the cranium. The internal carotid artery supplies intracranial structures and is the source of the **ophthalmic artery** (of-**thal**-mik), which supplies the eye, orbit, and lacrimal gland (see Figure 2-6).

EXTERNAL CAROTID ARTERY

As with the internal carotid artery, the **external carotid artery** begins at the superior border of the thyroid cartilage, at the termination of the common carotid artery and the carotid sheath. The external carotid artery travels superiorly in a more medial position in relationship to the internal carotid artery after arising from the common carotid artery (Figures 6-3 and 6-4). The external carotid artery supplies the extracranial tissue of the head and neck, including the oral cavity. The external carotid artery has four sets of branches grouped according to their location to the main artery: the anterior, medial, posterior, and terminal branches (Table 6-1).

ANTERIOR BRANCHES OF EXTERNAL CAROTID ARTERY

There are three anterior branches from the external carotid artery: the superior thyroid, lingual, and facial arteries (see Figure 6-4). The lingual and facial arteries divide serving areas of the head and neck and thus are of interest to dental professionals.

Superior Thyroid Artery. The **superior thyroid artery** (**thy**-roid) is an anterior branch from the external carotid artery (see Figures 6-3 and 6-5). The superior thyroid artery has four branches: the infrahyoid artery, sternocleidomastoid branch, superior laryngeal artery, and cricothyroid branch. These branches supply the structures inferior to the hyoid bone such as the infrahyoid muscles, SCM muscle, muscles of the larynx, and thyroid gland, respectively. The nearby **inferior thyroid artery** is a branch off the thyrocervical trunk

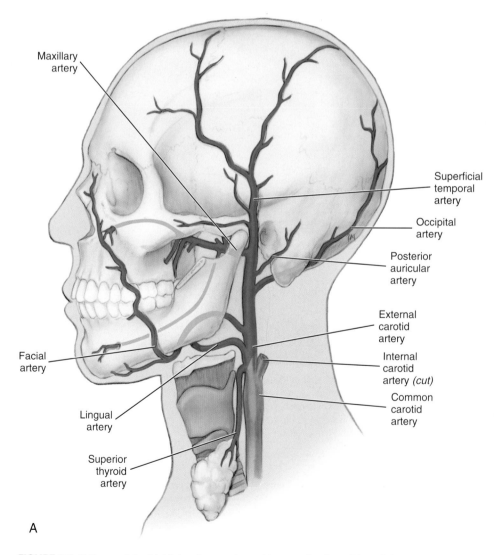

A

FIGURE 6-3 Pathway of the highlighted external carotid artery after branching off the common carotid artery. Note that the medial branch of external carotid artery, the ascending pharyngeal artery, cannot be seen **(A)**. See next page for part **B**.

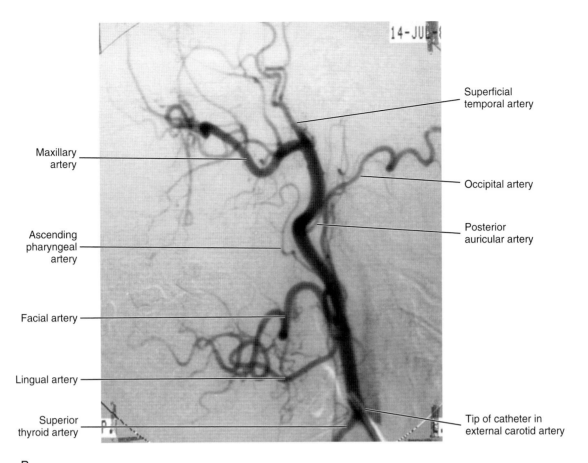

Maxillary artery

Ascending pharyngeal artery

Facial artery

Lingual artery

Superior thyroid artery

Superficial temporal artery

Occipital artery

Posterior auricular artery

Tip of catheter in external carotid artery

B

FIGURE 6-3, cont'd Lateral projection arteriogram of external carotid artery **(B)**. (**B** *from Logan BM, Reynolds PA: McMinn's color atlas of head and neck anatomy, ed 4, St Louis, 2010, Elsevier.)*

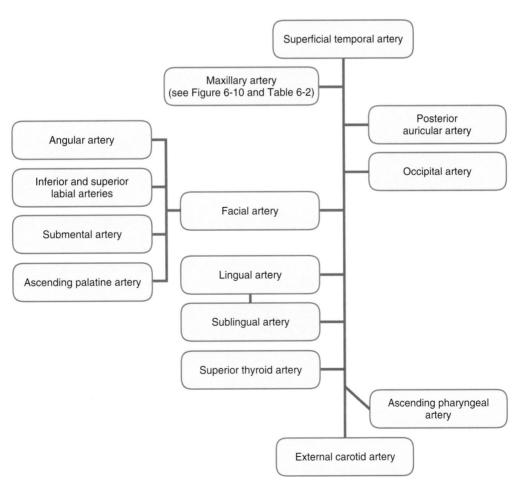

FIGURE 6-4 Branches of the external carotid artery.

TABLE 6-1	External Carotid Artery Branches		
BRANCHES OF EXTERNAL CAROTID ARTERY	**POSITION OF BRANCHES**	**FURTHER BRANCHES**	
Superior thyroid artery	Anterior	Infrahyoid artery	Infrahyoid muscles
		Sternocleidomastoid branch	Sternocleidomastoid muscle
		Superior laryngeal artery	Muscles of the larynx
		Cricothyroid branch (along with the inferior thyroid artery from subclavian artery)	Thyroid gland
Lingual artery	Anterior	Dorsal lingual arteries	Posterior dorsal surface of tongue
		Deep lingual artery	Ventral surface to apex of tongue
		Sublingual artery	Mylohyoid muscle, sublingual salivary gland, and floor of the mouth as well as lingual periodontium and gingiva of mandibular teeth
		Suprahyoid branch	Suprahyoid muscles
		Tonsillar branches	Lingual tonsils and soft palate
Facial artery	Anterior	**CERVICAL BRANCHES**	
		Ascending palatine artery with its tonsillar branches	Soft palate, palatine muscles, and palatine tonsils
		Submental artery	Submandibular lymph nodes, mylohyoid and digastric muscles*
		Glandular branches	Submandibular salivary gland
		FACIAL BRANCHES	
		Inferior labial artery	Lower lip area
		Superior labial artery	Upper lip area
		Angular artery	Lateral side of naris
Ascending pharyngeal artery	Medial	Pharyngeal artery with its pharyngeal, meningeal, and tonsillar branches	Pharyngeal walls, soft palate, meninges, and pharyngeal tonsils
Occipital artery	Posterior	Sternocleidomastoid branch	Sternocleidomastoid muscle
		Muscular branches	Suprahyoid muscles
		Auricular branch	Auricular region
		Meningeal branch	Meninges
		Descending branches	Trapezius muscle
Posterior auricular artery	Posterior	Auricular branch	Auricular region
		Stylomastoid artery	Mastoid process
Superficial temporal artery	Terminal	Transverse facial artery	Parotid salivary gland
		Middle temporal artery	Temporalis muscle
		Frontal branch	Frontal region scalp
		Parietal branch	Parietal region scalp
Maxillary artery	Terminal	See Table 6-2 and Figure 6-10	

*Can in some lesser number of cases supply lingual periodontium and gingiva of mandibular teeth either alone or with sublingual artery.

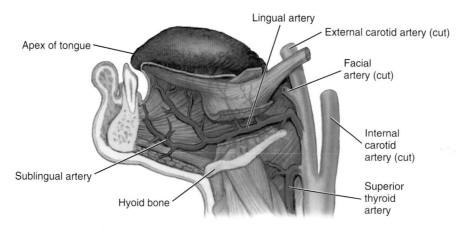

FIGURE 6-5 Pathways of the lingual artery and superior thyroid artery are highlighted.

of the subclavian artery but anastomoses with the superior thyroid artery to also supply the thyroid gland as well as other nearby structures such as the thymus gland. In a small number of cases, there is an additional supplying artery present, the **thyroid ima artery**. This variable artery comes from the brachiocephalic trunk of the arch of aorta, supplying the thyroid's anterior surface and isthmus.

Lingual Artery. The **lingual artery** (**ling**-gwuhl) is an anterior branch from the external carotid artery and arises superior to the superior thyroid artery at the level of the hyoid bone (Figure 6-5 and see Figure 6-3). The artery does not accompany the corresponding nerve throughout its course. Instead the lingual artery travels anteriorly to the apex of the tongue by way of its inferior surface. The lingual artery supplies the structures superior to the hyoid bone including the suprahyoid muscles and floor of the mouth by the dorsal lingual arteries, deep lingual artery, sublingual artery, and suprahyoid branch.

The tongue is also supplied by branches of the lingual artery including several small **dorsal lingual arteries** to the posterior dorsal surface as well as the **deep lingual artery**, the terminal part of the lingual artery, from the ventral surface to the apex. The lingual artery also has tonsillar branches to the lingual tonsils and soft palate.

The **sublingual artery** (sub-**ling**-gwuhl) supplies the mylohyoid muscle, sublingual salivary gland, and oral mucosa of the floor of the mouth as well as the lingual periodontium and gingiva of the mandibular teeth in most cases. The small **suprahyoid branch** (**soo**-pruh-**hi**-oid) supplies the suprahyoid muscles.

Facial Artery. The **facial artery** is the final anterior branch from the external carotid artery (Figure 6-6 and see Figure 6-3). The facial artery arises slightly superior to the lingual artery as it branches off anteriorly; however, in some cases the facial and lingual arteries share a common trunk. The facial artery has a complicated path as it runs medial to the mandible, superior to the submandibular salivary gland, and then near the mandible's inferior border at its lateral side.

From the inferior border of the mandible, the facial artery runs anteriorly and superiorly near the labial commissure and along the lateral side of the naris of the nose. The facial artery terminates at the medial canthus of the eye (see Figure 2-6). Thus the facial artery supplies the face in the oral, buccal, zygomatic, nasal, infraorbital, and orbital regions.

The facial artery is mainly parallel to the facial vein in the head area, although both blood vessels do not run adjacent to each other (see Figure 6-12). In the neck, the artery is separated from the vein by the posterior belly of the digastric muscle, stylohyoid muscle, and submandibular salivary gland. The facial artery's major branches include: the ascending palatine artery, tonsillar branches, submental artery, glandular branches, inferior labial artery, superior labial artery, and angular artery.

The **ascending palatine artery** (**pal**-uh-tine) is the first branch from the facial artery but since it is located near the neck region it is considered a cervical branch of the artery (see Figure 6-6). The ascending palatine artery supplies the soft palate, palatine muscles, and palatine tonsils by way of the tonsillar branches. This artery can be the source of serious blood loss or hemorrhage if it is injured during tonsillectomy (blood vessel pathology is discussed later).

Also considered cervical branches off the facial artery are the **submental artery** (sub-**men**-tuhl) that supplies the submandibular lymph nodes as well as the mylohyoid and digastric muscles and the glandular branches that supply the submandibular salivary gland and also nearby muscles. In a lesser number of cases it also supplies the lingual periodontium and gingiva of the mandibular teeth, either alone or with the sublingual artery.

In contrast, the other branches off the facial artery are considered facial branches since they are located more within the face. The **inferior labial artery** (**lay**-be-al) from the facial artery supplies the lower lip area including the area's muscles of facial expression such as the depressor anguli oris muscle. The **superior labial artery** is also a branch from the facial artery that supplies the upper lip area and similarly the area's muscles of facial expression. The **angular artery** (**ang**-u-lar) is the terminal branch of the facial artery and supplies the lateral side of the naris of the nose (see Figures 2-7 and 6-6).

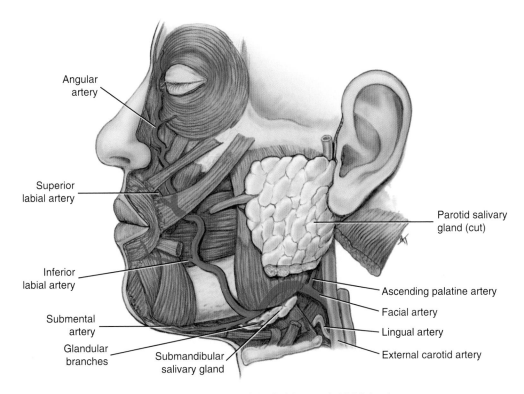

FIGURE 6-6 Pathway of the facial artery is highlighted.

MEDIAL BRANCH OF EXTERNAL CAROTID ARTERY

There is only one medial branch from the external carotid artery, the small **ascending pharyngeal artery** (fuh-**rin**-je-uhl) that arises close to the origin of the external carotid artery and thus cannot be viewed in most lateral views of the head and neck (see Figure 6-3, *B*). The ascending pharyngeal artery has many small branches that include: the **pharyngeal branch** and meningeal branch (muh-**nin**-je-uhl). These branches supply the pharyngeal walls (where they anastomose with the ascending palatine artery) as well as the soft palate and meninges, respectively. It also has tonsillar branches that supply the pharyngeal tonsils, which can be an additional source of serious blood loss or hemorrhage during a tonsillectomy.

POSTERIOR BRANCHES OF EXTERNAL CAROTID ARTERY

There are two posterior branches of the external carotid artery: the occipital and posterior auricular arteries (Figure 6-7).

Occipital Artery. The **occipital artery** (ok-**sip**-i-tuhl), a posterior branch of the external carotid artery, arises from the external carotid artery as it passes superiorly just deep to the ascending mandibular ramus and then travels to the posterior part of the scalp (see Figure 6-7). At its origin, the occipital artery is adjacent to the twelfth cranial or hypoglossal nerve. The occipital artery supplies the SCM muscle by way of the **sternocleidomastoid branch** (stir-no-kli-doh-**mass**-toid) and other muscles such as the suprahyoid muscles by way of its muscular branches. The artery also supplies the auricular regions and meninges by way of the auricular branch (aw-**rik**-u-luhr) and

meningeal branch, respectively. The descending branches supply the trapezius muscle. Branches of the occipital artery undergo anastamoses between the external carotid and the subclavian artery to provide regional collateral circulation.

Posterior Auricular Artery. The small **posterior auricular artery** is also a posterior branch of the external carotid artery (see Figure 6-7). The posterior auricular artery arises superior to the occipital artery and stylohyoid muscle at approximately the level of the tip of the temporal bone's styloid process (see Figure 3-18). The posterior auricular artery supplies the internal ear by its auricular branch and the mastoid process by the **stylomastoid artery** (sty-lo-**mass**-toid).

TERMINAL BRANCHES OF EXTERNAL CAROTID ARTERY

The two terminal branches of the external carotid artery include: the superficial temporal and maxillary arteries (Figures 6-8 to 6-10). The external carotid artery splits into these terminal branches within the parotid salivary gland. In addition, both terminal branches give rise to significant arteries in the head and neck area.

Superficial Temporal Artery. The **superficial temporal artery** (**tem**-puh-ruhl) is the smaller terminal branch of the external carotid artery (see Figure 6-8). The artery arises within the parotid salivary gland. This artery can be visible under the skin covering the temporal region in the patient. The superficial temporal artery has several branches including: the transverse facial artery, middle temporal artery, frontal branch, and parietal branch.

The small **transverse facial artery** (trans-**vurs**) supplies the parotid salivary gland duct and nearby facial area. The equally small **middle temporal artery** supplies the temporalis muscle. The frontal branch

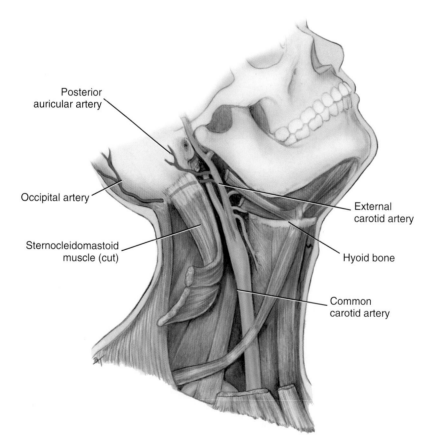

FIGURE 6-7 Pathways of the occipital artery and posterior auricular artery are highlighted.

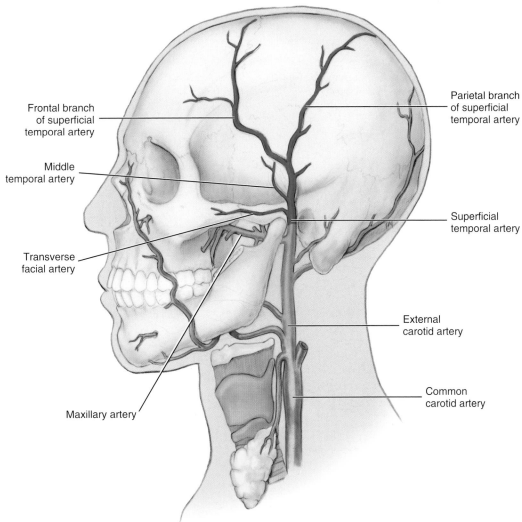

FIGURE 6-8 Pathway of the superficial temporal artery is highlighted.

(**frun**-tuhl) and parietal branch (pah-**ri**-uh-tuhl) both supply parts of the scalp in the frontal and parietal regions, respectively.

Maxillary Artery. The **maxillary artery** (**mak**-sil-lare-ee) is the largest terminal branch of the external carotid artery. This artery arises inferior to the temporomandibular joint (TMJ) and turns anteromedially to the neck of the mandibular condyle to travel deep to the structures of the face. There it courses between the muscles of mastication and ascends toward and enters the pterygopalatine fossa.

The course of the maxillary artery has three parts designated by location (see Table 6-2 and Figures 6-9 to 6-11). The *first part* (or mandibular part) of the maxillary artery begins at its origin at the neck of the mandibular condyle within the parotid salivary gland (see Figure 5-3). It then passes horizontally forward, between the neck of the mandibular condyle and the sphenomandibular ligament, where it lies parallel to and a little inferior to the auriculotemporal nerve; it then crosses the inferior alveolar nerve.

The *second part* (or pterygoid part) of the maxillary artery runs between the mandible and the sphenomandibular ligament, either superficial or deep to the lateral pterygoid muscle; when it reaches the gap between the two heads of origin of this muscle it enters the pterygopalatine fossa through the pterygomaxillary fissure (see Figure 3-61).

The *third part* (or pterygopalatine part) of the maxillary artery is also associated with the pterygopalatine fossa and will be discussed later.

Maxillary Artery: First Part. Arising from the first part of the maxillary artery are the **deep auricular artery**, which passes by the TMJ to enter the external acoustic meatus and the **anterior tympanic artery**, which passes into the tympanic cavity; both arteries supply the auricular region as well as the tympanic region, respectively.

The first part of the maxillary artery also gives rise to the middle meningeal, accessory middle meningeal, and inferior alveolar arteries. The **middle meningeal artery** supplies the dura mater of the brain and cranial bones by way of the foramen spinosum, which is located on the inferior surface of the skull (see Figure 6-9). The **accessory middle meningeal artery** helps to supply the dura mater and cranial bones as well as structures in the infratemporal fossa. This artery reaches the interior of the cranial cavity by way of the foramen ovale; however, this artery can be directly derived from the middle meningeal artery.

The **inferior alveolar artery** (al-**vee**-uh-luhr) also arises from the first part of maxillary artery within the infratemporal fossa (see Figures 6-9 and 9-38). The artery turns inferiorly to enter the mandibular foramen and then the mandibular canal, along with the inferior alveolar nerve and vein (discussed later). The inferior alveolar

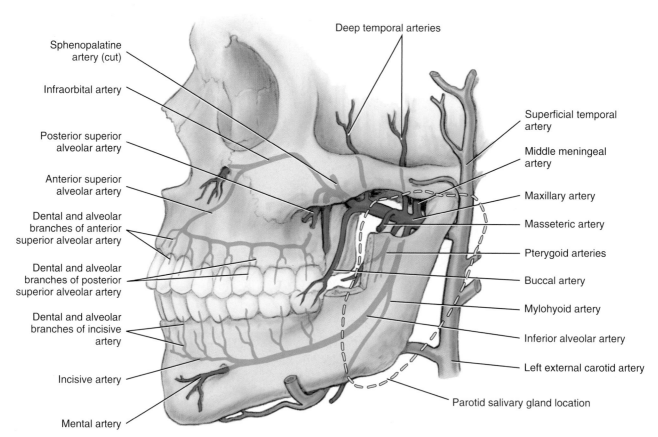

FIGURE 6-9 Pathway of the maxillary artery is highlighted. Note that the branches to nasal cavity and palate are not noted; see instead Figure 6-11.

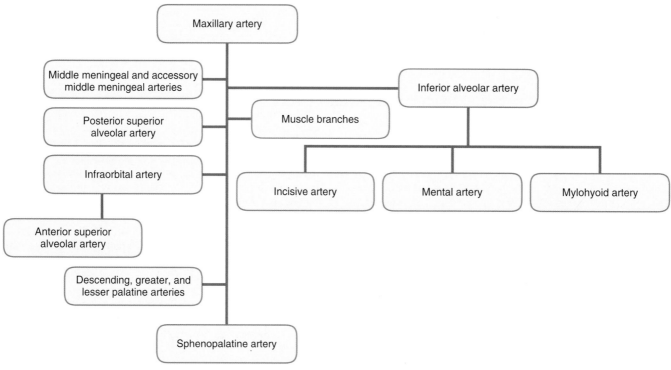

FIGURE 6-10 Branches of the maxillary artery; see also Table 6-2.

TABLE 6-2	Maxillary Artery Branches	

MAJOR BRANCHES OF MAXILLARY ARTERY WITH PART NOTED	FURTHER BRANCHES	STRUCTURES SUPPLIED
FIRST PART		
Deep auricular artery		Auricular region and outer surface of tympanic membrane
Anterior tympanic artery		Tympanic region and inner surface of tympanic membrane
Middle meningeal artery		Dura mater of brain and cranial bones
Accessory middle meningeal artery		Same as middle meningeal and also infratemporal fossa structures
Inferior alveolar artery	Dental and alveolar branches	Mandibular posterior teeth with buccal periodontium and gingiva
	Mylohyoid artery	Floor of the mouth and mylohyoid muscle
	Mental artery	Mental region
	Incisive artery with dental and alveolar branches	Mandibular anterior teeth with labial periodontium and gingiva
SECOND PART		
Deep temporal arteries	Anterior and posterior branches	Temporal region and temporalis muscle
Pterygoid arteries		Lateral and medial pterygoid muscles
Masseteric artery		Masseter muscle
Buccal artery		Buccinator muscle and buccal region
THIRD PART		
Posterior superior alveolar artery	Dental and alveolar branches	Maxillary posterior teeth and with buccal periodontium and gingiva and maxillary sinus
Infraorbital artery	Orbital and terminal branches	Orbital region and infraorbital region
	Anterior superior alveolar artery with dental and alveolar branches	Maxillary anterior teeth with labial periodontium and gingiva
	Middle superior alveolar artery, if present	Maxillary premolars with buccal periodontium and gingiva
Descending palatine artery	Greater and lesser palatine(s) arteries	Posterior hard palate with palatal periodontium and gingiva of maxillary posterior teeth and soft palate
Sphenopalatine artery	Posterior lateral nasal and septal branches	Nasal region and nasal cavity
	Nasopalatine branch	Anterior hard palate with palatal periodonitum and gingiva of maxillary anterior teeth

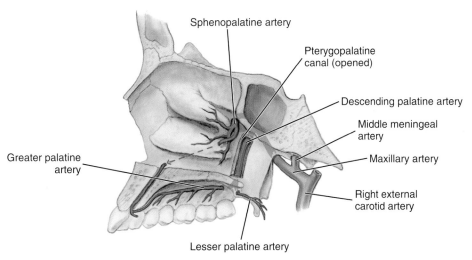

FIGURE 6-11 Pathways of the greater palatine artery, lesser palatine artery, and sphenopalatine artery branching off the maxillary artery are highlighted.

block has a high rate of positive aspiration with administration due to the nearness of the inferior alveolar artery to the inferior alveolar nerve exiting the mandibular foramen, which is the target area for the block.

The **mylohyoid artery** (my-lo-**hi**-oid) arises from the inferior alveolar artery before the main artery enters the mandibular canal by way of the mandibular foramen (see Figure 6-9). The mylohyoid artery travels with the mylohyoid nerve in the mylohyoid groove on the medial surface of the mandible and supplies the floor of the mouth and the mylohyoid muscle.

Within the mandibular canal, the inferior alveolar artery gives rise to dental and alveolar branches (see Figures 3-52 and 6-9). The dental branches of the inferior alveolar artery supply the pulp of the mandibular posterior teeth by way of each tooth's apical foramen. The alveolar branches of the inferior alveolar artery supply the buccal periodontium and gingiva of the mandibular posterior teeth. The inferior alveolar artery then branches into two arteries within the mandibular canal, the mental and incisive arteries.

The **mental artery** (**men**-tuhl) arises from the inferior alveolar artery and exits the mandibular canal by way of the mental foramen along with the mental nerve (see Figure 6-9). The mental foramen is located on the lateral surface of the mandible, usually inferior to the apices of the mandibular premolars (see Figure 3-51). After the mental artery exits the canal, the artery supplies the chin within the mental region and anastomoses with the inferior labial artery from the facial artery.

The **incisive artery** (in-**sy**-siv) branches off the inferior alveolar artery and remains within the mandibular canal along with the incisive nerve where it divides into dental and alveolar branches (see Figures 3-52 and 6-9). The dental branches of the incisive artery supply the pulp of the mandibular anterior teeth by way of each tooth's apical foramen. The alveolar branches of the incisive artery supply the labial periodontium and gingiva of the mandibular anterior teeth, and anastomose with the alveolar branches of the incisive artery on the contralateral side.

In addition, both the mental and incisive blocks have a high rate of positive aspiration with administration due to the nearness of both the mental artery and incisive artery to the mental and incisive nerves in the area of the mental foramen, respectively, which is the target area for both blocks (see Figure 9-43).

Maxillary Artery: Second Part. The second part of the maxillary artery has branches that are located near the muscle they supply (see Figure 6-9). These arteries all accompany branches of the mandibular nerve (or third division) of the fifth cranial or trigeminal nerve. The **deep temporal arteries** supply both the anterior and posterior parts of the temporalis muscle by two separate smaller branches as well as the surrounding temporal region. The **pterygoid arteries** (**ter**-i-goid) supply the lateral and medial pterygoid muscles. The **masseteric artery** (mass-i-**tare**-ik) supplies the masseter muscle. The **buccal artery** (**buk**-uhl) passes to the buccal mucosa to supply the buccinator muscle and the buccal region.

Maxillary Artery: Third Part. Just after the maxillary artery leaves the infratemporal fossa and enters the pterygopalatine fossa, it gives rise as the third part to the **posterior superior alveolar artery** (see Figures 6-9 and 9-7). This artery emerges from the ptergomaxillary fissure and then enters the posterior superior alveolar foramina along with the posterior superior alveolar nerve branches on the outer posterior surface of the maxilla, where it gives rise to dental branches and alveolar branches (see Figure 3-47). The posterior superior alveolar block has a high rate of positive aspiration with administration due to the nearness of the posterior superior alveolar artery to the posterior superior alveolar nerve as they both travel through the posterior superior alveolar foramina, which is the target area for the block (see Figure 9-3).

The posterior alveolar superior alveolar artery also anastomoses with the anterior superior alveolar artery. The dental branches of the posterior superior alveolar artery supply the pulp of the maxillary posterior teeth by way of each tooth's apical foramen. The alveolar branches of the posterior superior alveolar artery supply the buccal periodontium and gingiva of the maxillary posterior teeth. Some branches also supply the mucous membranes of the maxillary sinus.

After traversing the infratemporal fossa, the maxillary artery then enters the pterygopalatine fossa by way of the ptergomaxillary fissure continuing as the third part (see Figure 3-61). Inferior and deep to the eye, the **infraorbital artery** (in-fruh-**or**-bi-tuhl) also branches from the third part of the maxillary artery in the pterygopalatine fossa but may share a common trunk with the posterior superior alveolar artery (see Figure 6-9). The infraorbital artery then enters the orbit through the inferior orbital fissure (see Figure 3-7). While in the orbit, the infraorbital artery travels in the infraorbital canal. Within the infraorbital canal, the infraorbital artery provides orbital branches to the orbit and gives rise to the anterior superior alveolar artery that travels nearby to the anterior superior alveolar nerve.

Thus the **anterior superior alveolar artery** arises from the infraorbital artery and then gives rise to dental and alveolar branches (see Figure 6-9). The anterior superior alveolar artery also anastomoses with the posterior superior alveolar artery. The dental branches of the anterior superior alveolar artery supply the pulp of the maxillary anterior teeth by way of each tooth's apical foramen. The alveolar branches of the anterior superior alveolar artery supply the labial periodontium and gingiva of the maxillary anterior teeth.

A middle superior alveolar artery is also often present and supplies the buccal periodontium and gingiva of the maxillary premolars. When present, it branches from the infraorbital artery within the infraorbital canal and runs inferiorly along the lateral wall of the maxillary sinus traveling along with the middle superior alveolar nerve (if also present) toward the region of the maxillary canine and lateral incisors and anastomoses with both the anterior and posterior superior alveolar arteries.

After giving off these branches in the infraorbital canal, the infraorbital artery emerges onto the face from the infraorbital foramen on the outer surface of the maxilla along with the infraorbital nerve (see Figures 3-45 and 6-9). The infraorbital foramen is located inferior to the midpoint of the infraorbital rim of the orbit. The infraorbital artery's terminal branches supply parts of the orbital and infraorbital regions of the face and anastomose with the facial artery.

Also in the pterygopalatine fossa, the third part of the maxillary artery gives rise to the **descending palatine artery**, which travels to the palate through the pterygopalatine canal and then terminates in both the **greater palatine artery** and **lesser palatine artery** that travel along with the greater palatine and lesser palatine nerve to exit by way of the greater and lesser palatine foramina to then supply the posterior hard palate with the palatal periodontium and gingiva of the maxillary posterior teeth and soft palate, respectively (Figure 6-11 and see Figure 3-44). The greater palatine foramen is usually superior to the apices of the maxillary second or third molars on the outer surface of the posterior hard palate, with the lesser palatine foramen nearby but located more posteriorly.

The maxillary artery ends at its third part by becoming the **sphenopalatine artery** (sfe-no-**pal**-uh-tine), its main terminal branch, which supplies the nasal cavity within the nasal region by way of the sphenopalatine foramen (see Figure 3-61). The sphenopalatine artery gives rise to the posterior lateral nasal branches and septal branches as well as a **nasopalatine branch** (nay-zo-**pal**-uh-tine) that accompanies the nasopalatine nerve through the incisive foramen on the maxillae to supply the anterior hard palate as well as the palatal periodontium and gingiva of the maxillary anterior teeth (see Figures 3-44 and 6-11). The incisive foramen is beneath the incisive papilla just palatal to the maxillary central incisors in the midline of the outer surface of the anterior hard palate (see Figure 2-15).

VENOUS DRAINAGE OF HEAD AND NECK

The veins of the head and neck start out as small venules and become larger as they near the base of the neck on their way to the heart. The veins of the head and upper neck are usually symmetric in their coverage on each side of the body but have a greater variability in location than do the arteries, anastomosing freely. Veins are also generally larger and more numerous than arteries in the same area.

The internal jugular vein drains the brain as well as most of the other structures of the head and neck (Table 6-3), whereas the external jugular vein drains only a small part of the extracranial structures. However, the two veins have many anastomoses. The beginnings of both veins are discussed initially and, later, their route to the heart is discussed.

TABLE 6-3	Veins of the Head	
REGION OR TRIBUTARIES DRAINED	**DRAINAGE VEINS**	**MAJOR VEINS/ SINUSES**
Meninges of brain (only dura mater) and cranial vault bones	Middle meningeal	Pterygoid plexus
Lateral scalp area	Superficial temporal and posterior auricular	Retromandibular and external jugular
Frontal region	Supratrochlear and supraorbital	Facial and ophthalmic
Orbital region	Ophthalmic(s)	Cavernous sinus and pterygoid plexus
Superficial temporal and maxillary veins	Retromandibular	External jugular
Upper lip area	Superior labial	Facial
Maxillary teeth with periodontium and gingiva	Posterior superior alveolar	Pterygoid plexus
Lower lip area	Inferior labial	Facial
Mandibular teeth with periodontium and gingiva and submental region	Inferior alveolar	Pterygoid plexus
Submental region	Submental	Facial
Lingual and sublingual regions	Lingual	Facial or internal jugular
Deep facial areas and posterior superior alveolar and inferior alveolar veins	Pterygoid plexus	Maxillary
Pterygoid plexus of veins	Maxillary	Retromandibular

FACIAL VEIN

The **facial vein** drains into the internal jugular vein, which is discussed later (Figure 6-12). The facial vein begins near the medial canthus of the eye with the junction of two veins from the frontal region, the **supratrochlear vein** (**soo**-pruh-**trok**-lere) and **supraorbital vein** (see Figure 2-6). The supraorbital vein also anastomoses with the ophthalmic veins. The **ophthalmic veins** drain the orbit. This anastomosis provides a direct communication with the cavernous sinus (see Figure 8-6). This communication as well as the one-way direction of the blood flow may allow the cavernous sinus to become fatally infected through the spread of dental infection (discussed later, see also Figure 12-9).

The facial vein receives branches from the same areas of the face that are supplied by the facial artery (see earlier discussion). The facial vein anastomoses with the deep veins such as the pterygoid plexus of veins in the infratemporal fossa and with the large retromandibular vein before joining the internal jugular vein at the level of the hyoid bone (discussed later).

The facial vein has some important tributaries in the oral region (see Figure 6-12). The **superior labial vein** drains the upper lip area; the **inferior labial vein** drains the lower lip area. The **submental vein** drains the mental region including the chin as well as the submandibular region.

One excellent example of the venous variability concerns the **lingual veins**. These include the **dorsal lingual veins** that drain the dorsal surface of the tongue, the highly visible branching blue **deep lingual vein** noted during an intraoral examination that drains the ventral surface of the tongue (see Figure 2-18), and the **sublingual vein** that drains the floor of the mouth. The lingual veins may join to form a single vessel or may empty into larger vessels separately; they also may drain indirectly into the facial vein or directly into the internal jugular vein. The lingual veins are important clinically as they are capable of rapid and direct topical drug absorption.

RETROMANDIBULAR VEIN

The **retromandibular vein** (ret-roh-man-**dib**-u-luhr) will form the external jugular vein from a part of its route. The retromandibular vein is formed from the merger of the superficial temporal vein and maxillary vein (Figure 6-13). The retromandibular vein emerges from the parotid salivary gland and courses inferiorly. This vein and its beginning venules drain areas similar to those supplied by the superficial temporal and maxillary arteries.

Inferior to the parotid salivary gland, the retromandibular vein usually divides into two parts (see Figure 6-13). The anterior division joins the facial vein, and the posterior division continues its inferior course on the surface of the SCM muscle. After being joined by the **posterior auricular vein** (aw-**rik**-u-luhr), which drains the lateral scalp posterior to the ear, the posterior division of the retromandibular veins becomes the external jugular vein (discussed later).

SUPERFICIAL TEMPORAL VEIN

The **superficial temporal vein** drains the lateral scalp and is superficially located in skin covering the temporal region and can sometimes be noted on a patient during an extraoral examination (see Figure 6-13). The superficial temporal vein goes on to drain into and form the retromandibular vein, along with the deeper maxillary vein.

MAXILLARY VEIN

The **maxillary vein** is deeper than the superficial temporal vein and begins within the infratemporal fossa by collecting blood from the

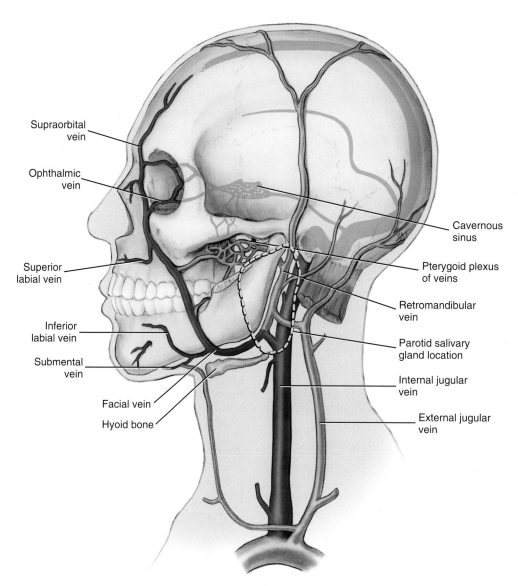

FIGURE 6-12 Pathways of the internal jugular vein and facial vein as well as the location of the cavernous sinus are highlighted.

pterygoid plexus of veins while accompanying the maxillary artery (see Figures 3-60 and 6-13). Through the pterygoid plexus of veins, the maxillary vein receives the middle meningeal, posterior superior alveolar, inferior alveolar veins, as well as other veins such as those from the nasal cavity and palate, which are served by the maxillary artery. After receiving these veins, the maxillary vein merges with the superficial temporal vein to drain into and form the retromandibular vein.

Pterygoid Plexus of Veins. The **pterygoid plexus of veins** is a collection of small anastomosing vessels surrounded by the lateral pterygoid muscle and surrounding the second part (or pterygoid part) of the maxillary artery on each side of the face within the infratemporal fossa (see Figure 6-13). This vascular plexus anastomoses with both the facial and retromandibular veins. The pterygoid plexus of veins protects the maxillary artery from being compressed during mastication; by either filling or emptying, the pterygoid plexus can accommodate changes in volume within the infratemporal fossa that occur when the mandible undergoes movement (see Chapter 5).

The pterygoid plexus of veins drains the veins from the deep parts of the face and then drains into the maxillary vein. The **middle**

meningeal vein also drains the blood from both the dura mater of the meninges (not the arachnoid or pia mater) and the bones of the cranial vault into the pterygoid plexus of veins.

Some parts of the pterygoid plexus of veins are located near the maxillary tuberosity, reflecting the drainage of both the maxillary and mandibular dental arches into the vascular plexus. Due to its location there is a possibility of piercing the pterygoid plexus of veins or possibly the nearby maxillary artery when a posterior superior alveolar block is incorrectly administered with the needle being overinserted (see Figure 9-7). When the pterygoid plexus of veins or maxillary artery is pierced as in this situation, a small amount of the blood escapes and enters the tissue, causing tenderness, swelling, and the discoloration of a hematoma or bruise (discussed later).

A spread of dental (or odontogenic) infection along the needle tract deep into the tissue can also occur when the posterior superior alveolar block is incorrectly administered with a contaminated needle. This may involve a serious spread of infection to the cavernous sinus (discussed later; and see also Chapter 12).

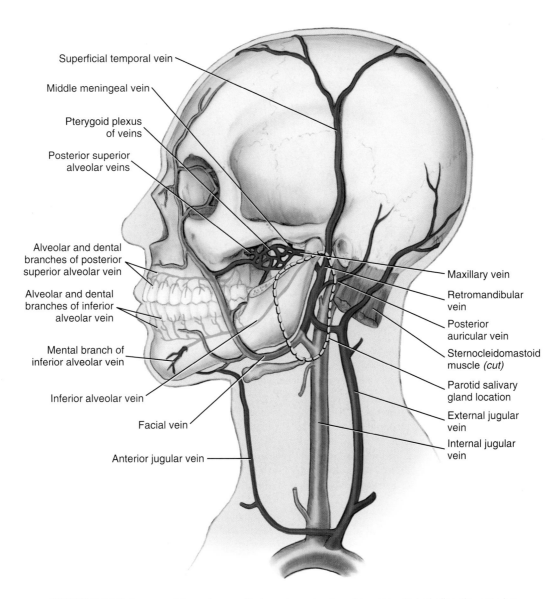

FIGURE 6-13 Pathways of the retromandibular vein and external jugular vein including the anterior jugular vein are highlighted.

Posterior Superior Alveolar Vein. The pterygoid plexus of veins also drains the **posterior superior alveolar vein**, which is formed by the merging of its dental and alveolar branches (see Figure 6-13). The dental branches of the posterior superior alveolar vein drain the pulp of the maxillary teeth by way of each tooth's apical foramen. The alveolar branches of the posterior alveolar vein drain the periodontium and gingiva of the maxillary teeth.

Inferior Alveolar Vein. The **inferior alveolar vein** forms from the merging of its dental branches, alveolar branches, and mental branches in the mandible, where they also drain into the pterygoid plexus of veins (see Figure 6-13). The dental branches of the inferior alveolar vein drain the pulp of the mandibular teeth by way of each tooth's apical foramen. The alveolar branches of the inferior alveolar vein drain the periodontium and gingiva of the mandibular teeth.

The mental branches of the inferior alveolar vein enter the mental foramen after draining the mental regions with the chin on the outer surface of the mandible, where they anastomose with branches of the facial vein. The mental foramen is on the outer surface of the mandible, usually inferior to the apices of the mandibular premolars (see Figure 3-52).

VENOUS SINUSES

The venous sinuses in the brain are located within the meninges. Specifically, these sinuses are within the dura mater, a dense connective tissue that lines the inner cranium (see Figure 8-4). These dural sinuses are channels by which blood is conveyed from the cerebral veins into the veins of the neck, particularly the internal jugular vein.

The venous sinus most important to dental care is the paired **cavernous sinus** (kav-er-nuhs). Each cavernous sinus is located on the lateral surfaces of the body of the sphenoid bone, at either side of the midline sella turcica (see Figures 3-34, 6-12, and 8-6). Each cavernous sinus communicates by anastomoses with its contralateral sinus and also with the pterygoid plexus of veins and superior ophthalmic vein, which anastomoses with the facial vein as discussed earlier. In addition, the paired intercavernous sinuses, with an anterior and a posterior position, connect the two cavernous sinuses across the midline.

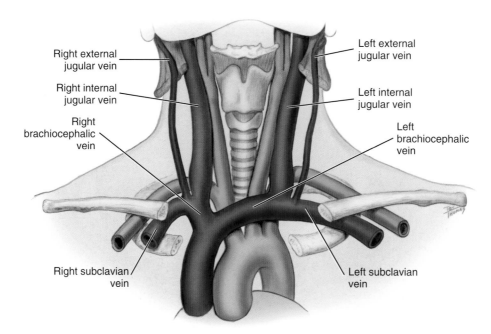

FIGURE 6-14 Pathways to the heart from the head and neck highlighting the venous drainage *(blue)* including the external and internal jugular veins, subclavian vein, brachiocephalic veins, and superior vena cava contrasted with the adjacent arterial supply *(red)*.

The internal carotid artery and certain cranial nerves (III, IV, V₁, V₂, and VI) or their branches pass through the blood-filled space of the cavernous sinus; it is the only anatomic location in which an artery travels completely through a venous structure. This sinus is important to dental professionals since the cavernous sinus may be involved with the spread of dental (or odontogenic) infection (see Figure 12-9).

INTERNAL JUGULAR VEIN

The **internal jugular vein** (**jug**-u-luhr) drains most of the structures of the head and neck (Figure 6-14 and see Figure 6-12). The internal jugular vein originates in the cranial cavity and leaves the skull through the jugular foramen. It receives many tributaries including the veins from the lingual, sublingual, and pharyngeal areas as well as the facial vein. The internal jugular vein runs with the common carotid artery and its branches as well as the tenth cranial or vagus nerve in the carotid sheath (see Figure 11-3). Within the carotid sheath, the deep cervical group of lymph nodes forms a chain along the internal jugular vein. The internal jugular vein descends in the neck to merge with the subclavian vein.

EXTERNAL JUGULAR VEIN

As mentioned earlier, the posterior division of the retromandibular vein becomes the **external jugular vein**. The external jugular vein continues the descent inferiorly along the neck, terminating in the subclavian vein (see Figures 6-13 and 6-14). Usually the external jugular vein is visible as it crosses the large SCM muscle; to increase its visibility, it can be distended by gentle supraclavicular digital pressure to block outflow (see Figure 4-2).

The **anterior jugular vein** drains into the external jugular vein (or directly into the subclavian vein) before it joins the subclavian vein (see Figure 6-13). The anterior jugular vein begins inferior to the chin, communicating with veins in the area, and descends near the midline within the superficial fascia, receiving branches from the superficial cervical structures. Only one anterior jugular vein may be present, but usually two veins are present, anastomosing with each other through a jugular venous arch.

PATHWAYS TO HEART FROM HEAD AND NECK

On each side of the body, the external jugular vein joins the subclavian vein from the arm, and then the internal jugular vein merges with the **subclavian vein** to form the **brachiocephalic vein** (see Figure 6-14). The brachiocephalic veins unite to form the **superior vena cava** (**vee**-nuh **kay**-vuh) and then travel to the heart. Because the superior vena cava is on the right side of the heart, the brachiocephalic veins are asymmetric. The right brachiocephalic vein is shorter and vertical in placement, and the left brachiocephalic vein is longer and horizontal in placement.

Clinical Considerations With Vascular System Pathology

The narrowing and blockage of the arteries can cause pathologic changes that impact the head and neck with dental care. This can be by a buildup of fatty **arterial plaque**, which consists of mainly cholesterol, as well as calcium, clotting proteins, and other substances, resulting in **atherosclerosis** (Figure 6-15). When this process occurs in the arteries leading to the heart, the result is cardiovascular disease. The process of atherosclerosis is now known to begin as early as childhood. However, even late in adulthood, lifestyle changes can reduce the onset or severity of coronary artery disease.

Blood vessels may also become compromised in certain disease processes such as high blood pressure, infection, traumatic injury, or endocrine pathology. These disease processes may lead to vascular lesions.

One of these lesions is a clot(s) or **thrombus** (plural, **thrombi**) that forms on the inner vessel wall (Figure 6-16). A thrombus (or thrombi) may dislodge from the inner vessel wall and travel as an **embolus** (plural, **emboli**) (Figure 6-17). Both of these vascular lesions can cause occlusion of the vessel in which the blood flow is blocked either partially or fully. Bacteria traveling in the blood can also cause **bacteremia**. Transient bacteremia can occur with dental treatment and can be a serious complication in certain medically compromised patients (see **Chapter 12**).

This occlusion of the blood vessel can hamper blood circulation and cause further complications such as stroke (such as with cerebrovascular accident), heart attack (such as with myocardial infarction), or tissue destruction (such as with gangrene), depending on the lesion's location. These thrombi may also be infected and spread infection by way of embolus formation, travelling to such areas as the cavernous sinus (see Figure 12-9). A dental professional needs to keep in mind the possibility of vascular vessel lesions when treating a patient with vascular disease or dental-related infections.

When a blood vessel is seriously traumatized, large amounts of blood can escape into surrounding tissue without clotting, causing a **hemorrhage**. This is a serious, life-threatening vascular lesion. Other vascular lesions can involve neoplastic or abnormal developmental growth of blood vessel tissue. A dental professional needs to be aware of the patient's medical history with regard to these serious vascular diseases.

Blood vessels may also undergo temporary localized traumatic injury such as bruising from the administration of intraoral local anesthetic. A bruise or **hematoma** results when a blood vessel is injured and a small amount of the blood escapes into the surrounding tissue and then clots. This escaped blood causes tenderness, swelling, and discoloration that will last until the inflammation subsides and the blood products are broken down by the body.

An extraoral hematoma may also result when administering a local anesthetic injection as the needle pierces the blood vessels adjacent to the target nerves. Blocks such as an inferior alveolar block may result in hematomas even when administered correctly (Figure 6-18). However, this can also occur with a posterior superior alveolar block that has been incorrectly administered too deep since its target area is superficial to the pterygoid plexus of veins and maxillary artery as discussed earlier (see Figure 6-19 and **Chapter 9**). These hematomas can vary in extent from minor bruising to major disfiguring lesions. Thus a dental professional needs to be aware of the location of larger blood vessels to prevent major injury of them during dental treatment such as with local anesthetic administration.

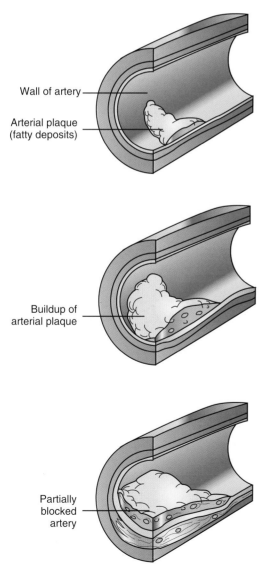

FIGURE 6-15 Fatty arterial plaque buildup in the walls of arteries that occurs with atherosclerosis. This change in the arteries can result in cardiovascular disease due to the partially blocked artery.

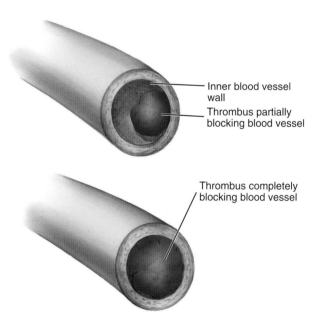

FIGURE 6-16 Thrombus forming on inner blood vessel walls, with partially and completely blocked blood vessels shown.

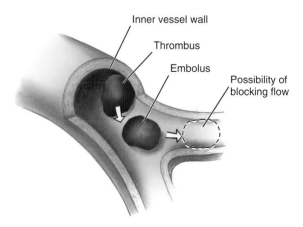

FIGURE 6-17 Dislodged thrombus from the inner vessel wall forming an embolus. The embolus can then travel in the blood vessel to create a blocked flow of blood.

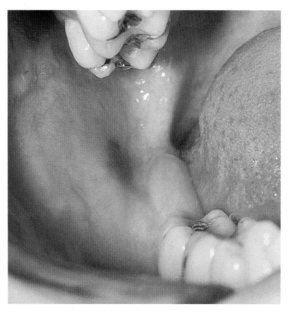

FIGURE 6-18 Small intraoral hematoma or bruise located within the soft tissue of the medial surface of the mandibular ramus of a patient. This occurred within a few hours after the administration of an inferior alveolar nerve block. Blood vessels in the region were pierced, which allowed blood to enter in the soft tissue. The discolored oral mucosa is from the broken-down red blood cells and hemoglobin pigment that remain in the surrounding soft tissue but most of the swelling has subsided along with the inflammatory process.

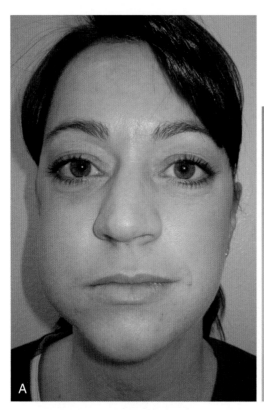
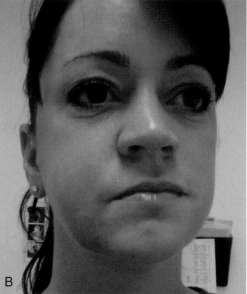

FIGURE 6-19 Initial swelling of an extraoral hematoma or bruise near the upper cheek, which has now become an ecchymosis since it is more than 10 mm in diameter. It resulted from an incorrect administration of the right posterior superior alveolar block from an overinsertion of the needle. This caused the deeper and larger blood vessels in the region to be pierced such as the pterygoid plexus of veins, which allowed blood to enter the soft tissue and the inflammatory process to begin **(A)**. Progression of the lesion 1 week following the initial swelling. The discolored skin is from the broken-down red blood cells and hemoglobin pigment that remain in the surrounding soft tissue in the lower half of the affected area due to gravity **(B)**. *(From Logothetis DD, editor: Local anesthesia for the dental hygienist, ed 2, St Louis, 2017, Elsevier.)*

REVIEW QUESTIONS

1. The posterior superior alveolar artery and its branches supply the
   - A. maxillary posterior teeth and periodontium.
   - B. mandibular posterior teeth and periodontium.
   - C. sternocleidomastoid muscle and thyroid gland.
   - D. temporalis muscle and parotid salivary gland.

2. Which of the following descriptions concerning the pterygoid plexus of veins is CORRECT?
   - A. Located around the infrahyoid muscles
   - B. Protects the superficial temporal artery
   - C. Drains the maxillary and mandibular dental arches
   - D. Can be pierced resulting in xerostomia

3. Which of the following veins results from the merger of the superficial temporal vein and maxillary vein?
   - A. Facial
   - B. Retromandibular
   - C. Internal jugular
   - D. External jugular
   - E. Brachiocephalic

4. Which of the following arteries arises from the inferior alveolar artery before the artery enters the mandibular canal?
   - A. Mylohyoid artery
   - B. Incisive artery
   - C. Mental artery
   - D. Posterior superior alveolar artery
   - E. Submental artery

5. Which of the following artery and transmitting foramen pairs below is a CORRECT match?
   - A. Buccal artery–infraorbital foramen
   - B. Middle meningeal artery–foramen spinosum
   - C. Incisive artery–mental foramen
   - D. Inferior labial artery–mandibular foramen
   - E. Submental artery–mental foramen

6. Which of the following arteries supplies the oral mucosa and glands of BOTH the hard and soft palates?
   - A. Greater and lesser palatine arteries
   - B. Posterior superior alveolar artery
   - C. Anterior superior alveolar artery
   - D. Infraorbital artery

7. Which of the following vascular lesions may result when a clot on the inner blood vessel wall becomes dislodged and travels in the vessel?
   - A. Hematoma
   - B. Venous sinus
   - C. Embolus
   - D. Hemorrhage

8. Which of the following descriptions concerning the maxillary artery is CORRECT?
   - A. Arises from the internal carotid artery
   - B. Enters the pterygopalatine fossa and forms terminal branches
   - C. Arises from the zygomaticofacial foramen to emerge on the face
   - D. Has mandibular, maxillary, nasal, palatine, and occipital branches

9. A venous sinus within the vascular system is a
   - A. network of blood vessels.
   - B. clot on the inner vessel wall.
   - C. blood-filled space between two tissue layers.
   - D. smaller vein or venule.

10. Which of the following arteries is a branch from the facial artery?
   - A. Superior labial
   - B. Ascending pharyngeal
   - C. Posterior auricular
   - D. Transverse facial

11. Which of the following structures is a smaller vessel that branches off an arteriole to supply blood directly to tissue?
   - A. Artery
   - B. Capillary
   - C. Vein
   - D. Venule

12. The carotid pulse can be palpated by emergency medical service personnel at the level of the
   - A. thyroid cartilage.
   - B. hyoid bone.
   - C. angle of the mandible.
   - D. supraclavicular fossa.

13. The tongue is MAINLY supplied by a branch from the
   - A. internal carotid artery.
   - B. external carotid artery.
   - C. sublingual artery.
   - D. facial artery.

14. Which of the following arteries can sometimes be visible under the skin of the temporal region on a patient?
   - A. Maxillary
   - B. Transverse facial
   - C. Middle temporal
   - D. Superficial temporal

15. Which of the following arteries anastomoses with the anterior superior alveolar artery?
   - A. Mylohyoid artery
   - B. Posterior superior alveolar artery
   - C. Facial artery
   - D. Maxillary artery

16. Which of the following vascular lesions results in a small amount of blood escaping into the surrounding tissue and clotting?
   - A. Hemorrhage
   - B. Hematoma
   - C. Embolus
   - D. Thrombus

17. For the left side of the body, the common carotid and subclavian arteries arise directly from the
   - A. aorta.
   - B. brachiocephalic artery.
   - C. internal carotid artery.
   - D. external carotid artery.

18. Which of the following is the larger terminal branch of the external carotid artery?
   - A. Superficial temporal artery
   - B. Ascending palatine artery
   - C. Facial artery
   - D. Maxillary artery
   - E. Lingual artery

19. The two brachiocephalic veins unite to form the
   - A. subclavian veins.
   - B. external jugular veins.
   - C. internal jugular veins.
   - D. superior vena cava.
   - E. aorta.

20. Which of the following structures is contained within the carotid sheath?
   - A. Facial nerve
   - B. Internal jugular vein
   - C. Aorta
   - D. Superficial lymph nodes

Identification Exercises

Identify the structures on the following diagrams by filling in each blank with the correct anatomic term. You can check your answers by looking back at the figure indicated in parentheses for each identification diagram.

1. (Figure 6-1)

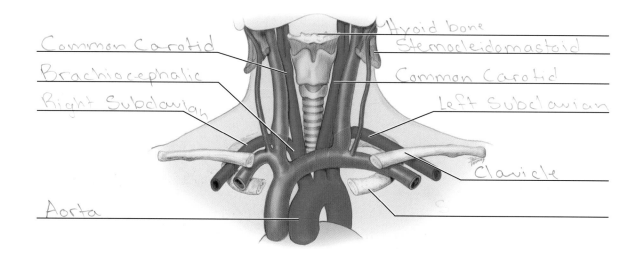

Common Carotid

Brachiocephalic

Right Subclavian

Aorta

Hyoid bone

Sternocleidomastoid

Common Carotid

Left Subclavian

Clavicle

2. (Figure 6-3, *A*)

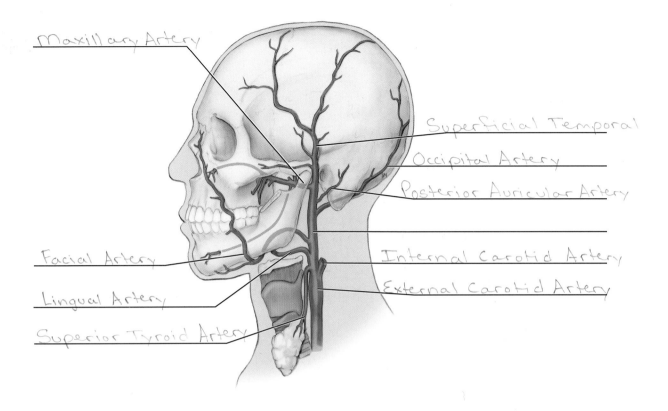

Maxillary Artery

Superficial Temporal

Occipital Artery

Posterior Auricular Artery

Facial Artery

Internal Carotid Artery

Lingual Artery

External Carotid Artery

Superior Tyroid Artery

3. (Figure 6-5)

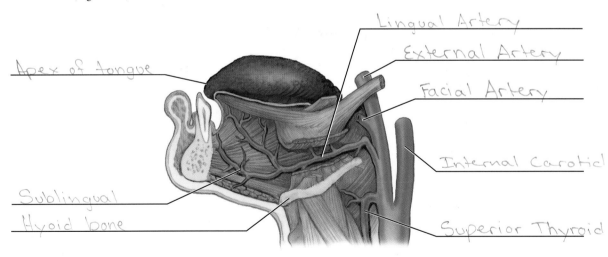

Lingual Artery

External Artery

Apex of tongue

Facial Artery

Internal Carotid

Sublingual

Hyoid bone

Superior Thyroid

4. (Figure 6-6)

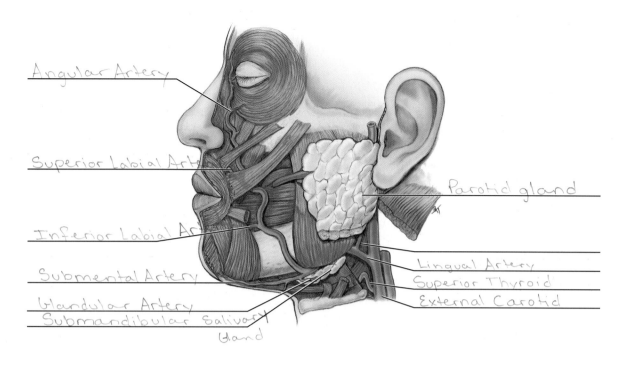

Angular Artery

Superior Labial Art

Inferior Labial Ar

Submental Artery

Glandular Artery

Submandibular Salivary
Gland

Parotid gland

Lingual Artery

Superior Thyroid

External Carotid

5. (Figure 6-8)

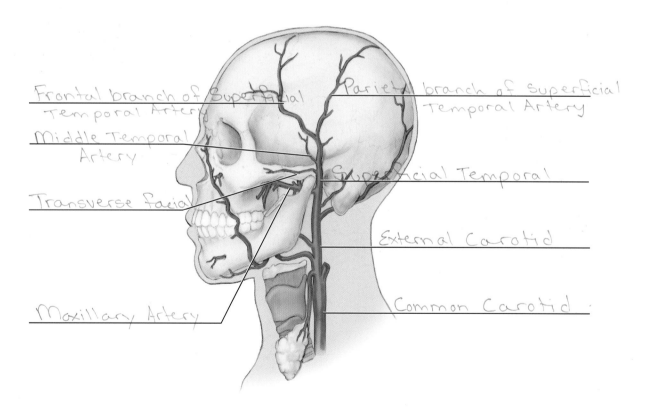

Frontal branch of Superficial
Temporal Artery

Middle Temporal
Artery

Transverse facial

Maxillary Artery

Parietal branch of Superficial
Temporal Artery

Superficial Temporal

External Carotid

Common Carotid

6. (Figure 6-9)

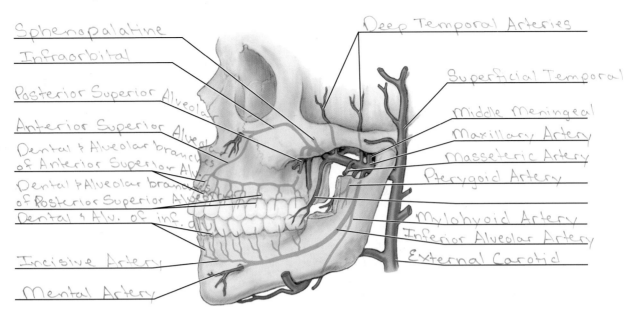

Sphenopalatine
Infraorbital
Posterior Superior Alveolar
Anterior Superior Alveolar
Dental & Alveolar branches of Anterior Superior Alv.
Dental & Alveolar branches of Posterior Superior Alveolar
Dental & Alv. of inf. a
Incisive Artery
Mental Artery

Deep Temporal Arteries
Superficial Temporal
Middle Meningeal
Maxillary Artery
Masseteric Artery
Pterygoid Artery
Mylohyoid Artery
Inferior Alveolar Artery
External Carotid

7. (Figure 6-11)

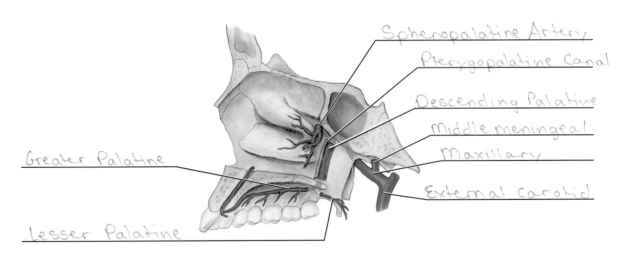

Sphenopalatine Artery
Pterygopalatine Canal
Descending Palatine
Middle meningeal
Maxillary
External Carotid
Greater Palatine
Lesser Palatine

8. (Figure 6-12)

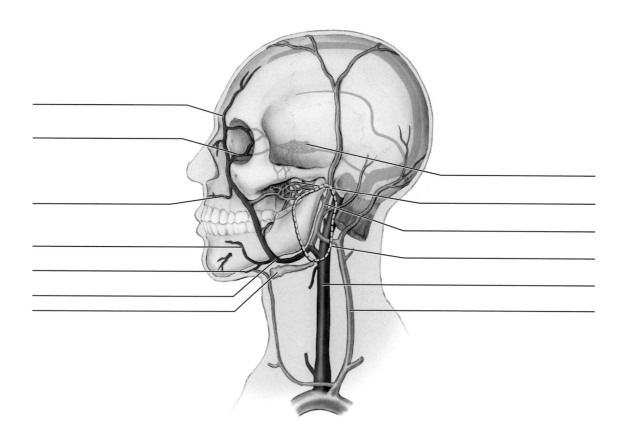

9. (Figure 6-13)

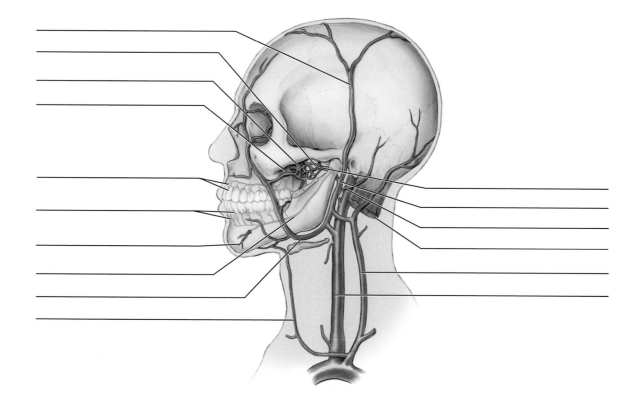

10. (Figure 6-14)

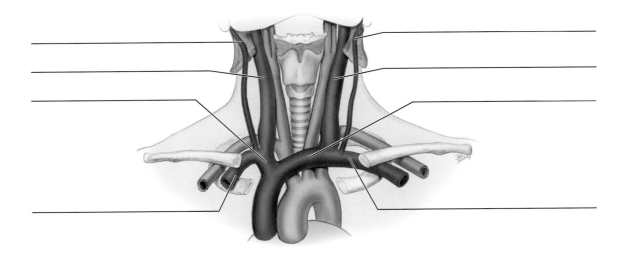

Glandular Tissue

1. Define and pronounce the **key terms** and **anatomic terms** in this chapter.
2. Locate and identify the glands and associated structures in the head and neck on a diagram, skull, and patient.
3. Discuss the glandular pathology associated with the head and neck.
4. Correctly complete the review questions and activities for this chapter.
5. Integrate an understanding of the head and neck glands during clinical dental practice.

● ● ● KEY TERMS

Dry eye syndrome (DES) Lacrimal glands produce less lacrimal fluid.

Duct Passageway to carry secretion from the exocrine gland to set location.

Endocrine gland (en-doh-krin) Ductless gland with secretion being poured directly into vascular system.

Exocrine gland (ek-soh-krin) Gland with associated duct serving as passageway

for secretion to be emptied directly into site of use.

Gland Structure producing chemical secretion necessary for body functioning.

Glandular tissue In the head and neck area includes lacrimal, salivary, thyroid, parathyroid, and thymus.

Goiter (goi-tuhr) Enlarged thyroid gland due to disease process.

Hyposalivation (hi-poh-sal-i-vay-shuhn) Reduced saliva production by salivary glands.

Mumps Contagious viral infection usually involving enlargement of both parotid salivary glands.

Salivary stone Formation of stone within a salivary gland.

Xerostomia (zeer-oh-stoh-me-uh) Dry mouth.

GLANDULAR TISSUE OVERVIEW

The **glandular tissue** in the head and neck area includes: the lacrimal, salivary, thyroid, parathyroid, and thymus glands. A **gland** is a structure that produces a chemical secretion necessary for body functioning. An **exocrine gland** is a gland that has a duct associated with it. A **duct** is a passageway that allows the secretion to be emptied directly into the location where the secretion is to be used. An **endocrine gland** is a ductless gland, with the secretion being poured directly into the vascular system, which then carries the secretion to the region in which it is to be used. Motor nerves associated with both types of glands help regulate the flow of the secretion, and sensory nerves are also present.

A dental professional needs to be able to locate and identify these glands and their innervation, lymphatic drainage, and vascular supply as well as examine them extraorally and possibly intraorally (Table 7-1 and see Appendix B). This information will help the dental professional determine if the glands are involved in a disease process and, if so, the extent of the involvement.

LACRIMAL GLANDS

The **lacrimal glands (lak-**ri-muhl) are paired almond-shaped exocrine glands that secrete lacrimal fluid or tears (see Figure 2-6). Its structure is similar to the salivary glands but it is unique in that it is composed of both epithelial and lymphatic tissue. Lacrimal fluid is a watery fluid that lubricates the conjunctiva lining the inside of the eyelids and the front of the eyeball. The lacrimal gland is divided into two parts that are continuous: the palpebral and orbital parts. The smaller palpebral part lies close to the eye, along the inner surface of the eyelid; if the upper eyelid is everted, the palpebral part can be seen. The larger orbital part is connected by way of the levator palpebrae superioris muscle.

LOCATION

Each gland is located within the lacrimal fossa formed from the frontal bone (see Figure 3-25). The lacrimal fossa is just inside the lateral part of the supraorbital rim within the orbit. The nasolacrimal duct is formed at the junction of the lacrimal bone and maxilla.

TABLE 7-1	Head and Neck Glands			
GLAND	**LOCATION**	**ASSOCIATED INNERVATION**	**LYMPHATIC DRAINAGE**	**BLOOD SUPPLY**
Lacrimal gland with lacrimal ducts	Lacrimal fossa of frontal bone	Greater petrosal of seventh cranial nerve and lacrimal nerve	Superficial parotid nodes	Lacrimal artery; superior ophthalmic vein
Parotid salivary gland with parotid duct	Parotid space posterior to the mandibular ramus, anterior and inferior to ear	Lesser petrosal of ninth cranial nerve and auriculotemporal nerve of mandibular nerve of fifth cranial nerve	Deep parotid nodes	Branches of external carotid artery; retromandibular vein
Submandibular salivary gland with submandibular duct	Submandibular space inferior and posterior to the body of mandible	Chorda tympani nerve of seventh cranial nerve	Submandibular nodes	Branches of facial and lingual arteries; mainly by anterior facial vein
Sublingual salivary gland with sublingual duct(s)	Sublingual space inferior to floor of mouth, medial to body of mandible	Chorda tympani nerve of seventh cranial nerve	Submandibular nodes	Submental and sublingual arteries; parallel venous return
Minor salivary glands with ducts	Buccal, labial, and lingual mucosa; soft and hard palate; floor of mouth; and base of circumvallate lingual papillae	Various nerves depending on location	Various nodes depending on location	Depending on location: various arteries; with parallel venous return
Thyroid gland	Inferior to hyoid bone, junction of larynx and trachea	Cervical sympathetic ganglia	Superior deep cervical nodes	Superior and inferior thyroid arteries, possibly thyroid ima artery; superior, middle, and inferior thyroid veins
Parathyroid glands	Close to or within thyroid	Cervical sympathetic ganglia	Superior deep cervical nodes	Superior and inferior thyroid arteries, possibly thyroid ima artery; superior, middle, and inferior thyroid veins
Thymus gland	In thorax, inferior to hyoid bone, superficial and lateral to trachea, and deep to sternum	Tenth cranial nerve and cervical spinal nerves	Within gland	Inferior thyroid and internal thoracic arteries; veins in posterior surface of gland that run directly into innominate vein

DUCTS

The larger orbital part of the gland contains the **lacrimal ducts.** At first, fine interlobular ducts unite to form approximately three to five main excretory ducts, which then join approximately five to seven ducts in the palpebral part before the secreted fluid may enter on the surface of the eye. Tears secreted collect in the fornix conjunctiva, the folds of the conjunctiva, and pass over the eye surface to the **lacrimal punctum** (plural, **puncta**) (**punk**-tum, **punk**-tah), a small hole found at the medial canthus of both the upper and lower eyelids (see Figure 2-6).

Any lacrimal fluid that passes over the eye surface ends up in the **nasolacrimal sac** (nay-so-**lak**-ri-muhl), a thin-walled structure behind each medial canthus. From the nasolacrimal sac, the lacrimal fluid continues into the nasolacrimal duct, ultimately draining into the inferior nasal meatus within the nasal cavity (see Figure 3-38). This connection of eye to nasal cavity explains why crying leads to a runny nose.

INNERVATION

The glands are innervated by parasympathetic fibers from the greater petrosal nerve, which is a branch of the seventh cranial or facial nerve. These preganglionic fibers synapse at the pterygopalatine ganglion, and postganglionic fibers reach the gland through maxillary branches of the fifth cranial or trigeminal nerve (see Figure 8-21). The lacrimal nerve also serves as an afferent nerve for the gland.

LYMPHATIC DRAINAGE

The glands drain into the superficial parotid lymph nodes.

BLOOD SUPPLY

The glands are supplied by the lacrimal artery, which is a branch of the ophthalmic artery of the internal carotid artery. Venous blood returns by way of the superior ophthalmic vein.

SALIVARY GLANDS

The **salivary glands** (sal-i-vare-ee) produce **saliva** (suh-**ly**-vuh), which is part of the defenses of the immune system as well as the beginning of breakdown of food products as part of the digestive system. Saliva lubricates and cleanses the oral cavity and helps in digestion. These glands are controlled by the autonomic nervous system (see Chapter 8).

The glands are divided by size into major and minor glands. However, both the major and minor salivary glands are exocrine glands and thus have ducts associated with them. These ducts help drain the saliva directly into the oral cavity where the saliva can function. The major salivary glands are palpated during an extraoral examination along with the other regional structures (see Appendix B); minor salivary glands are palpated during an intraoral examination if there is pathology present that increases their size due to inflammation or scarring. Salivary biomarkers for factors involved with systemic diseases, as well as periodontal disease, are now being effectively used.

MAJOR SALIVARY GLANDS

The **major salivary glands** are large paired glands and have named ducts associated with them. The three major salivary glands include: the parotid, submandibular, and sublingual salivary glands (Figure 7-1).

Parotid Salivary Gland. The **parotid salivary gland** (puh-**rot**-id) is the largest encapsulated major salivary gland but only contributes approximately 25% of the total salivary volume (Figure 7-2).

The salivary product from the parotid is only a serous type of secretion. The gland is divided into two lobes: the superficial and deep lobes.

Location. The parotid salivary gland occupies the parotid space, an area posterior to the mandibular ramus, anterior and inferior to the ear (see Figures 7-1 and 11-6). The gland extends irregularly from the zygomatic arch to the angle of the mandible.

The parotid salivary gland is effectively palpated bilaterally during an extraoral examination. Start anterior to each ear, moving to the zygomatic arch, and then inferior to the angle of the mandible (Figure 7-3).

Ducts. The duct associated with the parotid salivary gland is the **parotid duct** or *Stensen duct*. This long duct emerges from the anterior border of the gland, superficial to the masseter muscle. The duct pierces the buccinator muscle, and then opens up into the oral cavity on the inner surface of the buccal mucosa of the cheek, usually opposite the maxillary second molar (see Figure 9-4). The parotid papilla is a small elevation of tissue that marks the opening of the parotid duct on the inner surface of the cheek; its functioning is checked during an intraoral examination (see Figure 2-12).

Innervation. The parotid salivary gland is innervated by the efferent (parasympathetic) nerves of the otic ganglion of the ninth cranial or glossopharyngeal nerve by way of the lesser petrosal nerve, as well as by the afferent from the auriculotemporal nerve of the mandibular nerve of the fifth cranial or trigeminal nerve. However, the seventh cranial or facial nerve and its branches travel through the parotid salivary gland between its superficial and deep lobes to serve as a divider but are not involved in its innervation (see Figures 8-21 and 8-22).

Lymphatic Drainage. The gland drains into the deep parotid lymph nodes.

Blood Supply. The gland is supplied by a branch off the external carotid artery, the transverse facial artery. Venous return is by the retromandibular vein.

Submandibular Salivary Gland. The **submandibular salivary gland** (sub-man-**dib**-u-luhr) is the second largest encapsulated major salivary gland and yet is the main contributor to total salivary

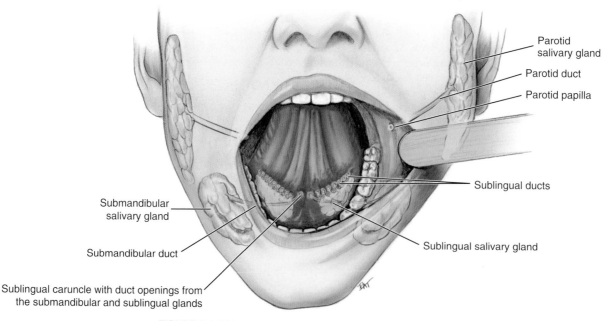

Parotid
salivary gland

Parotid duct

Parotid papilla

Sublingual ducts

Sublingual salivary gland

Submandibular
salivary gland

Submandibular duct

Sublingual caruncle with duct openings from
the submandibular and sublingual glands

FIGURE 7-1 Major salivary glands and associated structures.

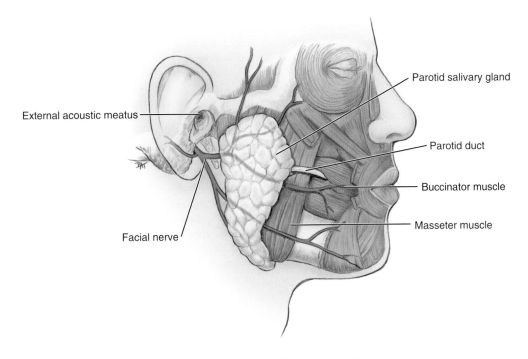

External acoustic meatus

Facial nerve

Parotid salivary gland

Parotid duct

Buccinator muscle

Masseter muscle

FIGURE 7-2 Parotid salivary gland and associated structures.

Clinical Considerations With Parotid Salivary Gland Pathology

The parotid salivary gland becomes enlarged and tender when a patient has **mumps**. This contagious viral infection usually involves inflammatory enlargement or *parotitis* (pare-o-**ty**-tis) of both glands, first one side and then the other, giving the characteristic "chipmunk" cheeks (Figure 7-4). The infection is rarely seen now because it can be prevented by childhood vaccination.

However, the parotid gland can be involved in cancer, which can also change the consistency of the gland to bony hard. In a lesser number of cases there is also unilateral facial pain on the involved side because the seventh or facial cranial nerve travels through the gland and undergoes perineural invasion; others may have related permanent facial nerve paralysis (see Figure 8-22). However, the most common presentation of parotid cancer is a painless, asymptomatic lump. The parotid salivary gland can also be pierced and the seventh cranial or facial nerve temporarily traumatized when an inferior alveolar block is incorrectly administered causing transient facial paralysis (see Figures 9-37 and 9-38).

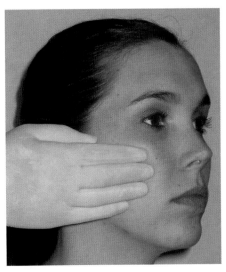

FIGURE 7-3 Demonstration of palpation of the parotid salivary gland during extraoral examination by starting in front of each ear, moving to the cheek area, and then inferior to the angle of the mandible. *(Courtesy of Margaret J. Fehrenbach, RDH, MS.)*

volume at approximately 60% to 65% (Figure 7-5). The saliva from the submandibular gland is a mixed salivary product that has both serous and mucous secretions.

Location. The submandibular salivary gland occupies the submandibular fossa in the submandibular space, mainly in its posterior part (see Figures 3-54, 7-1, and 11-12). Most of the gland is a larger lobe superficial to the mylohyoid muscle, but a smaller and deeper lobe wraps around the posterior border of the muscle. The submandibular gland is also located posterior to the sublingual gland.

The submandibular salivary gland is effectively bilaterally palpated inferior and posterior to the body of the mandible during an extraoral examination, moving inward from the inferior border of the mandible

near its angle as the patient lowers the head to feel its roundness (Figures 7-6).

Ducts. The duct associated with this gland is the **submandibular duct** or *Wharton duct*. This long duct travels along the anterior floor of the mouth then opens into the oral cavity at the sublingual caruncle, a small papilla near the midline of the floor of the mouth on each side of the lingual frenum (see Figure 2-19). The duct's tortuous travel for a considerable distance in a superior manner may be the reason the gland is the most common salivary gland to be involved in forming salivary stones as well as its mucous salivary product (see later discussion).

The submandibular duct arises from the deep lobe of the gland and remains medial to the mylohyoid muscle. The duct lies close to the large lingual nerve, a branch of the fifth cranial or trigeminal nerve, which can be injured in surgery performed to remove salivary stones from the duct (see Figure 8-20).

Innervation. The gland is innervated by the efferent (parasympathetic) fibers of the chorda tympani nerve and the submandibular ganglion of the seventh cranial or facial nerve (see Figure 8-21).

Lymphatic Drainage. The gland drains into the submandibular lymph nodes.

Blood Supply. The gland is supplied by the glandular branches off the facial artery. Venous return of the gland is mainly by the facial vein.

Sublingual Salivary Gland. The **sublingual salivary gland** (sub-**ling**-gwuhl) is the smallest, most diffuse, and only unencapsulated major salivary gland. The gland only contributes approximately 10% of the total salivary volume (Figure 7-7). The saliva from the sublingual gland is a mixed salivary product, but with the mucous secretion predominating.

Location. This gland occupies the sublingual fossa in the sublingual space at the floor of the mouth (see Figures 3-54, 7-1, and 11-12). This gland is superior to the mylohyoid muscle and medial to the body of the mandible. The sublingual gland is also located anterior to the submandibular gland.

The sublingual salivary gland is effectively palpated on the floor of the mouth posterior to each mandibular canine during an extraoral examination. Placing one index finger intraorally and the index finger of the opposite hand extraorally, the compressed gland is manually palpated between the fingers (Figure 7-8).

Ducts. The main duct associated with the gland is the **sublingual duct** or *Bartholin duct*. The sublingual duct then opens directly into the oral cavity through the same opening as the submandibular duct, the sublingual caruncle. The sublingual caruncle is a small papilla near the midline of the floor of the mouth on each side of the lingual frenum. Other smaller ducts of the gland open along the sublingual

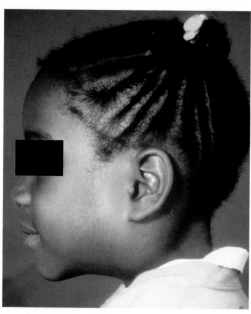

FIGURE 7-4 Enlarged bilateral parotid salivary glands noted on a patient with mumps. *(From Reynolds PA, Abrahams PH: McMinn's interactive clinical anatomy: head and neck, ed 2, London, 2001, Elsevier.)*

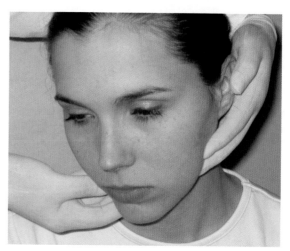

FIGURE 7-6 Demonstration of palpation of the submandibular salivary gland during extraoral examination by starting inward from the inferior border of the mandible near its angle as the patient lowers the head. *(Courtesy of Margaret J. Fehrenbach, RDH, MS.)*

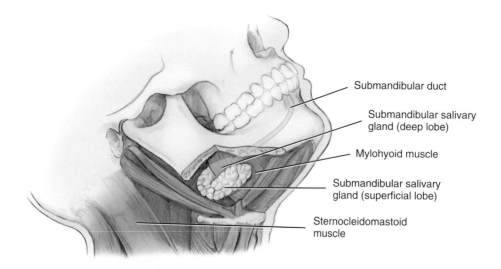

Submandibular duct

Submandibular salivary gland (deep lobe)

Mylohyoid muscle

Submandibular salivary gland (superficial lobe)

Sternocleidomastoid muscle

FIGURE 7-5 Submandibular salivary gland and associated structures.

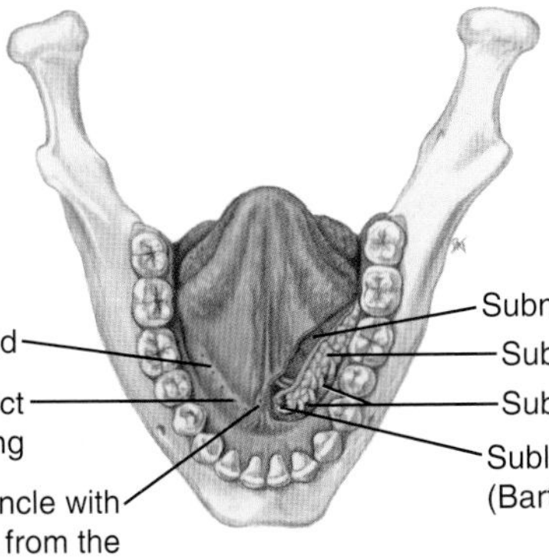

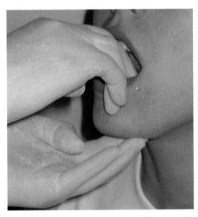

Sublingual fold

Sublingual duct opening

Sublingual caruncle with duct openings from the submandibular and sublingual glands

Submandibular duct

Sublingual gland

Sublingual ducts

Sublingual duct (Bartholin duct)

FIGURE 7-7 Sublingual salivary gland and associated structures. *(From Fehrenbach MJ, Popowics T:* Illustrated dental embryology, histology, and anatomy, *ed 4, St Louis, 2016, Elsevier.)*

FIGURE 7-8 Demonstration of palpation of the sublingual salivary gland during extraoral examination by starting at the floor of mouth behind each mandibular canine, with one hand placed intraorally and one hand placed extraorally. *(Courtesy of Margaret J. Fehrenbach, RDH, MS.)*

fold, a fold of tissue on each side of the floor of the mouth, and are collectively called the *ducts of Rivinus*. The functioning of these ducts associated with the sublingual gland is checked during an intraoral examination (see Figure 2-19).

Innervation. The sublingual salivary gland has the same innervation as submandibular salivary gland, which is by the efferent (parasympathetic) fibers of the chorda tympani nerve and the submandibular ganglion of the seventh cranial or facial nerve (see Figure 8-21).

Lymphatic Drainage. The gland drains into the submandibular lymph nodes.

Blood Supply. The gland is supplied by the sublingual artery off the lingual artery, with venous return paralleling the arterial supply.

MINOR SALIVARY GLANDS

The **minor salivary glands** are smaller than the larger major salivary glands but are more numerous; however, they are not individually encapsulated but surrounded by connective tissue within the submucosa. There are approximately 600 to 1,000 minor salivary glands, ranging in size from approximately 1 to 5 mm, that line the oral mucosa of the oral cavity and oropharynx. The minor salivary glands contribute less than 10% of total salivary volume; thus the major glands predominate in salivary secretions.

Location. Most of the minor salivary glands are mainly scattered throughout the oral cavity in the buccal, labial, and lingual mucosa, the soft palate, the posterior part of the lateral zones of the hard palate, and the floor of the mouth. In addition, minor salivary glands, the **von Ebner glands** (eeb-nuhr), are associated with the base of the large circumvallate lingual papillae on the posterior part of the tongue's dorsal surface (see Figure 2-17). The minor salivary glands are also found in lesser numbers along the mucosa of the tonsils, supraglottis region, and paranasal sinuses as well as between the muscle fibers of the tongue. They are not found in the gingival tissue and the anterior part of the lateral zones of the hard palate or its medial zone.

Most minor salivary glands secrete a mainly mucous type of salivary product, with some serous secretion. The exception is von Ebner glands, which secrete only a serous type of salivary product.

Ducts. Each minor salivary gland has a single duct that secretes saliva directly into the oral cavity since they are exocrine glands like the major salivary glands. But the unnamed ducts of the minor salivary glands are shorter than those of the major salivary glands.

Innervation. The minor salivary glands are innervated by various nerves depending on location.

Lymphatic Drainage and Blood Supply. The minor salivary glands drain into various lymph nodes and are supplied by various arteries depending on location, with venous return paralleling the arterial supply.

Clinical Considerations With Salivary Gland Pathology

Salivary glands may become enlarged, tender, and possibly firmer due to various disease processes. They may also become involved in the formation of a **salivary stone** (or sialolith) within the gland, blocking the drainage of saliva from the duct, especially with the submandibular gland. This can cause gland enlargement and tenderness in the major glands (with a ranula) or minor glands (with a mucocele) (Figures 7-9 and 7-10).

Salivary stones are uncomfortable but not dangerous, and can involve one or more enlarged, tender salivary glands. The clinician may also be able to palpate the stony hard salivary stone(s) during an examination. Facial radiographs or computed tomography (CT) can confirm the diagnosis. Salivary stones are usually removed manually or with minor surgery. With repeated stone formation or related infection, the affected salivary gland(s) may need to be also surgically removed.

Certain medications, disease, or destruction of salivary tissue by radiation therapy may result in **hyposalivation** by the salivary glands, which is a reduced production of saliva. This can result in **xerostomia** or dry mouth, which may be associated with DES since they have similar etiology (discussed earlier). Xerostomia can result in increased trauma to a nonprotected oral mucosa, increased cervical caries, problems in eating, speech and mastication, and bad breath or halitosis. Treatment is based on protecting the soft and hard tissue of the oral cavity, such as with salivary replacements, mineralization treatments, and lowering infection risk.

THYROID GLAND

The **thyroid gland (thy**-roid) is the largest endocrine gland (Figure 7-11). Because it is ductless, the gland produces and secretes **thyroxine (thy-rok**-sin) directly into the vascular system. Thyroxine is a hormone that stimulates the metabolic rate of the body. The gland consists of two lateral lobes, right and left, connected anteriorly by a midline isthmus.

LOCATION

The thyroid gland is located in the anterolateral regions of the neck. The gland is inferior to the thyroid cartilage at the midline of the neck, which is at the junction of the larynx and trachea (see Figure 2-24). The gland is also within a visceral compartment of the neck, along with the hyoid bone, larynx, trachea, esophagus, and pharynx. The entire visceral compartment is encased in previsceral fascia that is firmly adhered to the superior part of the trachea (see Figure 11-14).

In a healthy patient the thyroid gland is not visible, yet can be palpated as a soft mass during an extraoral examination. Examination of the thyroid gland is carried out by first locating the thyroid cartilage. Then pass the fingers up and down the gland examining it for abnormal masses as well as overall size of the gland. Then place one hand on each side of the trachea and gently displace the thyroid tissue to the contralateral side of the neck for each side, while the other hand manually palpates the displaced glandular tissue (Figure 7-12). Having the patient flex the neck slightly to the side when being palpated may help in this examination.

Next, the two lobes of the gland should be compared for size and texture using visual inspection, as well as manual or bimanual palpation. Finally, ask the patient to swallow to check for mobility of the

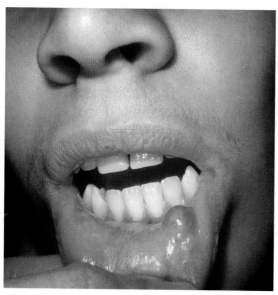

FIGURE 7-9 Mucocele of minor salivary gland in labial mucosa on a patient from blockage of saliva due to severance of the duct from trauma caused by a lip bite. *(Courtesy of Margaret J. Fehrenbach, RDH, MS.)*

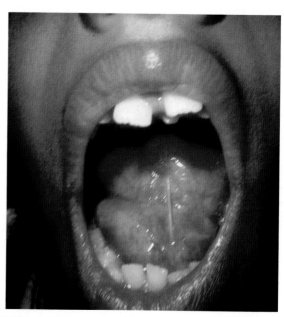

FIGURE 7-10 Ranula of submandibular salivary gland on a patient due to blockage of saliva by stone formation. *(Courtesy of Margaret J. Fehrenbach, RDH, MS.)*

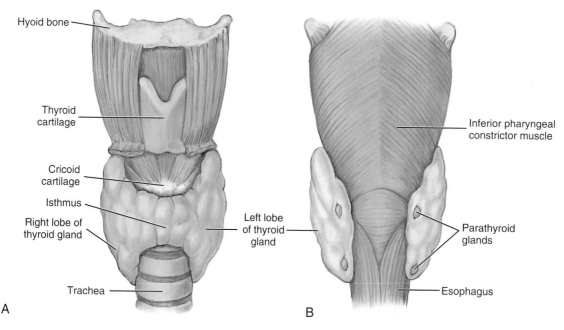

A — Hyoid bone, Thyroid cartilage, Cricoid cartilage, Isthmus, Right lobe of thyroid gland, Trachea

B — Inferior pharyngeal constrictor muscle, Left lobe of thyroid gland, Parathyroid glands, Esophagus

FIGURE 7-11 Thyroid gland with parathyroid glands noted from an anterior view **(A)** and from a posterior view **(B)**.

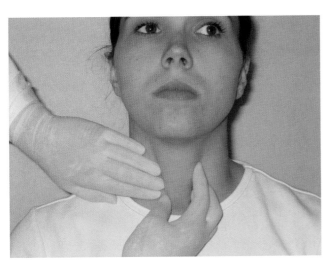

FIGURE 7-12 Demonstration of palpation of the thyroid gland during extraoral examination by placing one hand on one side of the trachea and gently displacing thyroid tissue to the contralateral side of the neck, while the other hand palpates displaced gland tissue. *(Courtesy of Margaret J. Fehrenbach, RDH, MS.)*

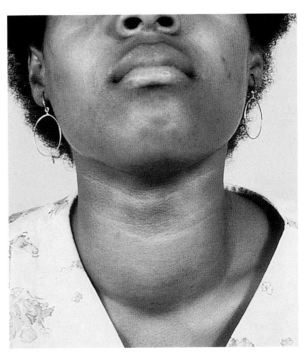

FIGURE 7-13 Enlarged thyroid or goiter on a patient. *(From Fehrenbach MJ, Popowics T: Illustrated dental embryology, histology, and anatomy, ed 4, St Louis, 2016, Elsevier.)*

gland; many clinicians find that having the patient swallow water helps this part of the examination. In a healthy state, the gland is mobile when swallowing occurs due its fascial encasement. Thus when the patient swallows, the gland moves superiorly, as does the whole larynx. With pathology, the thyroid gland can lose this mobility and become fixated (see discussion next).

INNERVATION

The gland is innervated by sympathetic nerves through the cervical ganglia. However, these nerves do not control endocrine secretion; the release of hormones by the thyroid gland is regulated by the pituitary gland.

LYMPHATIC DRAINAGE

The gland drains into the superior deep cervical lymph nodes.

BLOOD SUPPLY

The gland is supplied by both the superior and inferior thyroid arteries, the former by way of its cricothyroid branch. In a small number of cases, there is an additional supplying artery present, the thyroid ima artery. This variable artery comes from the brachiocephalic trunk of the arch of aorta, supplying the anterior surface and isthmus. Venous return is by the superior, middle, and inferior thyroid veins, which form a venous plexus. The superior and middle thyroid veins drain into the internal jugular veins, whereas the inferior thyroid vein drains into the brachiocephalic vein.

PARATHYROID GLANDS

The **parathyroid glands** (pare-uh-**thy**-roid) usually consist of four small endocrine glands, two on each side (see Figure 7-11, *B*). Because the glands are ductless, they produce and secrete parathyroid hormone directly into the vascular system to regulate calcium and phosphorus levels. In addition, the parathyroid glands may alter the function of the thyroid gland if they are involved in a disease process. The parathyroid glands have a distinct, encapsulated, smooth surface that

Clinical Considerations With Thyroid Gland Pathology

During a disease process involving the gland, the thyroid may become enlarged and partially visible during extraoral examination. This enlarged thyroid gland is considered a **goiter** (Figure 7-13). A goiter may be firm and tender when palpated during an extraoral examination and may contain hard masses and may or may not be associated with endocrine disease.

In addition, a diseased gland may lose its mobility and become fixated, not moving upward when the patient swallows as asked for during an extraoral examination, indicating a neoplastic growth. The gland may be partially or fully removed by surgery during treatment of various disease processes. Finding out whether the patient had the thymus gland irradiated as an infant is also important; this outdated procedure can cause thyroid cancer (discussed later). The patient should have a medical consultation if there are any undiagnosed changes in the gland.

differs from the thyroid gland, which has a more lobular surface, and lymph nodes, which are more pitted in appearance.

LOCATION

The parathyroid glands are usually adjacent to or within the thyroid gland on its posterior surface. Thus the parathyroid glands are not visible or palpable during extraoral examination of a patient.

INNERVATION

These glands are innervated by the same nerves that innervate the surrounding thyroid gland: the sympathetic nerves through the cervical ganglia.

LYMPHATIC DRAINAGE

These glands drain into the superior deep cervical lymph nodes, as does the surrounding thyroid gland.

BLOOD SUPPLY

These glands are primarily supplied by the inferior thyroid arteries, as is the surrounding thyroid gland, or possibly by an anastomotic branch between both the inferior thyroid and the superior thyroid artery by way of its cricothyroid branch. Venous return is by the superior, middle, and inferior thyroid veins; this is also true for the surrounding thyroid gland.

THYMUS GLAND

The **thymus gland** (**thy**-mus) is an endocrine gland and therefore ductless (Figure 7-14). However, it is also part of the immune system that fights disease processes; the T-cell lymphocytes, white blood cells of the immune system, mature in the gland in response to stimulation by thymus hormones. The gland grows from birth to puberty while performing this task.

After puberty, the gland stops growing and starts to shrink, undergoing involution. Thus by adulthood, the gland has almost disappeared and returned to its low weight present at birth, making it mainly a temporary structure. The adult gland consists of two lateral lobes, right and left, connected by an isthmus at the midline; other associated lobular structures may also be present.

LOCATION

The gland is located in the thorax (chest) and the anterior region of the base of the neck, inferior to the thyroid gland. The gland is also superficial and lateral to the trachea and deep to the sternum and origins of the sternohyoid and sternothyroid muscles (see Figure 4-24). The thymus may extend superiorly to the inferior part of the thyroid gland. The thymus gland is attached to the lobes of the thyroid gland by the thyrothymic ligament, which represents the remnants of the embryologic path of descent of the thymus gland and may contain some of the parathyroid glands. However, unlike the thyroid gland, the thymus gland is not easily palpated during an extraoral examination.

INNERVATION

This gland is innervated by branches of the tenth cranial or vagus nerve and cervical spinal nerves.

LYMPHATIC DRAINAGE

The lymphatic system of the gland arises within the substance of the gland and terminates in the internal jugular vein; thus the gland does not have any afferent vessels.

BLOOD SUPPLY

The gland is supplied by the inferior thyroid and internal thoracic arteries. The main venous return is by veins in the posterior surface of the gland that run directly into the innominate vein that is formed by the union of the internal jugular and subclavian veins.

Considerations With Thymus Gland Pathology

The thymus gland is a temporary gland until adulthood, but its involvement in various disease processes may alter the health of the patient while it is present. Some older patients may have mistakenly been given high levels of radiation therapy in childhood to shrink the thymus gland to keep the gland from cutting off the breathing, but which could possibly result in cancer of the adjacent thyroid gland (see earlier discussion). It is now known that the larger thymus gland of a child is only temporary and unrelated to sudden infant death syndrome as was formerly thought.

Additionally, a rare developmental variation exists known as *thymic rests*, which are ectopic accessory thymic tissue anywhere along the path of descent as the result of failure of descent, sequestration, or failure to involute. Thus the accessory gland tissue can be found in the vicinity of the superior vena cava, brachiocephalic vessels, and aorta. Rarely, it may be found in the posterior mediastinum or even in the dermis. Sometimes the gland tissue may present as a neck mass, which can be mistaken for a pathologic process.

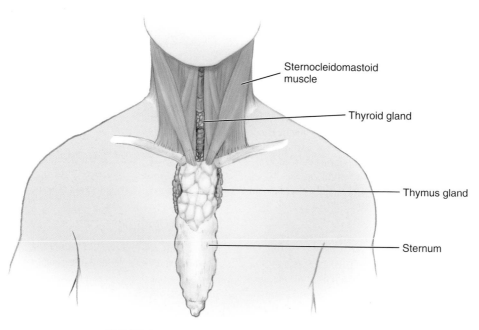

Sternocleidomastoid muscle

Thyroid gland

Thymus gland

Sternum

FIGURE 7-14 Thymus gland and associated structures.

REVIEW QUESTIONS

1. The sublingual salivary gland is located
   A. anterior to the submandibular gland.
   B. inferior to the mylohyoid muscle.
   C. lateral to the body of the mandible.
   D. within the mandibular vestibule fornix.

2. Which of the following glands has BOTH a superficial lobe and deep lobe?
   A. Thymus gland
   B. Parotid gland
   C. Thyroid gland
   D. Sublingual gland
   E. Lacrimal gland

3. Which of the following nerves innervates BOTH the submandibular and sublingual salivary glands?
   A. Trigeminal nerve
   B. Chorda tympani nerve
   C. Hypoglossal nerve
   D. Vagus nerve

4. Which of the following nerves travels through the parotid salivary gland but is NOT involved in its innervation?
   A. Trigeminal nerve
   B. Facial nerve
   C. Vagus nerve
   D. Glossopharyngeal nerve

5. Which of the following glands shrinks in size as a person undergoes maturation to an adult?
   A. Thymus gland
   B. Parotid gland
   C. Thyroid gland
   D. Sublingual gland
   E. Submandibular gland

6. Which of the following glands has a duct that usually opens on the inner surface of the cheek, opposite the maxillary second molar?
   A. Thymus gland
   B. Parotid gland
   C. Thyroid gland
   D. Sublingual gland
   E. Submandibular gland

7. Which oral landmark marks the opening of the submandibular duct?
   A. Parotid raphe
   B. Lingual frenum
   C. Parotid papilla
   D. Sublingual caruncle
   E. Nasolacrimal duct

8. The thyroid gland as part of the endocrine system is located
   A. anterior to the larynx.
   B. superior to the hyoid bone.
   C. posterior to the surrounding pharynx.
   D. in the posterior and medial neck region.

9. Which of the following blood vessels supplies the parotid salivary gland?
   A. Facial artery
   B. Lingual artery
   C. Internal carotid artery
   D. External carotid artery

10. As endocrine glands, the parathyroid glands are known to
    A. have one primary duct.
    B. have multiple secondary ducts.
    C. drain directly into blood vessels.
    D. drain directly into the thyroid gland.

11. The lacrimal gland ultimately drains into the
    A. lacrimal fossa.
    B. inferior nasal meatus.
    C. parotid salivary gland.
    D. internal carotid artery.

12. Which of the following can block the drainage of saliva from the duct?
    A. Excessive amounts of secretion
    B. Stone formation
    C. Lacrimal gland drainage
    D. Inflammation of blood vessels

13. Which of the following statements concerning minor salivary glands is CORRECT?
    A. Minor glands are smaller and less numerous than the major glands
    B. Minor glands secrete only mucous saliva
    C. Minor glands have longer ducts than major glands
    D. Minor glands are located in the buccal, labial, and lingual mucosa

14. In a healthy patient, the thyroid gland is known to
    A. consist of two lobes that are connected by an isthmus.
    B. not move with the thyroid cartilage when swallowing.
    C. secrete thyroxine, which slows down the metabolic rate.
    D. be clearly visible and easily palpated.

15. When examining the thyroid gland on a patient, it is important to
    A. ask the patient to swallow.
    B. ask the patient to cough.
    C. palpate the tissue directly over the trachea.
    D. move the gland superiorly and then inferiorly.

16. Into which structure does the lacrimal fluid initially end up after passing over the eye surface?
    A. Sublingual caruncle
    B. Nasolacrimal sac
    C. Nasolacrimal duct
    D. Parathyroid glands

17. Which of the following is a significant feature noted with the thymus gland?
    A. Maturation of immune system T-cells
    B. Regulation of calcium and phosphorus levels
    C. Stimulation of metabolic rate
    D. Cleansing of oral cavity and helping in digestion

18. Which of the following do NOT contain minor salivary glands?
    A. Labial mucosa
    B. Paranasal sinuses
    C. Attached gingiva
    D. Tonsils

19. Which of the following lesions is due to an enlarged thyroid gland?
    A. Mucocele
    B. Ranula
    C. Goiter
    D. Mumps

20. The primary lymphatic drainage of the sublingual salivary gland is by the
    A. submental nodes.
    B. malar nodes.
    C. superior deep cervical nodes.
    D. submandibular nodes.

Identification Exercises

Identify the structures on the following diagrams by filling in each blank with the correct anatomic term. You can check your answers by looking back at the figure indicated in parentheses for each identification diagram.

1. (Figure 7-1)

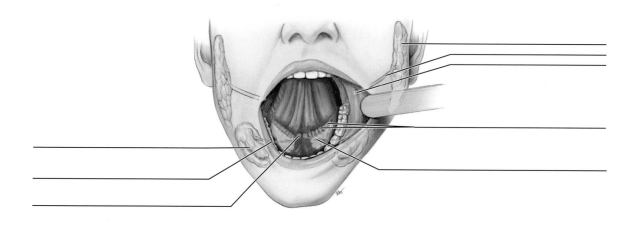

2. (Figure 7-2)

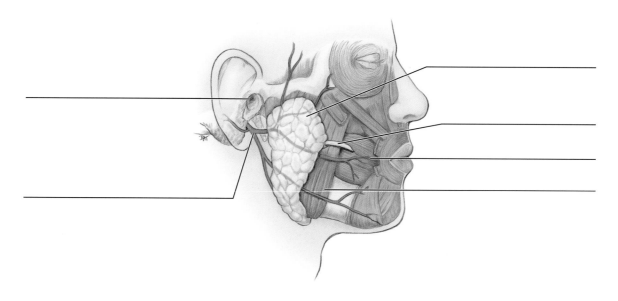

3. (Figure 7-5)

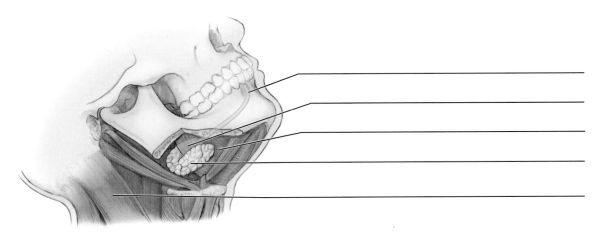

4. (Figure 7-7)

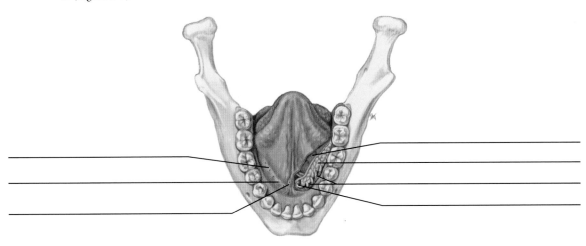

5. (Figure 7-11, *A*)

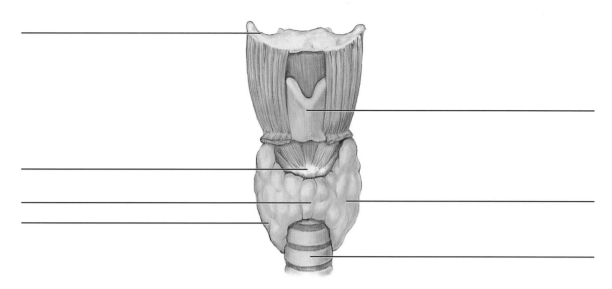

6. (Figure 7-14)

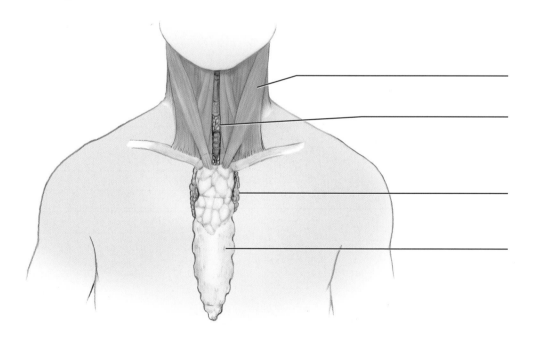

CHAPTER 8

Nervous System

●●● LEARNING OBJECTIVES

1. Define and pronounce the **key terms** and **anatomic terms** in this chapter.
2. Describe the components of the nervous system and outline the actions of nerves.
3. Discuss the divisions of the central and peripheral nervous systems.
4. Identify and trace the routes of the cranial nerves on a diagram and skull.
5. Discuss the structure innervated by each of the cranial nerves.
6. Identify and trace the routes of the nerves to the oral cavity and associated structures

of the head and neck on a diagram, skull, and patient.
7. Describe the structures innervated by each of the nerves of the head and neck.
8. Discuss the nervous system pathology associated with the head and neck region.
9. Correctly complete the review questions and activities for this chapter.
10. Integrate an understanding of head and neck nerves into clinical dental practice.

●●● KEY TERMS

Action potential (po-**ten**-shuhl) Rapid depolarization of cell membrane resulting in nerve impulse propagation along membrane.

Afferent nerve (**af**-uhr-uhnt) Sensory nerve carrying information from body periphery to brain or spinal cord.

Anesthesia (an-es-**thee**-zhuh) Loss of feeling or sensation resulting from use of certain drugs or gases.

Bell palsy (**pawl**-ze) Unilateral facial paralysis involving facial nerve.

Crossover-innervation Overlap of terminal nerve fibers from contralateral side of dental arch.

Dental plexus (**plek**-suhs) Network of nerves within both the maxillary and mandibular dental arches.

Efferent nerve (**ef**-uhr-uhnt) Motor nerve carrrying information away

from brain or spinal cord to body periphery.

Facial paralysis (puh-**ral**-i-sis) Loss of action of facial muscles.

Ganglion/Ganglia (**gang**-gle-on, **gang**-gle-uh) Accumulation of neuron cell bodies outside central nervous system.

Innervation (in-uhr-**vay**-shuhn) Supply of nerves to tissue, structures, or organs.

Nerve Bundle of neural processes outside the central nervous system; a part of the peripheral nervous system.

Nervous system Extensive, intricate network of structures that activates, coordinates, and controls all functions of the body.

Neuron (**noor**-on) Cellular component of the nervous system composed of cell body and neural processes.

Neurotransmitter (**noor**-o-**trans**-mit-uhr) Chemical agent from the neuron that is discharged with the arrival of the action potential, diffuses across the synapse, and binds to receptors on another cell's membrane.

Resting potential Charge difference between the fluid outside and inside cell resulting in differences in the distribution of ions.

Synapse (**sin**-aps) Junction between two neurons or between neuron and effector organ transmitting by electrical or chemical means.

Trigeminal neuralgia (TN) (try-**jem**-i-nuhl noo-**ral**-juh) Lesion of the trigeminal nerve involving facial pain.

NERVOUS SYSTEM OVERVIEW

The **nervous system** is an extensive, intricate network of neural structures that activates, coordinates, and controls all functions of the body. The nervous system causes muscles to contract resulting in facial expressions and joint movements, such as those involved in mastication and speech. The system also stimulates glands to secrete

and regulates other systems of the body such as the vascular system and digestive system. Finally, the nervous system allows sensation to be perceived, such as touch and even pain if present during dental treatment.

Understanding the nervous system and its components is important to the dental professional as this system allows for the function of the muscles, the temporomandibular joint, and the glands of the head and neck (see Chapters 4, 5, and 7). A thorough understanding of certain nerves is also important in pain management that involves administering local anesthesia during dental treatment (see Table 9-1 and Chapter 9). Finally, the dental professional must understand the pathology associated with nerves of the head and neck for effective dental care (discussed later).

The nervous system has two main divisions: the central and peripheral systems (Figures 8-1 and 8-2). These two divisions of the nervous system are constantly interacting. The **neuron** is the cellular component of the nervous system and is composed of a cell body and neural processes. A **nerve** is a bundle of neural processes outside the central nervous system and in the peripheral nervous system. A **synapse** is the junction between two neurons or between a neuron and an effector organ, where neural impulses are transmitted.

In order to function, most tissue, structures, and organs have **innervation**, a supply of nerves to the body part. A nerve allows information to be carried to and from the brain, which is the central information center. An accumulation of neuron cell bodies outside the central nervous system is a **ganglion** (plural, **ganglia**).

Nerves are of two types: afferent and efferent (see Figure 8-1). An **afferent nerve** or *sensory nerve* carries information away from the periphery of the body to the brain or spinal cord. Thus an afferent nerve carries sensory information to the brain such as taste, pain, and proprioception. Proprioception is information concerning the movement and position of the body. This sensory information is sent to the brain to be analyzed, acted on, associated with other information, and stored as memory.

An **efferent nerve** or *motor nerve* carries information away from the brain or spinal cord to the periphery of the body. Thus an efferent nerve carries motor information to the muscles in order to activate them, often in response to information received by way of the afferent nerves. One motor neuron with its branching process may control hundreds of muscle fibers.

The plasma membrane of a neuron, like all other cells, has an unequal distribution of ions and electric charges between the two sides of the membrane. The fluid outside of the membrane has a positive charge; the fluid inside has a negative charge. This charge difference is a **resting potential** and is measured in millivolts. Resting

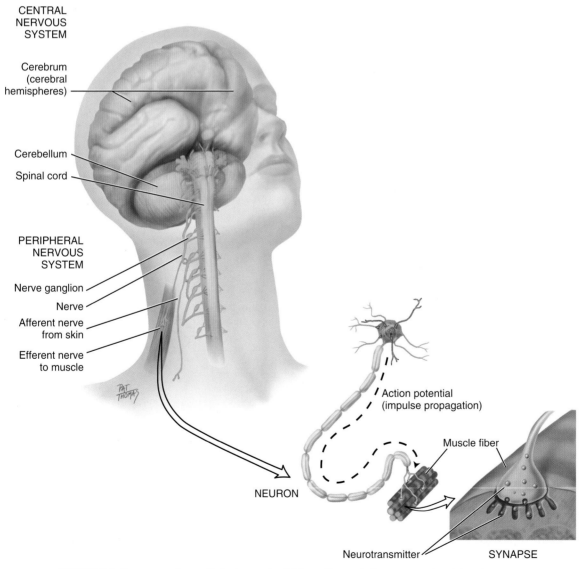

FIGURE 8-1 Nervous system with its two main divisions, the central nervous and peripheral nervous systems.

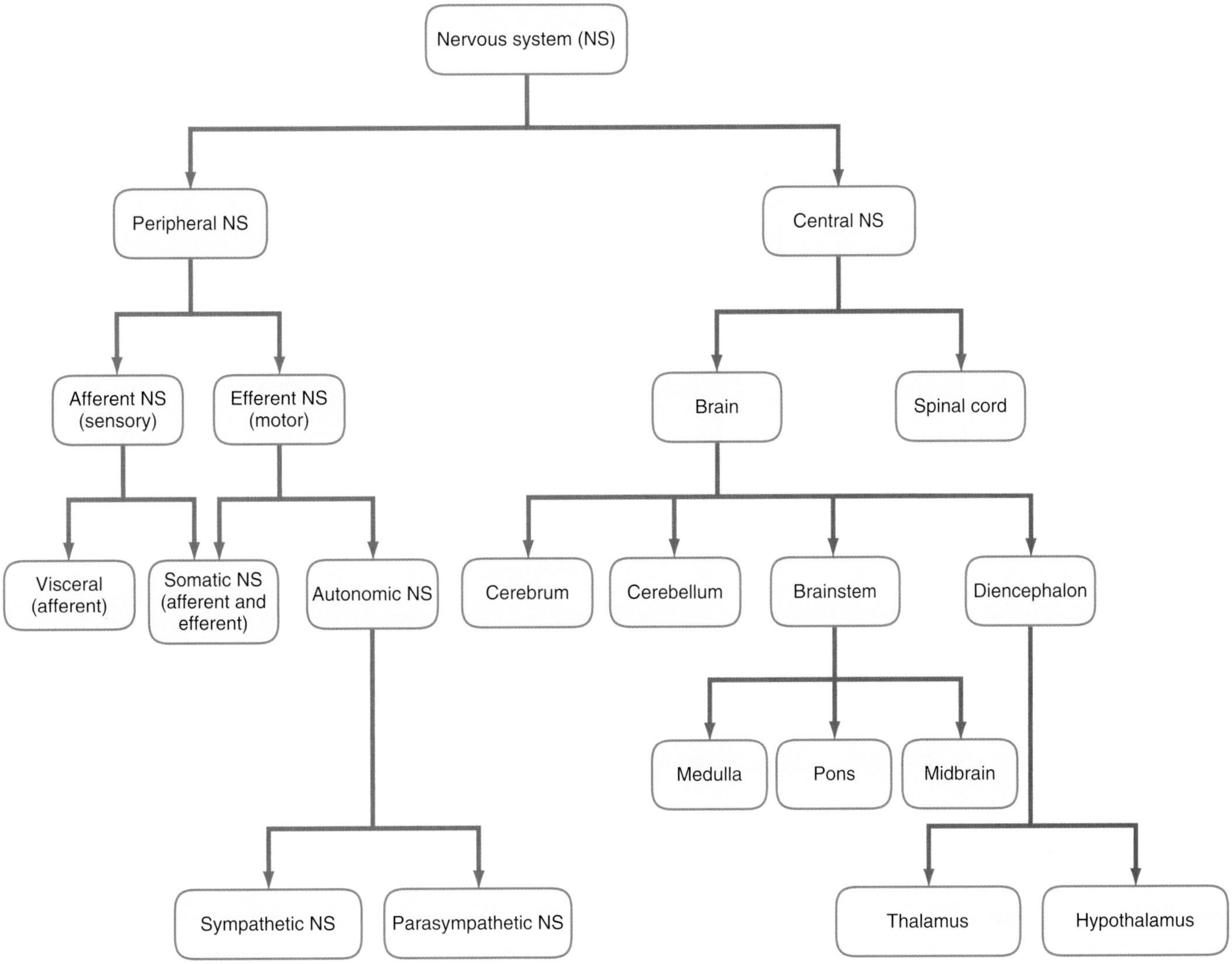

FIGURE 8-2 Divisions of the nervous system (*NS*).

potential results in part from differences in the distribution of positively charged ions (using sodium and potassium) and negatively charged ions in the cytoplasm and extracellular fluid. Sodium ions are more heavily concentrated outside the membrane, while potassium ions are more heavily concentrated inside the membrane. This imbalance is maintained by the active transport of ions against the concentration gradients by the sodium-potassium pump.

The rapid depolarization of the cell membrane results in an action potential, which then causes propagation of the nerve impulse along the membrane (see Figure 8-1). An **action potential** is a temporary reversal of the electric potential along the membrane for a brief period (less than a millisecond). Sodium gates suddenly open in the membrane to allow sodium ions to pour in, bringing a positive charge. At the height of the membrane potential reversal, sodium gates close and potassium channels open to allow potassium ions to pass to the outside of the membrane, reestablishing the resting potential. The changed ionic distributions must be reset by the continuously running sodium-potassium pump.

The action potential begins at one spot on the membrane but spreads to adjacent areas of the membrane, propagating the impulse along the length of the cell membrane. After passage of the action potential, there is a brief period—the refractory period—during which the membrane cannot be stimulated. This prevents the impulse from being transmitted backward along the membrane. By means of the action potential, nerve impulses travel the length of the neuron.

To have the impulse cross the synapse to another cell requires the actions of chemical agents from the neuron that are considered **neurotransmitters**. The neurotransmitters are discharged with the arrival of the action potential. Released neurotransmitters then diffuse across the synapse and bind to receptors on the membrane of the other cell. Neurotransmitters cause ion channels to open or close in the second cell, prompting changes in the excitability of that cell's membrane. In most organs, excitatory neurotransmitters such as acetylcholine and norepinephrine make it more likely that an action potential will be triggered in the second cell. Inhibitory neurotransmitters such as dopamine and serotonin make an action potential in the second cell less likely. Later neurotransmitters are either destroyed by specific enzymes, diffuse away, or are reabsorbed by the neuron.

Neurotransmitters tend to be small molecules; some are even hormones. Certain neurologic diseases (e.g., Parkinson, Huntington, and Alzheimer diseases) are associated with imbalances of neurotransmitters. In addition, some symptoms of Parkinson disease (e.g., rigidity) are due to a dopamine deficiency, and some symptoms of Huntington disease also may be caused by loss of a different inhibitory neurotransmitter.

Alzheimer disease is accompanied by a loss of acetylcholine-producing neurons, which may explain the memory problems that result. In addition, depression in Alzheimer disease can in some cases be linked to low levels of excitatory neurotransmitters, with drug therapy for depression altering those levels. Among the drugs that generally affect neurotransmitter function is cocaine, which blocks the uptake of norepinephrine while stimulating the uptake of dopamine.

Special neurotransmitters involved with the sensation of pain in the central nervous system are endorphins, natural opioids that produce elation and reduction of pain, as do synthetic neurotransmitters such as opium and heroin. Local anesthetic agents such as lidocaine, as used in dentistry, mimic inhibitory neurotransmitters by decreasing sensory neurons' ability to generate an action potential, thus producing localized anesthesia. **Anesthesia** is the loss of feeling or sensation resulting from the use of certain drugs or gases that serve as inhibitory neurotransmitters. With damage to the nerves, there can be abnormal sensation or paresthesia in a region involving trauma or agent toxicity (see Chapter 9) or infection (see Chapter 12).

CENTRAL NERVOUS SYSTEM

One of the major divisions of the nervous system, the **central nervous system (CNS)** includes: the brain and spinal cord (see Figures 8-2 and 8-4). The CNS is surrounded by bone, either the skull or vertebrae, and a system of membranes containing cerebrospinal fluid; both the bone and membranes serve to protect it. The system of membranes is the **meninges** (**muh**-nin-jez), which has three layers: dura mater, arachnoid mater, and pia mater. The dura mater also surrounds and supports the large venous channels (dural sinuses) carrying blood from the brain toward the heart (see Figure 6-12).

The major divisions of the **brain** include: the cerebrum, cerebellum, brainstem, and diencephalon (Figure 8-3). The **cerebrum** (suh-**ree**-bruhm) is the largest division of the brain and consists of two cerebral hemispheres. The cerebrum coordinates sensory data and motor functions and governs many aspects of intelligence and reasoning,

learning, and memory. The **cerebellum** (suhr-uh-**bel**-uhm) is the second largest division of the brain after the cerebrum. It functions to produce muscle coordination and maintains the usual level of muscle tone and posture as well as coordinates balance.

The **brainstem** has a number of divisions that include: the medulla, pons, and midbrain (Figure 8-4). The **medulla** (muh-**dul**-uh) is closest to the spinal cord and is involved with the regulation of heartbeat, breathing, vasoconstriction (blood pressure), and reflex centers for vomiting, coughing, sneezing, swallowing, and hiccupping. The cell bodies of the motor neurons for the tongue are located in the medulla. The **pons** (ponz) connects the medulla with the cerebellum and with higher brain centers. Cell bodies for cranial nerves V and VII are found in the pons. The **midbrain** includes relay stations for hearing, vision, and motor pathways.

Superior to the brainstem, the **diencephalon** (dy-uhn-**sef**-uh-lon) primarily includes: the thalamus and hypothalamus (see Figure 8-4). The **thalamus** (**thal**-uh-muhs) serves as a central relay point for incoming nerve impulses. The **hypothalamus** (hi-poh-**thal**-uh-muhs) regulates homeostasis; it has specific regulatory areas for thirst, hunger, body temperature, water balance, and blood pressure; all these regulatory areas help to link the nervous system to the endocrine system.

The other component of the CNS, the **spinal cord**, runs along the dorsal side of the body and links the brain to the rest of the body (see Figure 8-4). The spinal cord in adults is encased in a series of bony vertebrae that comprise the vertebral column. The spinal column consists of two components of brain substance: gray and white matter. The gray matter of the spinal cord consists mostly of unmyelinated cell bodies and dendrites. The surrounding white matter is made up of tracts of axons, insulated in sheaths of myelin, formed from a combination of lipids and proteins. Some tracts are ascending (charged with carrying messages to the brain), and others are descending (charged with carrying messages from the brain). The spinal cord is also involved in reflexes that do not immediately involve the brain.

PERIPHERAL NERVOUS SYSTEM

The other major division of the nervous system, the **peripheral nervous system (PNS)** (puh-**rif**-uhr-uhl), is composed of all the nerves creating pathways among the CNS and the receptors, muscles, and glands of the body (see Figure 8-2). The PNS is further divided into: the **afferent nervous system** or *sensory nervous system*, which carries information from receptors to the brain or spinal cord, and the **efferent nervous system** or *motor nervous system*, which carries information from the brain or spinal cord to muscles or glands. As an example: A nerve cell leading from the eye to the brain and carrying visual information is a part of the afferent nervous system. In contrast, a nerve cell leading from the brain to the muscles controlling the eye's movement is a part of the efferent nervous system. The efferent division of the PNS is further subdivided into: the somatic nervous system and autonomic nervous system.

SOMATIC NERVOUS SYSTEM

The **somatic nervous system (SNS)** (so-**mat**-ik) is a subdivision of the efferent division of the peripheral nervous system and includes all nerves controlling the muscular system and external sensory receptors. The SNS involves both receptors and effectors. External sense organs (including skin) are receptors; muscle fibers and gland cells are effectors. First, the sensory input taken in by the PNS is processed by the CNS. After this CNS initial processing, the responses are sent by the PNS from the CNS to the organs of the body. The motor

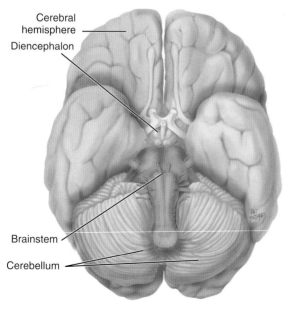

FIGURE 8-3 Ventral view of the gross brain with the brainstem highlighted.

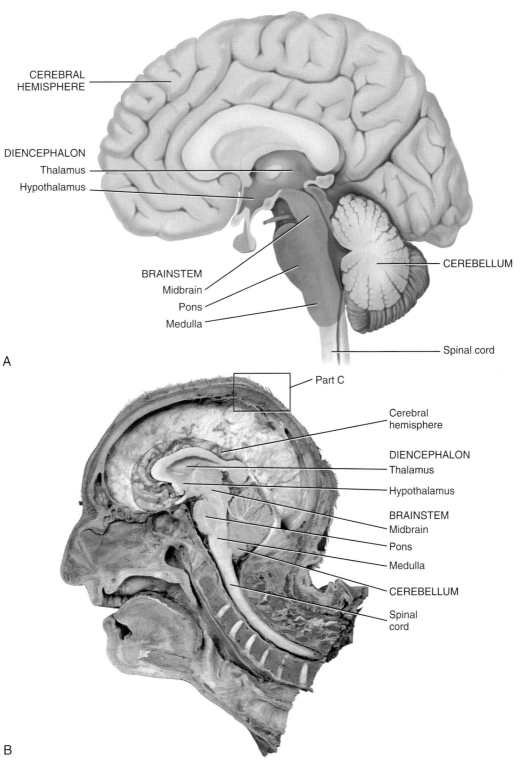

FIGURE 8-4 The brain with the brainstem highlighted in a sagittal section **(A)** and with dissection **(B)**. See the next page for parts **C** and **D**.

Continued

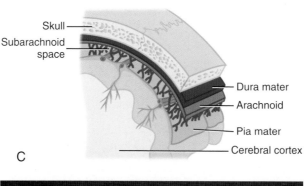

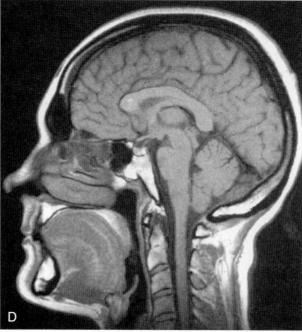

FIGURE 8-4, cont'd The brain with its layers of meninges **(C)**, and with magnetic resonance imaging of the head and neck **(D)**. *(B and D from Reynolds PA, Abrahams PH:* McMinn's interactive clinical anatomy: head and neck, *ed 2, London, 2001, Elsevier.)*

neurons of the somatic system are distinct from those of the autonomic system. Inhibitory signals cannot be sent through the motor neurons of the somatic system.

AUTONOMIC NERVOUS SYSTEM

The **autonomic nervous system (ANS)** (aw-toh-**nom**-ik) is the other subdivision of the efferent division of the peripheral nervous system. This system operates without any conscious control as a considerate caretaker of the body. Autonomic fibers are efferent nerves, and they always occur in two-nerve chains: the first nerve carries autonomic fibers to a ganglion, where they terminate near the cell bodies of the second nerve. The ANS itself has two nervous system subdivisions: sympathetic and parasympathetic nervous systems. Most tissue, structures, and organs are supplied by both of the divisions of the ANS. However, the sympathetic and parasympathetic systems generally work in opposition to each other: one stimulates an organ and the other inhibits it.

The **sympathetic nervous system** (sim-puh-**thet**-ik) is involved in "fight-or-flight" responses such as occur with the shutdown of salivary

gland secretion. Thus such a response by the sympathetic system leads to the reduced level of saliva with hyposalivation, which can cause dry mouth or xerostomia (see Chapter 7). This condition can be mimicked when taking certain medications that cause hyposalivation with xerostomia.

Sympathetic nerves arise in the spinal cord and relay in ganglia arranged like a chain running up the neck close to the vertebral column on both sides. Therefore all the sympathetic neurons in the head have already relayed in a ganglion. Sympathetic fibers reach the cranial tissue they supply by traveling with the arteries.

The **parasympathetic nervous system** (pare-uh-sim-pah-**thet**-ik) is involved in "rest-or-digest" responses such as occur when there is stimulation of salivary gland secretions, the exact opposite of the earlier discussion. Thus such a response by the parasympathetic system leads to the salivary flow to aid in digestion when being stimulated by food.

Parasympathetic fibers associated with the glands of the head and neck region are carried within various cranial nerves and are briefly described here, as well as in greater detail later. The ganglia are located in the head, and therefore parasympathetic neurons in this region may be either preganglionic neurons (before relaying in the ganglion) or postganglionic neurons (after relaying in the ganglion).

The principal parasympathetic outflow for glands in the head and neck is carried within both the seventh and ninth cranial nerves (see Figure 8-21 and Chapter 7). The seventh cranial or facial nerve has two branches involved in glandular secretion. The greater petrosal nerve is associated with the pterygopalatine ganglion, and the lacrimal gland is the major target organ. The chorda tympani nerve is associated with the submandibular ganglion, and the target organs are the submandibular and sublingual salivary glands. The lesser petrosal nerve, which is a branch of the ninth cranial or glossopharyngeal nerve, is associated with the otic ganglion, and the target organ is the parotid salivary gland.

CRANIAL NERVES

The **cranial nerves** (**kray**-nee-uhl) are an important part of the PNS. The paired twelve cranial nerves are connected to the brain at its base and pass through the skull by way of fissures or foramina (Figures 8-5 and 8-6 and Table 8-1 and see Chapter 3 and Table 3-3). The cranial nerves serve to innervate structures in the head or neck. In addition, the tenth cranial or vagus nerve descends through the neck and into the thorax (chest) and abdomen where it innervates internal organs.

Certain cranial nerves are either afferent or efferent, and others have both types of neural processes. The cranial nerves are numbered according to their location in regards to the brain, going from the anterior of the brain to its posterior. Both Roman numerals (I to XII)

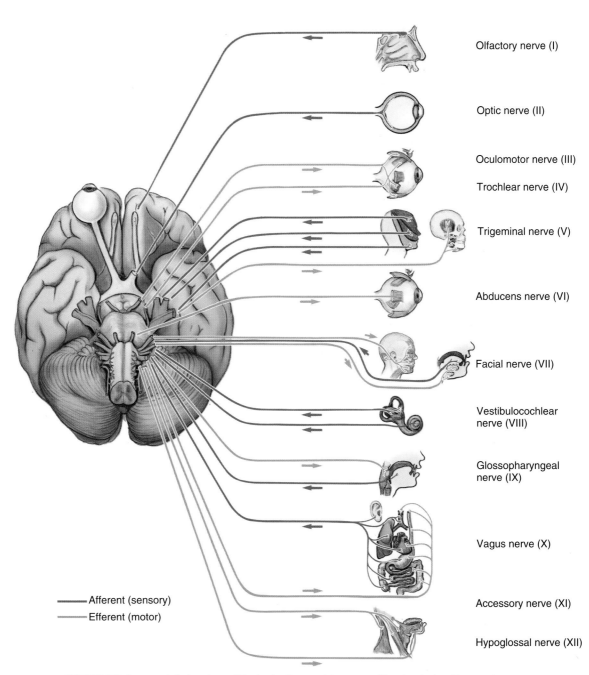

FIGURE 8-5 From an inferior view of the brain, the cranial nerves with color designations and arrows of innervation as well as structures innervated.

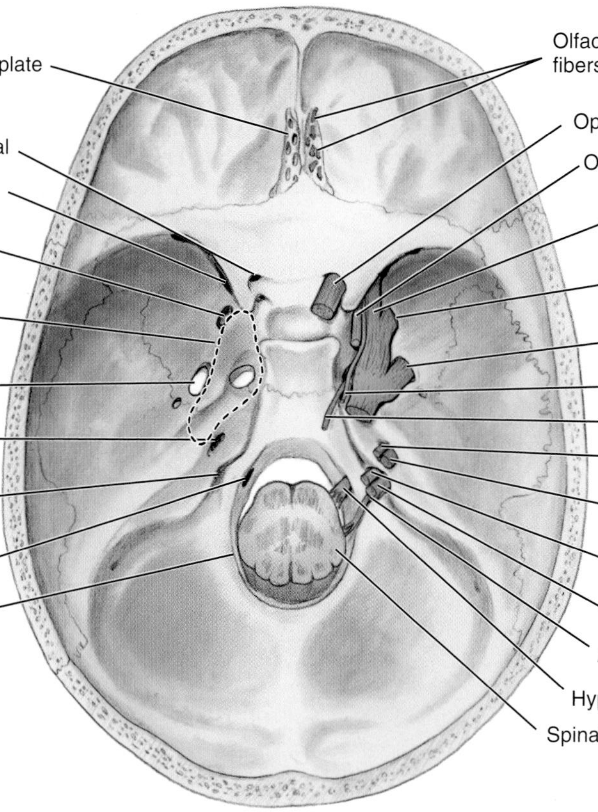

FIGURE 8-6 Superior view of the internal skull noting the highlighted cranial nerves exiting (on the right). Note also the openings in the bones of the skull for these cranial nerves (on the left).

TABLE 8-1		**Cranial Nerve Innervations**
NERVE		**NERVE TYPES AND STRUCTURES INNERVATED**
I	Olfactory	Afferent: nasal mucosa
II	Optic	Afferent: retina of the eye
III	Oculomotor	Efferent: eye muscles including some smooth muscles (parasympathetic)
IV	Trochlear	Efferent: one eye muscle
V	Trigeminal	Efferent: muscles of mastication and other cranial muscles Afferent: face and head skin, teeth, oral cavity, and most general sensation for tongue
VI	Abducens	Efferent: one eye muscle
VII	Facial	Efferent: muscles of facial expression, other cranial muscles, lacrimal gland and submandibular, sublingual, and minor salivary glands (parasympathetic) Afferent: skin around ear and taste sensation for tongue
VIII	Vestibulocochlear	Afferent: inner ear
IX	Glossopharyngeal	Efferent: stylopharyngeus muscle and parotid salivary gland (parasympathetic), and respiratory mucosa of pharynx Afferent: skin around ear and taste and general sensation for tongue
X	Vagus	Efferent: most muscles of soft palate, pharynx, larynx, thoracic and abdominal organs (parasympathetic) Afferent: skin around ear and taste sensation for epiglottis
XI	Accessory	Efferent: muscles of neck
XII	Hypoglossal	Efferent: tongue muscles

and anatomic terms are used to designate the cranial nerves within this chapter. A general background of the 12 cranial nerves is discussed next.

CRANIAL NERVE I

The first (I) cranial or **olfactory nerve** (ol-**fak**-tuh-ree) transmits smell from the nasal mucosa to the brain and thus functions as an afferent nerve. The nerve enters the skull through the perforations in the cribriform plate of the ethmoid bone to join the olfactory bulb in the brain (see Figures 3-36 and 9-24).

CRANIAL NERVE II

The second (II) cranial or **optic nerve** (**op**-tik) transmits sight from the retina of the eye to the brain and thus functions as an afferent nerve. The nerve enters the skull through the optic canal of the sphenoid bone on its way from the retina (see Figure 3-19). In the skull, both the right and left optic nerves join at the optic chiasma, where many of the fibers cross to the contralateral side before continuing into the brain as the optic tracts.

CRANIAL NERVE III

The third (III) cranial or **oculomotor nerve** (ok-u-lo-**moh**-tuhr) serves as an efferent nerve to some of the eye muscles that move the eyeball. The nerve also carries preganglionic parasympathetic fibers to the ciliary ganglion near the eyeball. The postganglionic fibers innervate small muscles within the eyeball. The nerve lies within the lateral wall of the cavernous sinus and exits the skull through the superior orbital fissure of the sphenoid bone on its way to the orbit (see Figure 3-19).

CRANIAL NERVE IV

The small fourth (IV) cranial or **trochlear nerve** (**trok**-lere) also serves as an efferent nerve for one eye muscle, as well as proprioception, similar to the oculomotor nerve but without any parasympathetic fibers. Similar to the oculomotor nerve, the trochlear nerve runs in the lateral wall of the cavernous sinus and exits the skull

through the superior orbital fissure of the sphenoid bone on its way to the orbit (see Figure 3-19).

CRANIAL NERVE V

The fifth (V) cranial or **trigeminal nerve** (try-**jem**-i-nuhl) has both an efferent component for the muscles of mastication (as well as some other cranial muscles) and an afferent component for the teeth, tongue, and oral cavity, as well as most of the skin of the face and head. Although the trigeminal nerve has no preganglionic parasympathetic fibers, many postganglionic parasympathetic fibers travel along with its branches.

The trigeminal nerve is the largest cranial nerve and has two roots: sensory and motor (see Figures 8-5 and 8-6). The sensory root of the trigeminal nerve has three nerve divisions: the ophthalmic, maxillary, and mandibular nerves (Figure 8-7). The ophthalmic nerve (first division of nerve) provides sensation to the upper face and scalp. The maxillary nerve (second division of nerve) and mandibular nerve (third division of nerve) provide sensation to the middle and lower face, respectively.

Each of the three nerves or divisions of the sensory root of the trigeminal nerve enters the skull in one of three different fissures or foramina in the sphenoid bone (see Figure 8-7). The ophthalmic nerve or first division enters through the superior orbital fissure. The maxillary nerve or second division enters by way of the foramen rotundum. The mandibular nerve or third division passes through the skull by way of the foramen ovale.

The motor root of the trigeminal nerve accompanies the mandibular nerve of the sensory root and also exits the skull through the foramen ovale of the sphenoid bone.

The trigeminal nerve is the most significant cranial nerve to the dental professional because it innervates relevant tissue, structures, and organs of the head and neck (Table 8-2). The trigeminal nerve is discussed in greater detail later in this chapter, and the local anesthesia of its nerve branches is discussed in Chapter 9.

CRANIAL NERVE VI

The sixth (VI) cranial or **abducens nerve** (ab-**doo**-suhnz) or *abducent nerve* serves as an efferent nerve to one of the muscles that moves the

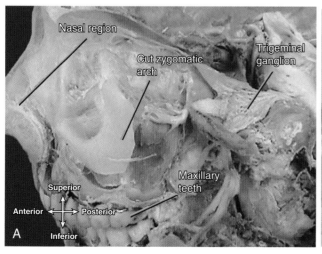
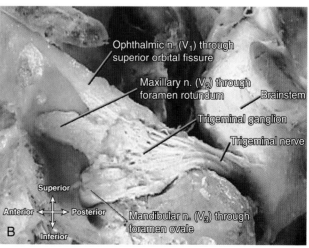

FIGURE 8-7 Dissection of the trigeminal ganglion **(A)**, and its three nerves or divisions **(B)**. *(Courtesy of Jeremy S. Melker, MD.)*

TABLE 8-2	Orofacial Structures Innervation
OROFACIAL STRUCTURES	**NERVES AND FIBER TYPE**
Maxillary anterior teeth and associated labial periodontium and gingiva	ASA of V_2: afferent
Maxillary posterior teeth and associated buccal periodontium and gingiva as well as maxillary sinus	MSA and PSA of V_2: afferent
Anterior hard palate and associated palatal periodontium and gingiva of maxillary anterior teeth as well as nasal septum	Nasopalatine of V_2: afferent
Posterior hard palate and associated palatal periodontium and gingiva of maxillary posterior teeth	Greater palatine of V_2: afferent
Soft palate and palatine tonsils	Lesser palatine of V_2, glossopharyngeal (IX): afferent Branches of V_3, accessory (XI), and vagus (X): efferent
Mandibular teeth and associated facial periodontium and gingiva of mandibular anterior teeth and premolars as well as labial mucosa	IA and its incisive and mental branches of V_3: afferent
Associated buccal periodontium and gingiva of mandibular molars as well as buccal mucosa	Buccal of V_3: afferent
Associated lingual periodontium and gingiva of mandibular teeth as well as floor of mouth	Lingual of V_3: afferent
Tongue—general sensation	Body, lingual of V_3; Base, glossopharyngeal (IX): afferent
Tongue—taste sensation	Body, chorda tympani of facial (VII); Base, glossopharyngeal (IX): afferent
Tongue muscles	Hypoglossal (XII): efferent
Parotid salivary gland	Otic ganglion Lesser petrosal of glossopharyngeal (IX) (parasympathetic) via auriculotemporal of V_3: efferent
Submandibular and sublingual salivary glands	Submandibular ganglion Chorda tympani of facial (VII) (parasympathetic) via lingual of V_3: efferent
Lacrimal gland	Pterygopalatine ganglion Greater petrosal nerve of facial (VII) (parasympathetic) via zygomatic of V_2 and lacrimal of V_1: efferent
Muscles of facial expression	Branches of facial (VII): efferent
Muscles of mastication	Medial pterygoid, deep temporal, masseteric, and lateral pterygoid of V_3: efferent
Trapezius and sternocleidomastoid muscles	Accessory (XI): efferent

ASA, Anterior superior alveolar; *IA*, inferior alveolar; *MSA*, middle superior alveolar; *PSA*, posterior superior alveolar; V_1, ophthalmic nerve; V_2, maxillary nerve; V_3, mandibular nerve.

eyeball, similar to the oculomotor and trochlear nerves. Similar to both of those cranial nerves, the nerve exits the skull through the superior orbital fissure of the sphenoid bone on its way to the orbit (see Figure 3-19).

However, the nerve has a somewhat different intracranial course. Rather than lying in the wall of the cavernous sinus, the nerve runs through the sinus, close to the internal carotid artery, and is often the first nerve affected by a serious infection of the sinus (see Chapter 12).

CRANIAL NERVE VII

The seventh (VII) cranial or **facial nerve** carries both efferent and afferent components. The nerve carries an efferent component for the muscles of facial expression and the posterior suprahyoid muscles, as well as for the preganglionic parasympathetic innervation of the lacrimal gland (relaying in the pterygopalatine ganglion) and the submandibular and sublingual salivary glands (relaying in the submandibular ganglion) (see Figures 8-5 and 8-6). The afferent

component serves a tiny patch of skin behind the ear and taste sensation with the taste buds of certain lingual papillae from the anterior two-thirds of the tongue.

The facial nerve leaves the cranial cavity by passing through the internal acoustic meatus, which leads to the facial canal within the temporal bone (see Figure 3-18). Finally, the nerve exits the skull by way of the stylomastoid foramen of the temporal bone. The facial nerve is significant to dental professionals because it innervates relevant tissue of the head and neck (see Table 8-2) and it travels through the parotid salivary gland. Thus the facial nerve can also be involved in complications with the administration of local anesthesia (see Chapters 7 and 9) and is discussed in greater detail later in this chapter.

CRANIAL NERVE VIII

The eighth (VIII) cranial or **vestibulocochlear nerve** (vuhs-tib-u-lo-**kok**-luhr) serves as an afferent nerve for hearing and balance. This nerve conveys signals from the inner ear to the brain. The inner ear is located within the temporal bone. The nerve enters the cranial cavity through the internal acoustic meatus of the temporal bone (see Figure 3-19).

The nerve supplies the two major parts of the inner ear: the cochlea and semicircular canals. The first part, the cochlea, serves the function of hearing and is supplied by the cochlear part of the vestibulocochlear nerve. The second part, the semicircular canals, serves the function of balance and is supplied by the vestibular part of the vestibulocochlear nerve.

CRANIAL NERVE IX

The ninth (IX) cranial or **glossopharyngeal nerve** (gloss-o-fuh-**rin**-je-uhl) carries an efferent component for the pharyngeal muscle and the stylopharyngeus muscle, and also provides the preganglionic gland parasympathetic innervation for the parotid salivary gland (relaying in the otic ganglion). In addition, the glossopharyngeal nerve also carries an afferent component for the oropharynx and for taste and general sensation from the base of the tongue, and thus is the afferent limb of the gag reflex.

The nerve passes through the skull by way of the jugular foramen, between the occipital bone and temporal bone (see Figure 3-19). The tympanic branch, with sensory fibers for the middle ear and preganglionic parasympathetic fibers for the parotid salivary gland, arises here and reenters the skull.

After supplying the ear, parasympathetic fibers leave the skull through the foramen ovale of the sphenoid bone as the **lesser petrosal nerve** (puh-**troh**-suhl) (see Figure 3-32). These preganglionic fibers then terminate in the **otic ganglion** (**ot**-ik) (see Figure 8-20). The otic ganglion is located near the medial surface of the mandibular nerve of the trigeminal or fifth cranial nerve, just inferior to the foramen ovale. Inferior branches of the glossopharyngeal nerve supply the carotid artery, oropharynx, and base of the tongue (afferent component), as well as the stylopharyngeus muscle. The glossopharyngeal nerve is significant to dental professionals because it innervates relevant tissue of the head and neck (see Table 8-2).

CRANIAL NERVE X

The tenth (X) cranial or **vagus nerve** (**vay**-guhs) carries a large efferent component for the muscles of the soft palate, pharynx, and larynx and for parasympathetic fibers (and associated visceral afferent fibers) to organs in the thorax and abdomen including the thymus gland, heart, and stomach. The nerve carries a smaller afferent component for a small amount of skin around the ear and for taste sensation for the epiglottis.

The nerve passes through the skull by way of the jugular foramen, between the occipital and temporal bones (see Figure 3-19). The vagus nerve is significant to dental professionals because it innervates relevant tissue of the head and neck (see Table 8-2).

CRANIAL NERVE XI

The eleventh (XI) cranial or **accessory nerve** functions as an efferent nerve for the trapezius and sternocleidomastoid muscles as well as for muscles of the soft palate and pharynx (see Figures 4-29 and 4-30). This nerve is only partly a cranial nerve and consists of two roots: one from the brain and one from the spinal cord. The accessory nerve exits the skull through the jugular foramen, between the occipital and temporal bones (see Figure 3-19). The accessory nerve is significant to dental professionals because it innervates relevant tissue of the head and neck (see Table 8-2).

CRANIAL NERVE XII

The twelfth (XII) cranial or **hypoglossal nerve** (hi-poh-**gloss**-uhl) functions as an efferent nerve for both the intrinsic and extrinsic muscles of the tongue (see Figure 4-28). The nerve exits the skull through the hypoglossal canal in the occipital bone (see Figure 3-19). The hypoglossal nerve is significant to dental professionals because it innervates the tongue (see Table 8-2).

NERVES TO HEAD AND NECK REGIONS AND ASSOCIATED STRUCTURES

The dental professional must understand the basic components of the nervous system, as well as the location of the major nerve supply of the head and neck because it adds to the general background of certain pathologies involving head and neck muscles (discussed later), the temporomandibular joint, and the salivary glands (see discussion in Chapters 5 and 7, respectively).

The management of dental pain using local anesthetic agents is key to providing effective dental care for patients. Thus the dental professional involved in the administration of local anesthesia in the oral cavity must have an understanding of the nervous system of the head and neck (see Chapter 9).

The two cranial nerves that primarily affect the head and neck structures, the trigeminal nerve and facial nerve, are discussed in greater detail in this chapter, with the stronger emphasis on the trigeminal nerve.

TRIGEMINAL NERVE

The dental professional must have a thorough understanding of the fifth (V) cranial or trigeminal nerve. Each trigeminal nerve is a short nerve trunk composed of two closely adapted roots (Figures 8-7 and 8-8). These roots of the nerve consist of a thicker sensory root and thinner motor root.

Within the skull, a bulge can be noted in the **sensory root of the trigeminal nerve**. This bulge is the **trigeminal ganglion** (semilunar or gasserian ganglion), which is located on the anterior surface of the petrous part of the temporal bone (see Figure 3-31). Anterior to the trigeminal ganglion, the sensory root arises from three nerves or divisions that pass into the skull by way of three different fissures or foramina in the sphenoid bone.

As discussed earlier and as detailed later, these three nerves or divisions of the sensory root include: the ophthalmic, maxillary, and mandibular nerves. The ophthalmic nerve and maxillary nerve of the sensory root carry only afferent nerve fibers. The ophthalmic nerve enters through the superior orbital fissure. The maxillary nerve enters by way of the foramen rotundum. In contrast, the entire motor root of the cranial nerve runs with the mandibular nerve and thus the mandibular nerve carries both afferent and efferent nerve fibers. Important to note is that the commonly used terms "V_1," "V_2," and "V_3" (pronounced "vee one," "vee two," and "vee three") are simply shorthand notation for these nerves or divisions of the fifth cranial or trigeminal nerve since "V" is the Roman number for five.

The **motor root of the trigeminal nerve** supplies the efferent nerves for the muscles of mastication as well as a few other cranial muscles. As part of the mandibular nerve, the motor root exits the skull at the foramen ovale of the sphenoid bone.

Ophthalmic Nerve. The first nerve division or V_1 of the sensory root of the trigeminal nerve is the **ophthalmic nerve** (of-**thal**-mik) (Figures 8-9 and 8-10). This smallest division serves as an afferent nerve for the conjunctiva, cornea, eyeball, orbit, forehead, and the

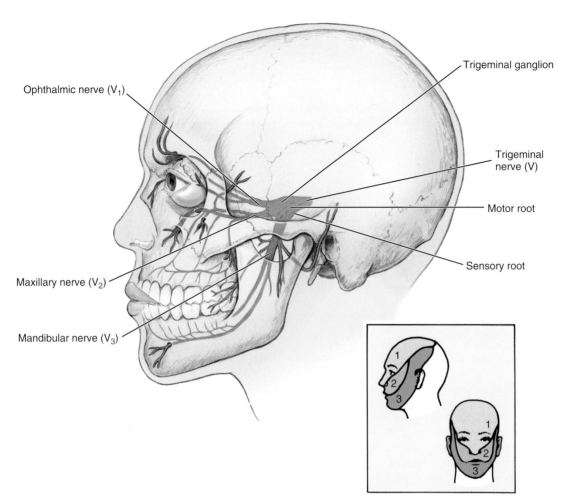

FIGURE 8-8 General pathway of the trigeminal or fifth cranial nerve and its motor and sensory roots. The three nerves or divisions of the cranial nerve are highlighted; note the innervation coverage for each nerve (*see inset*).

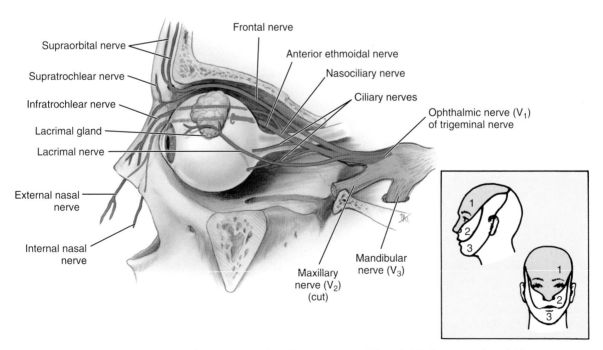

FIGURE 8-9 Lateral view of the cut-away orbit with the pathway of the ophthalmic nerve or first division of the trigeminal nerve highlighted; note the innervation coverage for the ophthalmic nerve (*see inset*).

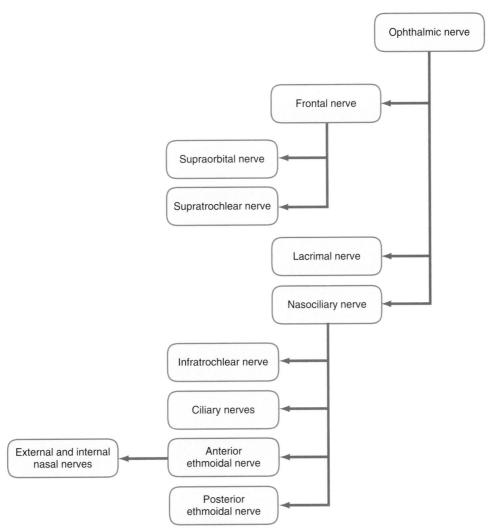

FIGURE 8-10 Ophthalmic nerve (V₁) and its branches to the facial region.

ethmoidal and frontal sinuses, plus a part of the dura mater and parts of the nasal cavity and nose.

The nerve carries this sensory information toward the brain by way of the superior orbital fissure of the sphenoid bone (see Figure 3-19). Other nerves that traverse this fissure include the third, fourth, and sixth cranial nerves. The ophthalmic nerve arises from three major nerves: the frontal, lacrimal, and nasociliary nerves.

Frontal Nerve. The **frontal nerve** is an afferent nerve located in the orbit and is composed of a merger of the **supraorbital nerve** (**soo**-pruh-**or**-bi-tuhl) from the forehead and anterior scalp and the **supratrochlear nerve** (**soo**-pruh-**trok**-lere) from the bridge of the nose and medial parts of the upper eyelid and forehead. The nerve courses along the roof of the orbit toward the superior orbital fissure of the sphenoid bone where it is joined by the lacrimal and nasociliary nerves to form V₁ (see Figure 3-25).

Lacrimal Nerve. The **lacrimal nerve** (**lak**-ri-muhl) serves as an afferent nerve for the lateral part of the upper eyelid, conjunctiva, and lacrimal gland. The nerve also delivers the postganglionic parasympathetic nerves to the lacrimal gland (see Figure 2-6 and Chapter 7). These nerves are responsible for the production of lacrimal fluid or tears. The nerve runs posteriorly along the lateral roof of the orbit and then joins the frontal and nasociliary nerves near the superior orbital fissure of the sphenoid bone to form V₁ (see Figure 3-25).

Nasociliary Nerve. Several afferent nerve branches converge to form the **nasociliary nerve** (nay-zo-**sil**-ee-a-re). These branches include the **infratrochlear nerve** (in-fruh-**trok**-lere) from the skin of the medial part of the eyelids and the side of the nose, **ciliary nerves** (**sil**-ee-a-re) to and from the eyeball, and **anterior ethmoidal nerve** (eth-**moy**-duhl) and **posterior ethmoidal nerve** from the nasal cavity and paranasal sinuses (see Figures 3-8, 3-9, and 9-24). The anterior ethmoidal nerve is formed by the **external nasal nerve** (**nay**-zuhl) from the skin of the ala and apex of the nose and the **internal nasal nerves** from the anterior part of the nasal septum and lateral wall of the nasal cavity.

The nasociliary nerve is an afferent nerve that runs within the orbit, superior to the second cranial or optic nerve, to join the frontal and lacrimal nerves near the superior orbital fissure of the sphenoid bone to form V₁.

Maxillary Nerve. The second nerve division or V₂ from the sensory root of the trigeminal nerve is the **maxillary nerve** (**mak**-sil-ar-ee), which is set between the other two divisions both in size and location (Figures 8-11 and 8-12). The afferent nerve branches of the maxillary nerve carry sensory information for the maxillae and its overlying skin, oral mucosa, maxillary sinuses, nasal cavity, palate, nasopharynx, and part of the dura mater.

The maxillary nerve is a nerve trunk formed within the pterygopalatine fossa by the convergence of many nerves; the largest

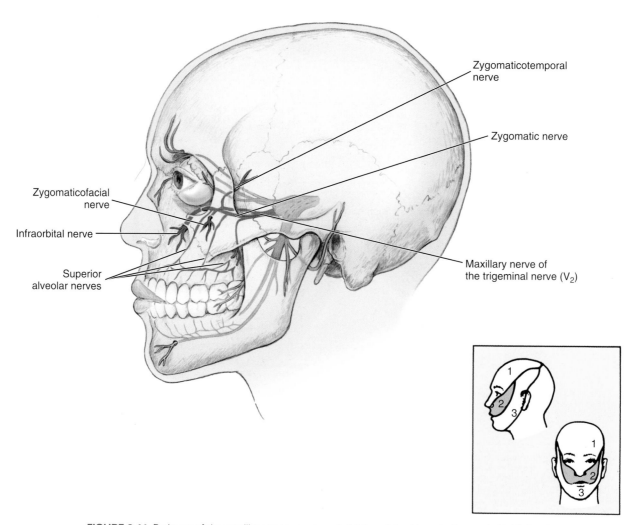

FIGURE 8-11 Pathway of the maxillary nerve or second division of the trigeminal nerve is highlighted; note the innervation coverage for the maxillary nerve (*see inset*).

contributor is the infraorbital nerve (see Figure 3-61). The tributaries of the infraorbital nerve or maxillary nerve trunk include: the zygomatic, the anterior, middle and posterior superior alveolar, the greater and lesser palatine, and the nasopalatine nerves.

After all these branches come together in the pterygopalatine fossa to form the maxillary nerve, the nerve enters the skull through the foramen rotundum of the sphenoid bone (see Figure 3-33). Small afferent meningeal branches from parts of the dura mater join the maxillary nerve as it enters the trigeminal ganglion.

A large ganglion, the **pterygopalatine ganglion** (ter-i-go-**pal**-uh-tine), lies just inferior to the maxillary nerve within the pterygopalatine fossa. This ganglion serves as a relay station for parasympathetic nerves that arise within the facial nerve (described later). Fibers from the ganglion (postganglionic) are then distributed to various types of tissue such as the minor salivary glands by the nerves of V₂. Because the pterygopalatine ganglion lies between the maxillary nerve and its tributaries from the palate, the sensory fibers actually pass through the ganglion. However, unlike the parasympathetic fibers just discussed, the sensory fibers do not synapse within the ganglion.

Zygomatic Nerve. The **zygomatic nerve** (zy-go-**mat**-ik) is an afferent nerve composed of the merger of the zygomaticofacial nerve and the zygomaticotemporal nerve in the orbit (see Figure 8-11). This nerve also conveys the postganglionic parasympathetic fibers for the

lacrimal gland to the lacrimal nerve (see earlier discussion). The zygomatic nerve courses posteriorly along the lateral orbit floor and enters the pterygopalatine fossa through the inferior orbital fissure, which is between the sphenoid bone and maxilla, to finally join V₂ (see Figure 3-47).

The rather small **zygomaticofacial nerve** (zygo-mat-i-ko-**fay**-shuhl) serves as an afferent nerve for the skin of the cheek. This nerve pierces the frontal process of the zygomatic bone at the zygomaticofacial foramen and enters the orbit through its lateral wall (see Figure 3-42). The zygomaticofacial nerve then turns posteriorly to join with the zygomaticotemporal nerve.

The other nerve, the **zygomaticotemporal nerve** (zy-go-mat-i-ko-**tem**-puh-ruhl), serves as an afferent nerve for the skin of the temporal region and pierces the temporal surface of the zygomatic bone at the zygomaticotemporal foramen (see Figure 3-42). The zygomaticotemporal nerve then traverses the lateral wall of the orbit to join the zygomaticofacial nerve, forming the zygomatic nerve.

Infraorbital Nerve. The **infraorbital nerve** (in-fruh-**or**-bi-tuhl) or *IO nerve* is an afferent nerve formed from the merger of cutaneous branches from the upper lip, the medial part of the cheek, side of the nose, and the lower eyelid (Figure 8-13). The IO nerve then passes into the infraorbital foramen of the maxilla, with its opening serving as a landmark for the administration of the infraorbital block, which

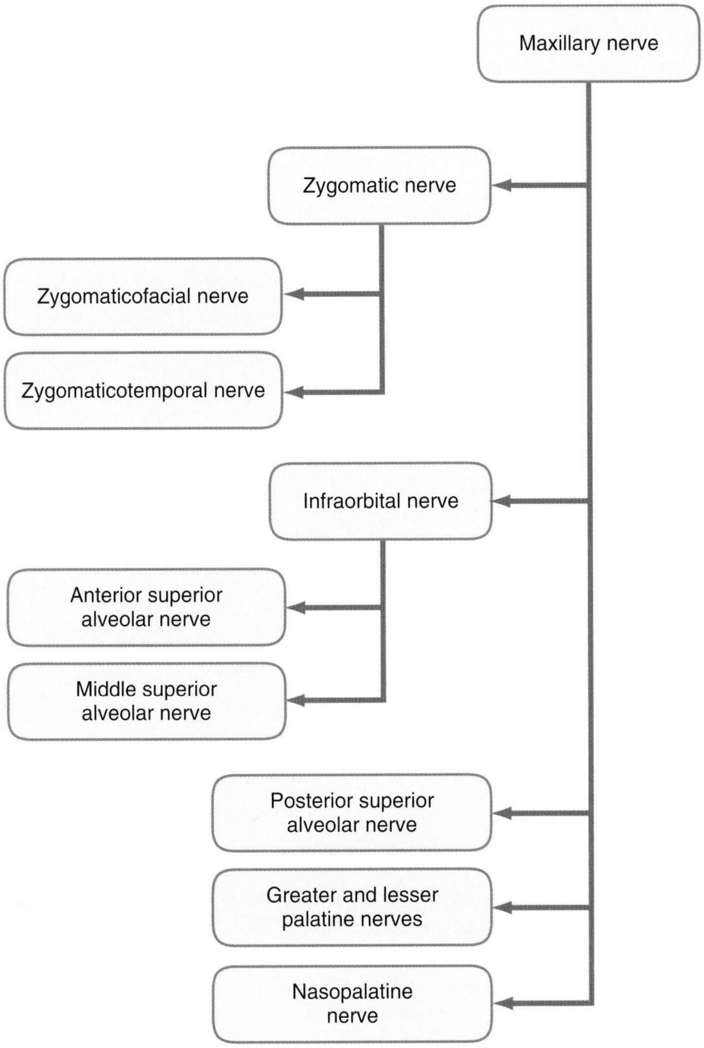

Maxillary nerve

Zygomatic nerve

Zygomaticofacial nerve

Zygomaticotemporal nerve

Infraorbital nerve

Anterior superior
alveolar nerve

Middle superior
alveolar nerve

Posterior superior
alveolar nerve

Greater and lesser
palatine nerves

Nasopalatine
nerve

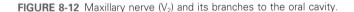

FIGURE 8-12 Maxillary nerve (V$_2$) and its branches to the oral cavity.

when administered, anesthetizes the IO nerve as well as both the anterior and middle superior alveolar nerves (see Figures 9-15 and 9-18 and Table 9-1).

The infraorbital foramen is located inferior to the midpoint of the inferior margin of the orbit, the infraorbital rim. Palpation of the infraorbital foramen during an extraoral examination or before an administration of a local anesthetic agent will cause transient soreness to the area due to the presence of the nerve (see Figure 9-16). Then the IO nerve travels posteriorly through the infraorbital canal, along with the infraorbital blood vessels where it is joined by the anterior superior alveolar nerve (see Figures 3-45 to 3-47).

From the infraorbital canal and groove, the IO nerve passes into the pterygopalatine fossa through the inferior orbital fissure. After it leaves the infraorbital groove and within the pterygopalatine fossa, the IO nerve receives the posterior superior alveolar nerve and joins with it or directly with the maxillary nerve.

Anterior Superior Alveolar Nerve. The **anterior superior alveolar nerve** (al-**vee**-uh-luhr) or *ASA nerve* serves as an afferent nerve for the maxillary central incisors, lateral incisors, and canines as well as associated labial periodontium and gingiva to the midline.

The ASA nerve originates from dental branches in the pulp of these teeth that exit through the apical foramina (see Figure 8-13). The ASA

nerve also receives interdental branches from the surrounding periodontium, which together become part of the superior dental plexus within the maxillary arch (see Figures 9-12 and 9-14). A **dental plexus** is a network of nerves within both the maxillary and mandibular dental arches. The superior dental plexus in the maxillary arch also receives interdental branches from other branches of the maxillary nerve, both the middle and posterior superior alveolar nerves (discussed next).

The ASA nerve then ascends along the anterior wall of the maxillary sinus to join the IO nerve within the infraorbital canal (see Figure 3-45). Thus the ASA nerve can be anesthetized by either the anterior superior alveolar block as discussed, or along with the middle superior alveolar nerve by the infraorbital block (discussed earlier and Table 9-1). The ASA nerve can also be anesthetized with the anterior middle superior alveolar block along with other maxillary nerve branches using a palatal technique.

The ASA nerve can also involve crossover-innervation to the contralateral side in a patient. **Crossover-innervation** is the overlap of terminal nerve fibers from the contralateral side of the dental arch. Crossover-innervation is important to consider when administering local anesthesia for the maxillary teeth and associated tissue with the ASA nerve as well as for the mandibular anterior teeth with the incisive nerve (see Chapter 9).

Middle Superior Alveolar Nerve. The **middle superior alveolar nerve** or *MSA nerve* serves as an afferent nerve for the maxillary premolars and the mesiobuccal root of the maxillary first molar and associated buccal periodontium and gingiva, if the nerve is present.

The MSA nerve if present originates from dental branches in the pulp that exit the teeth through the apical foramina, as well as interdental and interradicular branches from the periodontium (see Figure 8-13). The MSA nerve, like the ASA and posterior superior alveolar nerves, is part of the superior dental plexus in the maxillary arch as discussed earlier (see Figures 9-8, 9-9, and 9-11). The MSA nerve then ascends to join the IO nerve by running in the lateral wall of the maxillary sinus.

Thus the MSA nerve if present can be anesthetized by either the middle superior alveolar block as discussed, or along with the ASA nerve, the infraorbital block (discussed earlier and see Table 9-1). The MSA nerve can also be anesthetized by the anterior middle superior alveolar block along with other maxillary nerve branches using a palatal technique.

However, the MSA nerve is not always present in all patients; it is present only in approximately 28% of the population. If the MSA nerve is not present, the area is innervated by both the ASA and posterior superior alveolar nerves, but mainly by the ASA nerve. If the MSA nerve is present, there is also communication between the MSA nerve and both the ASA nerve and posterior superior alveolar nerve. These considerations are important when administering local anesthesia for the maxillary posterior teeth and associated tissue; however, the administration of both the posterior superior alveolar block as well as the middle superior alveolar block will provide complete coverage to the maxillary posterior teeth (see Chapter 9).

Posterior Superior Alveolar Nerve. The **posterior superior alveolar nerve** or *PSA nerve* joins the IO nerve (or maxillary nerve directly in some cases) in the pterygopalatine fossa (see Figures 8-13 and 9-3). The PSA nerve serves as an afferent nerve for the mucous membranes of the maxillary sinus and the maxillary molars with the associated buccal periodontium and gingiva in most cases unless the MSA nerve is present (see earlier discussion and see Table 9-1).

Thus some branches of the PSA nerve remain external to the posterior surface of the maxilla. These are the external branches that provide afferent innervation for the maxillary molars. Other afferent

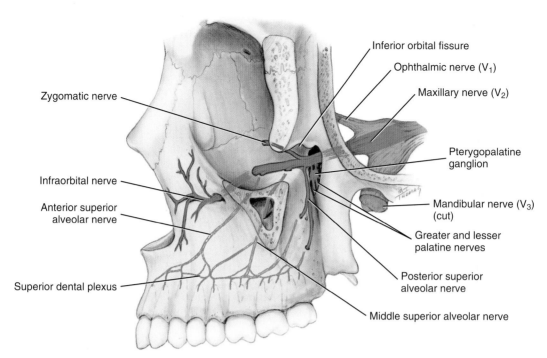

FIGURE 8-13 Lateral view of the skull with part of lateral wall of orbit removed; the branches of the maxillary nerve are highlighted.

nerve branches of the PSA nerve originate from dental branches in the pulp of the maxillary molars and exit the teeth by way of the apical foramina, as well as the interdental branches and interradicular branches from the periodontium. The PSA nerve, like the ASA and MSA nerves, is part of the superior dental plexus in the maxillary arch as discussed earlier.

All these internal branches of the PSA nerve enter the multiple posterior superior alveolar foramina on the surface of the maxilla. The posterior superior alveolar foramina are posterosuperior on the maxillary tuberosity as well as superior to the apex of the maxillary second molar. The posterior superior alveolar blood vessels also travel through these same foramina (see Figures 3-47 and 6-9). The openings of the posterior superior alveolar foramina and maxillary tuberosity are landmarks for the administration of the posterior superior alveolar block that anesthetizes the PSA nerve (see Figures 9-2, 9-4, and 9-7).

Both the external and internal branches of the PSA nerve then move superiorly together along the maxillary tuberosity, which forms the posterolateral wall of the maxillary sinus, to join either the IO nerve or maxillary nerve.

Greater and Lesser Palatine Nerves. Both palatine nerves join with the maxillary nerve from the palate (Figure 8-14). The **greater palatine nerve** (**pal**-uh-tine) or *GP nerve* (or anterior palatine nerve) is located between the mucoperiosteum and bone of the posterior hard palate (see Figures 3-16 and 3-44). The GP nerve serves as an afferent nerve for the posterior hard palate and the associated palatal periodontium and gingiva of the ipsilateral maxillary posterior teeth (see Table 9-1). Communication may also occur with the nasopalatine nerve terminal fibers in the associated palatal periodontium and gingiva of the maxillary first premolar, which may complicate the use of local anesthesia in the region (see Chapter 9).

Posteriorly, the GP nerve enters the greater palatine foramen in the horizontal plate of the palatine bone superior to the apices of the maxillary second or third molar to travel within the pterygopalatine

canal, along with the greater palatine blood vessels. The opening of the greater palatine foramen is a landmark for the administration of the greater palatine block that anesthetizes the GP nerve (see Figures 9-19, 9-20, and 9-22). The GP nerve can also be anesthetized with the anterior middle superior alveolar block along with other maxillary nerve branches using a palatal technique.

The **lesser palatine nerve** or *LP nerve* (or posterior palatine nerve) serves as an afferent nerve for the soft palate and palatine tonsils. The LP nerve enters the lesser palatine foramen in the palatine bone near its junction with the pterygoid process of the sphenoid bone, along with the lesser palatine blood vessels (see Figure 8-14). The LP nerve then joins the GP nerve within the pterygopalatine canal. When administering the greater palatine block, some patients may become uncomfortable and may gag if the soft palate becomes inadvertently and harmlessly anesthetized, which is possible given the proximity of the LP nerve and its foramen (see Chapter 9).

Both palatine nerves move superiorly through the pterygopalatine canal, toward the maxillary nerve in the pterygopalatine fossa. On the way, the palatine nerves are joined by **lateral nasal branches**, which are afferent nerves from the posterior nasal cavity.

Nasopalatine Nerve. The **nasopalatine nerve** (nay-zo-**pal**-uh-tine) or *NP nerve* originates in the mucosa of the anterior hard palate, palatal to the maxillary central incisors (see Figure 8-14). This nerve serves as an afferent nerve for the anterior hard palate and the associated palatal periodontium and gingiva of the maxillary anterior teeth bilaterally from maxillary canine to canine, as well as the nasal septal tissue.

Both the right and left NP nerves enter the incisive canal by way of the incisive foramen, located between the articulating palatine processes of the maxillae and deep to the incisive papilla, thus exiting the oral cavity (see Figures 2-15 and 3-48). The opening of the incisive foramen and overlying incisive papilla are both landmarks for the administration of the nasopalatine block that anesthetizes both the right and left NP nerves (see Figures 9-23 and 9-24 and Table 9-1).

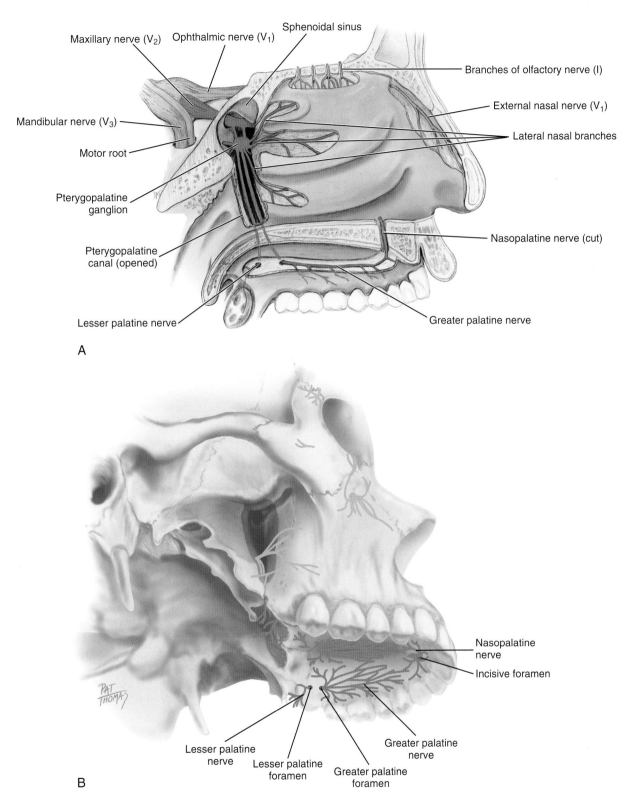

Maxillary nerve (V₂)   **Ophthalmic nerve (V₁)**   Sphenoidal sinus

Branches of olfactory nerve (I)

External nasal nerve (V₁)

Mandibular nerve (V₃)

Lateral nasal branches

Motor root

Pterygopalatine ganglion

Nasopalatine nerve (cut)

Pterygopalatine canal (opened)

Lesser palatine nerve

Greater palatine nerve

A

Nasopalatine nerve

Incisive foramen

Lesser palatine nerve

Lesser palatine foramen

Greater palatine nerve

Greater palatine foramen

B

FIGURE 8-14 Maxillary nerve and its palatine branches, which include the greater, lesser, and naso-palatine nerves, are highlighted from a medial view of the lateral nasal wall and opened pterygopalatine canal with the nasal septum removed, thus severing the nasopalatine nerve **(A)**. From an oblique lateral view of the skull and its hard palate **(B)**.

The NP nerves are also anesthetized with the anterior middle superior alveolar block along with other maxillary nerve branches using a palatal technique.

The NP nerve then travels along the nasal septum. Communication also occurs with the terminal fibers of the GP nerve in the associated palatal periodontium and gingiva of the maxillary canine, which may complicate the use of local anesthesia in the region (see Chapter 9).

Mandibular Nerve. The third nerve division or V₃ of the trigeminal nerve is the **mandibular nerve** (man-**dib**-u-luhr), which is a short main trunk formed by the merger of a smaller anterior trunk and a larger posterior trunk within the infratemporal fossa deep to the base of the skull, before the nerve passes through the foramen ovale of the sphenoid bone (Figures 8-15 to 8-17 and see Figure 3-32). The mandibular nerve then joins with the ophthalmic nerve and maxillary nerve to form the trigeminal ganglion of the trigeminal nerve. The mandibular nerve is the largest of the three nerve divisions that form the trigeminal nerve; the mandibular nerve is also a mixed nerve with both afferent and efferent nerves. Additionally, it contains the entire efferent part of the trigeminal nerve.

A few small branches arise from the V₃ trunk before its separation into the anterior and posterior trunks (see Figure 8-20). These branches from the undivided mandibular nerve include the **meningeal branches** (muh-**nin**-je-uhl), which are afferent nerves for parts of the dura mater. Also from the undivided mandibular nerve is the **medial pterygoid nerve** (**ter**-i-goid), which is an efferent nerve for the medial pterygoid and tensor veli palatini muscles as well as a muscle of the middle ear, the tensor tympani (see Figure 4-23).

Anterior Trunk of Mandibular Nerve. The anterior trunk or *anterior division* of the mandibular nerve is formed by the merger of the buccal nerve and additional muscular nerve branches (Figure 8-18). The anterior trunk has both afferent and efferent nerves.

Buccal Nerve. The **buccal nerve** (**buk**-uhl) (or long buccal nerve) serves as an afferent nerve for the skin of the cheek, buccal mucosa, as well as the associated buccal periodontium and gingiva of the mandibular molars. The buccal nerve is located on the surface of the

buccinator muscle (see Figures 4-11 and 8-17). The buccal nerve then travels posteriorly in the cheek, deep to the masseter muscle.

The buccal nerve then passes anteriorly to the anterior border of the mandibular ramus, distal and buccal to the most distal mandibular molar, and goes between the two heads of the lateral pterygoid

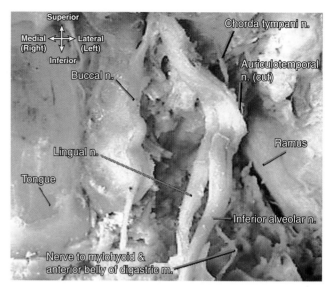

FIGURE 8-16 Dissection of the mandibular nerve of the trigeminal nerve. *(Courtesy of Jeremy S. Melker, MD.)*

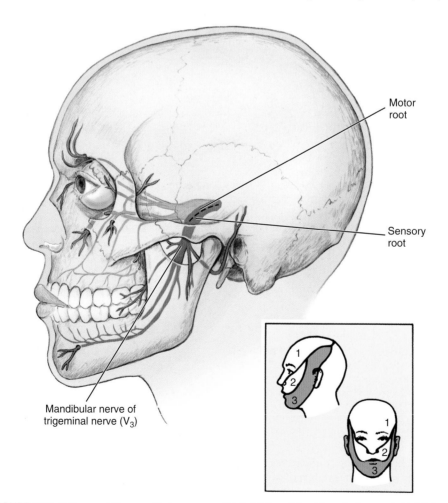

FIGURE 8-15 Pathway of the mandibular nerve or third division of the trigeminal nerve is highlighted; note the innervation coverage for the mandibular nerve *(see inset).*

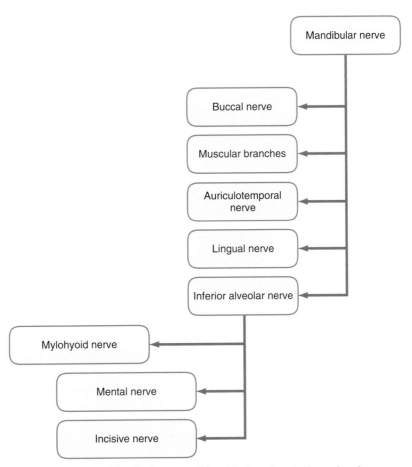

FIGURE 8-17 Mandibular nerve (V₃) and its branches to the oral cavity.

muscle to join the anterior trunk of V₃ (see Figure 8-18). The anterior border of the mandibular ramus is a landmark for the administration of the buccal block that anesthetizes the (long) buccal nerve (see Figures 9-39 and 9-41 and Table 9-1). The buccal nerve is also usually anesthetized with the Gow-Gates and Vazirani-Akinosi mandibular blocks along with other branches of the mandibular nerve (see Chapter 9). However, this nerve must not be confused with the buccal branch of the facial nerve, which is an efferent nerve that innervates the buccinator muscle.

Muscular Branches. Several muscular branches are part of the anterior trunk of V₃ (see Figures 8-17 and 8-18). They arise from the motor root of the trigeminal nerve. The **deep temporal nerves** (**tem**-puh-ruhl), usually two in number with both anterior and posterior nerves, are efferent nerves that pass between the sphenoid bone and the superior head of the lateral pterygoid muscle and turn around the infratemporal crest of the sphenoid bone to terminate in the deep surface of the temporalis muscle that they innervate (see Figure 4-22). The posterior deep temporal nerve may arise in common with the masseteric nerve, and the anterior deep temporal nerve may be associated at its origin with the buccal nerve.

The **masseteric nerve** (mass-i-**tare**-ik) is also an efferent nerve that passes between the sphenoid bone and the superior border of the lateral pterygoid muscle. The nerve then accompanies the masseteric blood vessels through the mandibular notch to innervate the masseter muscle (see Figure 4-19). A small sensory branch also goes to the temporomandibular joint. The **lateral pterygoid nerve**, after a short course, enters the deep surface of the lateral pterygoid muscle between the muscle's two heads of origin and serves as an efferent nerve for the lateral pterygoid muscle (see Figure 4-22).

Posterior Trunk of Mandibular Nerve. The posterior trunk or *posterior division* of the mandibular nerve is formed by the merger of the auriculotemporal, lingual, and inferior alveolar nerves (Figure 8-19). The posterior trunk has both afferent and efferent nerves.

Auriculotemporal Nerve. The **auriculotemporal nerve** (aw-**rik**-u-lo-**tem**-puh-ruhl) travels with the superficial temporal blood vessels and serves as an afferent nerve for the external ear, scalp, and temporomandibular joint (Figure 8-20 and see Figure 8-19). The nerve also carries postganglionic parasympathetic nerve fibers to the parotid salivary gland. Important to note is that these parasympathetic fibers arise from the lesser petrosal branch of the glossopharyngeal or ninth cranial nerve, joining the auriculotemporal nerve only after relaying in the otic ganglion near the foramen ovale.

Communication of the auriculotemporal nerve with the facial nerve near the ear also occurs. The auriculotemporal nerve courses deep to the lateral pterygoid muscle and neck of the mandible, then splits to encircle the middle meningeal artery, and finally joins the posterior trunk of V₃. The auriculotemporal nerve is anesthetized with the Gow-Gates mandibular block and also in some cases with the inferior alveolar block due to its proximity to the inferior alveolar nerve (see Figures 9-31 and 9-47).

Lingual Nerve. The **lingual nerve** (**ling**-gwuhl) is formed from afferent branches from the associated lingual periodontium and gingiva of mandibular teeth and from the body of the tongue. It first travels along the lateral surface of the tongue (see Figures 8-16 to 8-20). The nerve then passes posteriorly, passing from the medial to the lateral side of the duct of the submandibular salivary gland by going inferior to the duct.

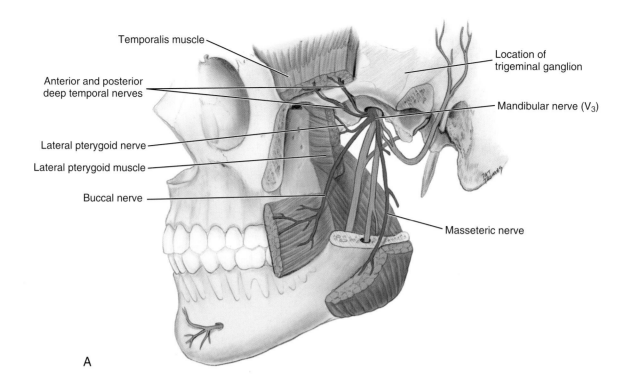

A

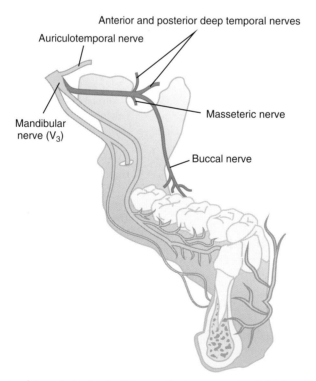

B

FIGURE 8-18 Pathway of the anterior trunk of the mandibular nerve or third division of the trigeminal nerve is highlighted from a lateral view **(A)** and from a medial view **(B)**.

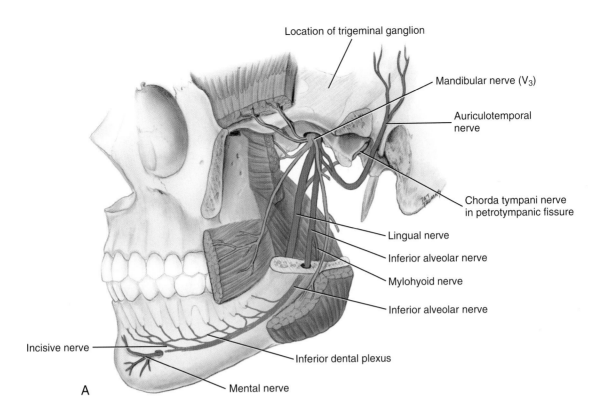

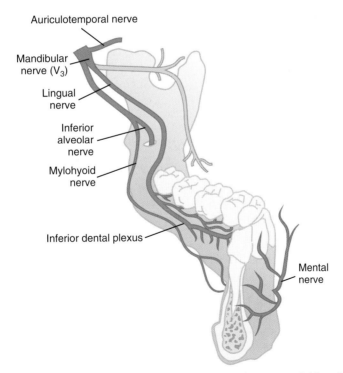

FIGURE 8-19 Pathway of the posterior trunk of the mandibular nerve or third division of the trigeminal nerve is highlighted from a lateral view **(A)** and from a medial view **(B)**.

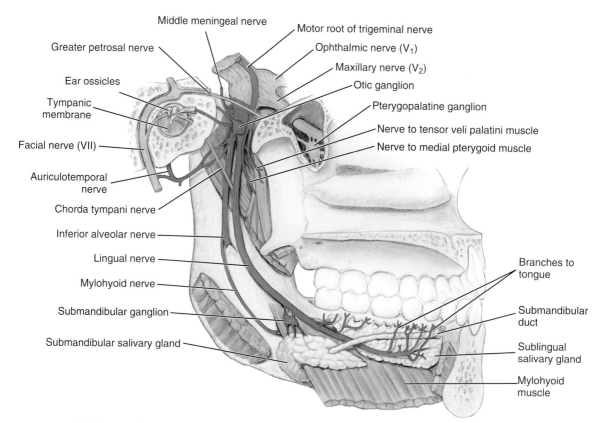

FIGURE 8-20 Medial view of the mandible with the motor and sensory branches of the mandibular nerve or third division highlighted.

The lingual nerve communicates with the **submandibular ganglion** (sub-man-**dib**-u-luhr) located superior to the deep lobe of the submandibular salivary gland (Figure 8-21 and see Figure 7-5). The submandibular ganglion is part of the parasympathetic system. Parasympathetic efferent innervation for the sublingual and submandibular salivary glands arises from the facial nerve (more specifically, the chorda tympani nerve, which is discussed later) but travels along with the lingual nerve (see Figure 8-21).

At the base of the tongue, the lingual nerve ascends and runs between the medial pterygoid muscle and the mandible, anterior and slightly medial to the inferior alveolar nerve. Thus the lingual nerve is anesthetized when administering an inferior alveolar block through diffusion of the local anesthetic agent within the pterygomandibular space (see Figures 9-31, 9-34, and 9-38). In addition, the Gow-Gates or Vazirani-Akinosi mandibular blocks can be used to anesthetize the lingual nerve along with other branches of the mandibular nerve (see Figure 9-47).

The lingual nerve is only a short distance posterior to the roots of the most distal mandibular molar and it can be endangered by dental procedures in this region such as the extraction of mandibular third molars and possibly trauma from local anesthetic injections.

The lingual nerve then continues to travel superiorly to join the posterior trunk of V₃. Thus the lingual nerve serves as an afferent nerve for general sensation for the body of the tongue, the floor of the mouth, and the associated lingual periodontium and gingiva of the mandibular teeth to the midline. Current thought has implicated most of the paresthesia of the mandible after local anesthesia administration with trauma to this nerve (see later discussion).

Inferior Alveolar Nerve. The **inferior alveolar nerve** or **IA nerve** is an afferent nerve formed from the merger of the mental nerve and

incisive nerve (see Figures 8-17 and 8-19). The mental and incisive nerves are discussed later in this section.

After forming from the merger of the two nerves, the IA nerve continues to travel posteriorly through the mandibular canal, along with the inferior alveolar artery and vein (see Figures 3-52 and 3-54). The IA nerve is joined by dental branches such as the interdental and interradicular branches from the surrounding periodontium to be part of the inferior dental plexus in the mandibular arch as discussed earlier.

The IA nerve then exits the mandible through the mandibular foramen, an opening of the mandibular canal on the medial surface of the mandibular ramus, in which also travels the inferior alveolar blood vessels. The IA nerve is then joined by the nearby mylohyoid nerve (discussed later). Although older sources give the location of the mandibular foramen as three-fourths along the mandibular ramus from the coronoid notch to the posterior border of the mandibular ramus, most recent research studies of skulls show the mandibular foramen position instead as approximately two-thirds the distance from the coronoid notch to the posterior border of the mandibular ramus, entirely within the pterygomandibular space; all these recent studies show that it is at least slightly posterior to the middle of the mandibular ramus (see Figure 11-8). The coronoid notch and pterygomandibular space are both oral landmarks for the administration of the inferior alveolar block due to their relationship to the mandibular foramen (see Figures 9-32 and 9-34 to 9-38 and Table 9-1).

The IA nerve then travels lateral to the medial pterygoid muscle, between the sphenomandibular ligament and mandibular ramus; this is posterior and slightly lateral to the lingual nerve. The IA nerve along

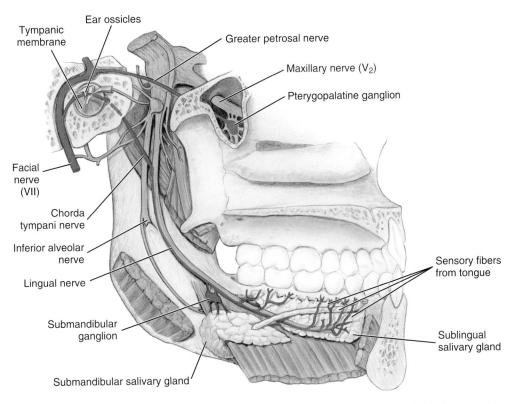

Tympanic membrane
Ear ossicles
Greater petrosal nerve
Maxillary nerve (V₂)
Pterygopalatine ganglion
Facial nerve (VII)
Chorda tympani nerve
Inferior alveolar nerve
Lingual nerve
Sensory fibers from tongue
Submandibular ganglion
Sublingual salivary gland
Submandibular salivary gland

FIGURE 8-21 Pathway of the trunk of the facial nerve, greater petrosal nerve, and chorda tympani nerve are highlighted; note relationship of the chorda tympani nerve with lingual nerve.

with the lingual nerve is anesthetized by the inferior alveolar block within the pterygomandibular space (see Figure 9-30).

The IA nerve then joins the posterior trunk of V₃ (see Figures 8-16, 8-19, and 8-20). The IA nerve carries afferent innervation for the mandibular teeth and associated facial periodontium and gingiva of the mandibular anterior teeth and premolars as well as labial mucosa through its incisive and mental branches to the midline. In addition, both the Gow-Gates or Vazirani-Akinosi mandibular blocks can be used to anesthetize the IA nerve along with other branches of the mandibular nerve at differing sites on the mandible (see Figure 9-47 and Table 9-1).

In some cases there are two nerves present on one side, creating bifid IA nerves. This situation can occur unilaterally or bilaterally and can be detected on a radiograph by the presence of a double mandibular canal. As discussed in Chapter 3, there can be more than one mandibular foramen, usually inferiorly placed, either unilaterally or bilaterally, along with the bifid IA nerves. These variations must be kept in mind when administering local anesthesia for the mandibular teeth and associated tissue (see Chapter 9).

Mental Nerve. The **mental nerve** (**men**-tuhl) is composed of external branches that serve as afferent nerves for the chin, lower lip, and labial mucosa as well as the associated facial periodontium and gingiva of the mandibular anterior teeth and premolars to the midline (see Figure 8-19 and Table 9-1). The mental nerve then enters the mental foramen on the lateral surface of the mandible, usually inferior to the apices of the mandibular premolars, in which the mental blood vessels also travel (see Figure 6-9). Palpation of the mental foramen during an extraoral examination or before an administration of a local anesthetic agent will cause transient soreness to the area due to the presence of the nerve (see Figure 9-44).

The opening of the mental foramen is a landmark for the administration of the mental block that anesthetizes the mental nerve. In addition, the inferior alveolar block, Gow-Gates mandibular block, or Vazirani-Akinosi mandibular block can be used to anesthetize the mental nerve along with other branches of the mandibular nerve from other target injection sites (see Figure 9-47).

After entering via the mental foramen and traveling a distance within the mandibular canal, the mental nerve merges with the incisive nerve to form the IA nerve within the mandibular canal but before the IA nerve exits by way of the mandibular canal (see Figures 3-52 and 3-54).

Incisive Nerve. The **incisive nerve** (in-**sy**-siv) is an afferent nerve composed of dental branches from the mandibular anterior teeth and premolars that originate in the pulp, exit the teeth through the apical foramina, and join with interdental branches from the surrounding periodontium to be part of the inferior dental plexus in the mandibular arch in the region as discussed earlier (see Figure 8-19). The incisive nerve serves as an afferent nerve for the mandibular anterior teeth and premolars and associated facial periodontium and gingiva to the midline (see Table 9-1).

The incisive nerve travels along with the incisive blood vessels (see Figure 6-9) within the mandibular incisive canal, which is an anterior continuation of the mandibular canal that runs bilaterally from the mental foramen usually to the region of the ipsilateral lateral incisor teeth. The incisive nerve then merges with the mental nerve, just posterior to the mental foramen. The incisive nerve either terminates as nerve endings within the mandibular anterior teeth or adjacent lingual cortical bone and soft tissue.

The mental foramen, as was discussed with the mental nerve, is usually located inferior to the apices of the mandibular premolars on the lateral surface of the mandible. Tiny lingual foramina are usually located on the medial side of the mandible inferior to the apices of the mandibular central incisors at the midline. Both the mental and lingual foramina can be noted on certain radiographs. The incisive nerve is anesthetized by the incisive block and has the same landmark as the mental block, the opening of the mental foramen (see Figures 9-43, 9-45, 9-46, and 9-47). The incisive nerve continues on to form the IA nerve within the mandibular canal before the IA nerve exits the mandibular canal (see Figures 3-52 and 3-54).

Crossover-innervation from the contralateral incisive nerve can also occur, which is an important consideration when administering local anesthesia for the mandibular anterior teeth and premolars and associated tissue (see Chapter 9). In addition, the incisive nerve can be anesthetized by the inferior alveolar block and either the Gow-Gates or Vazirani-Akinosi mandibular blocks, along with other branches of the mandibular nerve.

Mylohyoid Nerve. After the inferior alveolar nerve exits the mandibular foramen, a small branch occurs, the **mylohyoid nerve** (my-lo-**hi**-oid) (see Figures 4-25 and 8-16 to 8-20). This nerve pierces the sphenomandibular ligament and runs inferiorly and anteriorly in the mylohyoid groove and then onto the inferior surface of the mylohyoid muscle. The mylohyoid nerve serves as an efferent nerve to the mylohyoid muscle and anterior belly of the digastric muscle (the posterior belly of the digastric muscle is innervated by a branch from the facial nerve).

However, the mylohyoid nerve may in some cases also serve as an afferent nerve for the mandibular first molar, which needs to be considered when there is lack of clinical effectiveness of the inferior alveolar block (see Chapter 9). If there is concern, the mylohyoid nerve can be additionally anesthetized by administering a supraperiosteal injection for the tooth on the medial border of the mandible, or possibly a periodontal ligament injection directly into the periodontium of the tooth. The mylohyoid nerve is also anesthetized by either the Gow-Gates or Vazirani-Akinosi mandibular blocks along with other branches of the mandibular nerve (see Figure 9-47).

Clinical Consideration With Trigeminal Nerve Pathology

A dental professional needs to have an understanding of nervous system pathology associated with the head and neck. These lesions include the pathology that can occur to the trigeminal nerve such as trigeminal neuralgia.

Trigeminal neuralgia (TN) or *tic douloureux* also has no known etiology but involves the afferent nerve of the fifth cranial or trigeminal nerve. It usually unilaterally involves either the maxillary or mandibular nerve branches but not the ophthalmic branch. One theory is that this lesion is caused by pressure on the sensory root of the trigeminal ganglion by area blood vessels.

The patient may feel excruciating short-term pain on one side of the face when facial trigger zones are touched or even when speaking or masticating, setting off associated brief muscle spasms or tics in the area. These trigger zones vary among patients but can include areas around each eye or the ala of the nose. The right side of the face, along with its regions and structures, is affected more commonly than the left side. The pattern of pain follows along the pathway of the fifth cranial or trigeminal nerve branch involved.

Treatment for trigeminal neuralgia can include peripheral neurectomy by surgery or ultrasonic treatment in which the sensory root of the trigeminal nerve is sectioned, cutting off innervation to the tissue. Injection of the trigeminal nerve with various chemicals has also been used to cause necrosis of the nerve, as have systemic antidepressant and anticonvulsant drugs, with varying degrees of success.

FACIAL NERVE

The dental professional must also have an understanding of the seventh (VII) cranial or facial nerve. It carries both efferent and afferent nerves. The facial nerve emerges from the brain and enters the internal acoustic meatus in the petrous part of the temporal bone (see Figure 3-19). Within the temporal bone, the nerve gives off a small efferent branch to a muscle in the middle ear (stapedius) and two larger branches, the greater petrosal and chorda tympani nerves, both of which carry parasympathetic fibers (see Figure 8-21).

The main trunk of the facial nerve emerges from the skull through the stylomastoid foramen of the temporal bone and gives off two branches, the posterior auricular nerve and a branch to the posterior belly of the digastric muscle and stylohyoid muscle (Figure 8-22 and see Figure 3-31, *A*).

The facial nerve then passes into the parotid salivary gland and divides the gland into superficial and deep lobes. The trunk of the facial nerve itself divides into numerous branches to supply the muscles of facial expression (discussed in depth later), but does not innervate the parotid salivary gland itself (see Figure 7-2). Avoiding anesthesia of this nerve at this location within the parotid salivary gland is important when administering an inferior alveolar block or Vazirani-Akinosi mandibular block because it may result in transient facial paralysis if administered incorrectly (discussed later and see Figures 9-37 and 9-56). In addition, a neoplastic growth in the parotid salivary gland may be painful due to the presence of this nerve or cause facial paralysis (see Chapter 7).

GREATER PETROSAL NERVE

The **greater petrosal nerve** (puh-**troh**-suhl) is a branch off the facial nerve before it exits the skull (see Figure 8-21). The greater petrosal nerve carries efferent nerve fibers, which are preganglionic parasympathetic fibers to the pterygopalatine ganglion in the pterygopalatine fossa (see Figure 3-61).

The postganglionic fibers arising in the pterygopalatine ganglion then join with branches of the maxillary nerve of the trigeminal nerve to be carried to the lacrimal gland (via the zygomatic and lacrimal nerves), nasal cavity, and minor salivary glands of the hard and soft palate. The greater petrosal nerve also carries afferent nerve fibers for taste sensation in the palate.

CHORDA TYMPANI NERVE

This small branch of the facial nerve, the **chorda tympani nerve** (**kor**-duh **tim**-pan-ee), is a parasympathetic efferent nerve for the submandibular and sublingual salivary glands and also serves as an afferent nerve for taste sensation for the anterior two-thirds of the body of the tongue (see Figures 8-19 to 8-21).

After branching off the facial nerve within the petrous part of the temporal bone, the chorda tympani nerve crosses the medial surface of the tympanic membrane (eardrum), and then exits the skull by the petrotympanic fissure, located immediately posterior to the temporomandibular joint (see Figure 3-30). The chorda tympani nerve then travels with the lingual nerve along the floor of the mouth in the same nerve bundle.

In the submandibular triangle, the chorda tympani nerve, appearing as part of the lingual nerve, has communication with the submandibular ganglion. The submandibular ganglion is located superior to the deep lobe of the submandibular salivary gland, for which it supplies parasympathetic efferent innervation (see Figures 7-5 and 8-21).

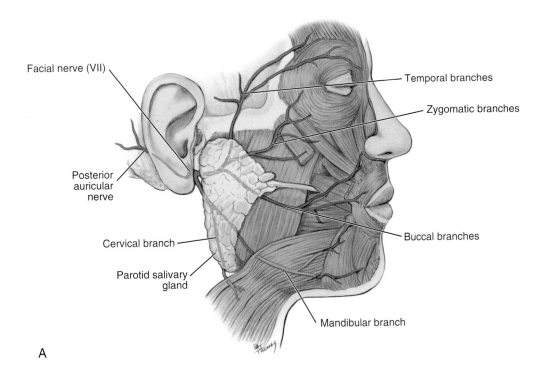

A

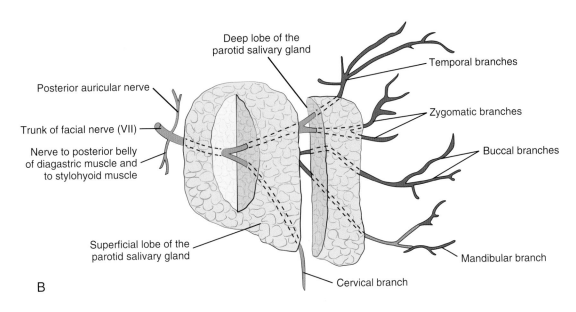

B

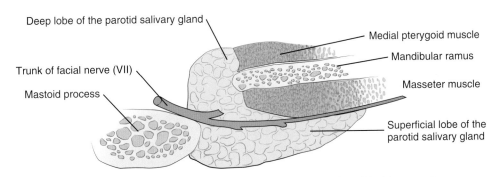

C

FIGURE 8-22 Pathway of the branches of the facial nerve to the muscles of facial expression are highlighted: lateral view with branches designated **(A)**, lateral view with parotid salivary gland sectioned **(B)**, and transverse section showing the superficial and deep lobes of the parotid salivary gland divided by the trunk of the facial nerve **(C)**.

POSTERIOR AURICULAR, STYLOHYOID, AND POSTERIOR DIGASTRIC NERVES

The **posterior auricular nerve** (aw-**rik**-u-luhr), **stylohyoid nerve** (sty-lo-**hi**-oid), and **posterior digastric nerve** (di-**gas**-trik) are branches of the facial nerve after it exits the stylomastoid foramen. All are efferent nerves. The posterior auricular nerve supplies the occipital belly of the epicranial muscle (see Figure 8-22). The other two nerves supply the stylohyoid muscle and the posterior belly of the digastric muscle, respectively.

BRANCHES TO MUSCLES OF FACIAL EXPRESSION

Additional efferent nerve branches of the facial nerve originate within the parotid salivary gland and pass to the muscles they innervate (see Figures 4-5 and 8-22). These branches to the muscles of facial expression include: the temporal, zygomatic, buccal, (marginal) mandibular, and cervical branches. However, these branches are rarely seen as five independent nerves; they may vary in number and connect irregularly. For convenience when studying, they are described as five simple branches.

The temporal branches supply the muscles anterior to the ear, frontal belly of the epicranial muscle, superior part of the orbicularis oculi muscle, and corrugator supercilii muscle.

The zygomatic branches supply the inferior part of the orbicularis oculi muscle and zygomatic major and minor muscles. The buccal branches supply the muscles of the upper lip and nose and buccinator, risorius, and orbicularis oris muscles. The zygomatic and buccal branches are usually closely associated, exchanging many fibers.

The (marginal) mandibular branch supplies the muscles of the lower lip and mentalis muscle. The mandibular branch should not be confused with the mandibular nerve or V₃. The cervical branch runs inferior to the mandible to supply the platysma muscle.

Clinical Considerations With Facial Nerve Pathology

A dental professional needs to have an understanding of nervous system pathology associated with the head and neck. This includes pathology that can occur to the facial nerve, such as facial paralysis and Bell palsy.

Facial paralysis is the loss of muscular action of the muscles of facial expression (see **Chapter 4**). This lesion can occur secondary to a brain injury by way of a stroke (cerebrovascular accident), with other muscles of the head and neck also affected. The lesion can also occur by directly injuring the nerve that supplies the efferent nerves to the muscles of facial expression, the seventh cranial or facial nerve. Facial paralysis can be unilateral or bilateral as well as transient or permanent depending on the nature of the nerve damage. These injuries can occur because the facial nerve branches are superficially located and vulnerable to trauma.

Transient facial paralysis can occur due to injection into the parotid salivary gland during an incorrectly administered inferior alveolar block or Vazirani-Akinosi mandibular block as discussed earlier (see Figures 9-37 and 9-56). The affected facial muscles temporarily lose tone on the involved side; the patient has a drooping eyebrow, eyelid, and labial commissure, with a dribbling of saliva as a result. There is also an inability to show normal expression, close the eye, or whistle on that same side. As a result, there can be secondary infection in the involved eye; speech and mastication are also difficult. The usual levels of muscle

---

Clinical Considerations With Facial Nerve Pathology—cont'd

movement and associated sensation return after a few hours unless there are further complications.

Bell palsy involves unilateral facial paralysis with no known cause, except that there is a loss of excitability of the involved facial nerve (see Figure 4-6). All or just some of the branches of the facial nerve may be affected. The onset of this paralysis is abrupt, and most symptoms reach the peak in two days. One theory of its cause is that the facial nerve becomes inflamed within the temporal bone, possibly with a viral etiology. Bell palsy may undergo remission or may become chronic depending on the amount of loss of facial nerve excitability. No specific treatment exists, but early injections of antiinflammatory or antiviral medications or physical therapy may be helpful.

The injury to the facial nerve can occur secondary to injury to the parotid salivary gland or surrounding region. If cancer (malignant neoplasm) occurs within the parotid salivary gland, the facial nerve can be injured because it travels through the gland. During facial surgery or due to a laceration (deep wound) to the parotid salivary gland region, the facial nerve within the tissue can also be traumatized (see **Chapter 7**).

REVIEW QUESTIONS

1. The brainstem of the central nervous system consists of which of the following structures?
   A. Cerebrum, cerebellum, pons, and medulla
   B. Medulla, cerebrum, midbrain, and pons
   C. Medulla, pons, and midbrain
   D. Midbrain, ganglia, and nerves
2. The central nervous system consists of which two of the following structures?
   A. Spinal cord and peripheral nervous system
   B. Brain and spinal cord alone
   C. Autonomic and somatic nervous systems
   D. Brain and autonomic nervous system
3. Which of the following is a CORRECT statement concerning neurotransmitters within the nervous system?
   A. Discharged with the arrival of the action potential
   B. Bind to red blood cells so as to prompt transmission of impulses
   C. Can initiate an action potential in an adjacent cell if inhibitory
   D. Destroyed by specific white blood cells while still active
4. To what division of the nervous system does a nerve cell belong if it leads from the eye to the brain carrying visual information?
   A. Central nervous system
   B. Medulla and pons
   C. Afferent nervous system
   D. Efferent nervous system
5. An efferent nerve with the nervous system is known to carry information
   A. from the periphery of the body to the brain or spinal cord.
   B. such as taste or pain to the spinal cord.
   C. such as proprioception to the brain.
   D. away from the brain or spinal cord to the periphery of the body.
6. Which of the following structures do the posterior superior alveolar nerve and its branches innervate?
   A. Frontal sinus
   B. Maxillary molars
   C. Parotid salivary gland
   D. Temporalis muscle

7. Through which of the following foramina does the facial nerve pass through the skull?
   A. Foramen rotundum
   B. Foramen ovale
   C. Jugular foramen
   D. Stylomastoid foramen
8. Which of the following cranial nerves is DIRECTLY involved in Bell palsy?
   A. Trigeminal nerve
   B. Facial nerve
   C. Glossopharyngeal nerve
   D. Vagus nerve
9. Which of the following nerve and muscle pairs is a CORRECT match?
   A. Long buccal nerve, buccinator muscle
   B. Accessory nerve, platysma muscle
   C. Hypoglossal nerve, intrinsic tongue muscles
   D. Auriculotemporal nerve, temporalis muscle
10. Which of the following nerve and innervation pairs is a CORRECT match?
    A. Facial nerve, parotid salivary gland
    B. Chorda tympani nerve, sublingual salivary gland
    C. Vagus nerve, temporomandibular joint
    D. Lingual nerve, base of tongue
11. Which of the following cranial nerves has fibers that provide crossover-innervation to the contralateral side in the skull before continuing into the brain?
    A. Facial nerve
    B. Optic nerve
    C. Trochlear nerve
    D. Vestibulocochlear nerve
12. Which of the following cranial nerves carries taste sensation for the base of the tongue?
    A. Trigeminal nerve
    B. Facial nerve
    C. Vagus nerve
    D. Glossopharyngeal nerve
13. In which of the following regions of the head and neck is the trigeminal ganglion located?
    A. Superior to the deep lobe of the submandibular salivary gland
    B. Anterior surface of the petrous part of the temporal bone
    C. Posterior surface of the maxillary tuberosity of the maxilla
    D. Anterior to the infraorbital foramen of the maxilla
14. Which of the following nerves supplies sensory information for the soft palate?
    A. Greater palatine nerve
    B. Lesser palatine nerve
    C. Nasopalatine nerve
    D. Posterior alveolar nerve
15. Which of the following nerves has branches that innervate the posterior belly of the digastric muscle?
    A. Facial
    B. Mylohyoid
    C. Buccal (long)
    D. Maxillary
16. Which of the following nerves within orofacial regions may show crossover-innervation from the contralateral side in a patient?
    A. Posterior superior alveolar nerve
    B. Anterior superior alveolar nerve
    C. Posterior auricular nerve
    D. Buccal nerve

17. Which of the following nerves listed below is considered part of the ophthalmic nerve?
    A. Nasociliary nerve
    B. Maxillary nerve
    C. Zygomaticotemporal nerve
    D. Zygomaticofacial nerve
18. Which of the following anatomic names is also used for cranial nerve X?
    A. Hypoglossal nerve
    B. Vagus nerve
    C. Glossopharyngeal nerve
    D. Accessory nerve
19. Which of the following nerves is located within the mandibular canal?
    A. Lingual nerve
    B. Mylohyoid nerve
    C. Inferior alveolar nerve
    D. Masseteric nerve
20. Which of the following nerves exits the foramen ovale of the sphenoid bone?
    A. Chorda tympani of the facial nerve
    B. Greater petrosal nerve of the facial nerve
    C. Ophthalmic nerve of the trigeminal nerve
    D. Motor root of the trigeminal nerve
21. Which of the following cranial nerves and its motor function is involved in pathology when a patient protrudes the tongue and a deviation to the right side is noted?
    A. V
    B. VII
    C. X
    D. XII
22. Which of the following nerves exits the skull through the foramen ovale?
    A. Facial
    B. Ophthalmic
    C. Maxillary
    D. Mandibular
    E. Glossopharyngeal
23. Which of the following nerves serves the pulp of the mandibular molars?
    A. Lingual nerve
    B. (Long) buccal nerve
    C. Mental nerve
    D. Incisive nerve
    E. Inferior alveolar nerve
24. Which of the following is considered the loss of feeling or sensation resulting from the use of certain drugs or gases that serve as inhibitory neurotransmitters?
    A. Paresthesia
    B. Bell palsy
    C. Trigeminal neuralgia
    D. Anesthesia
25. Which nerve may in some cases also serve as an afferent nerve for the mandibular first molar and needs to be considered when there is failure of the inferior alveolar local anesthetic block?
    A. Mylohyoid nerve
    B. Posterior superior alveolar nerve
    C. Anterior middle superior alveolar nerve
    D. Glossopharyngeal nerve

Identification Exercises

Identify the structures on the following diagrams by filling in each blank with the correct anatomic term. You can check your answers by looking back at the figure indicated in parentheses for each identification diagram.

1. (Figure 8-4, *A*)

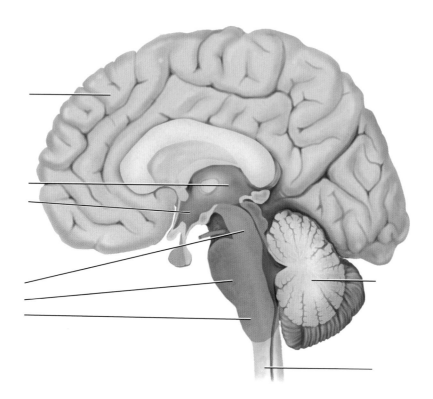

2. (Figure 8-5)

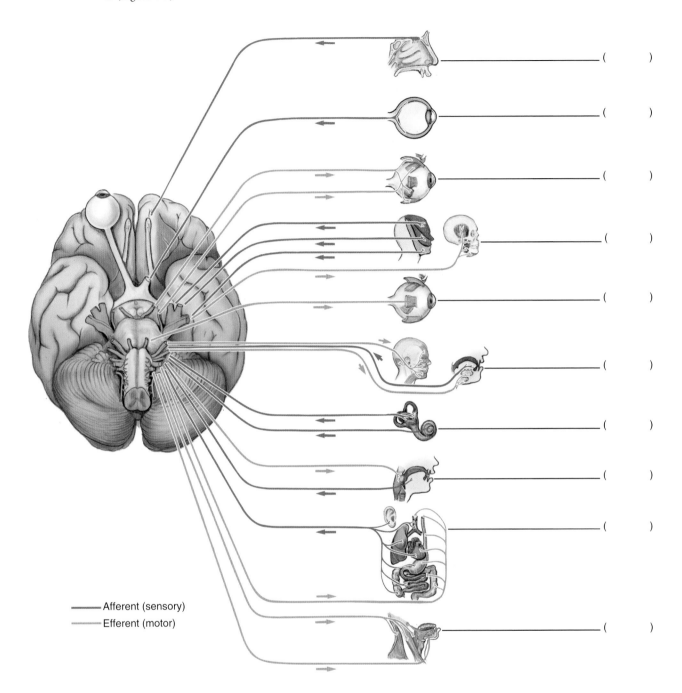

3. (Figure 8-6)

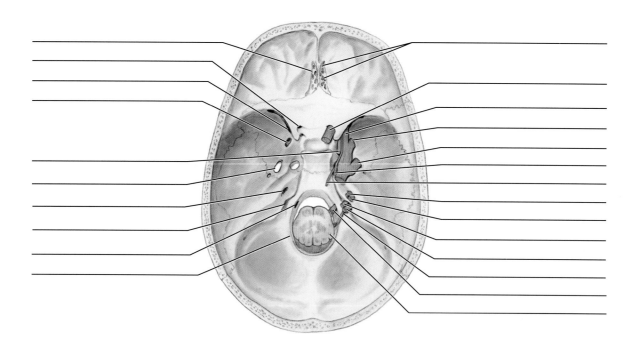

4. (Figures 8-8 and 8-11)

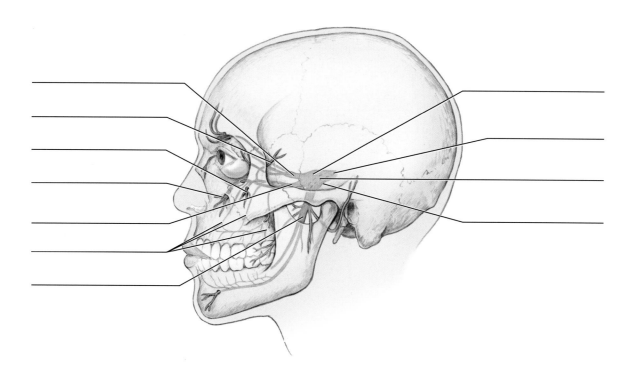

5. (Figure 8-13)

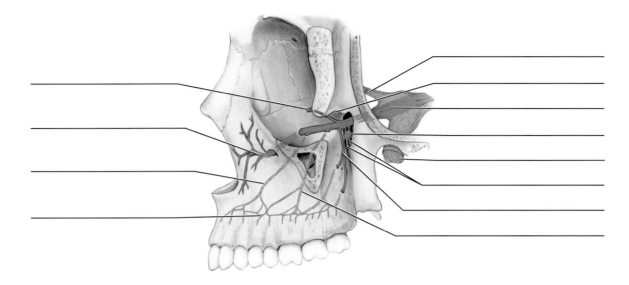

6. (Figure 8-14, *A*)

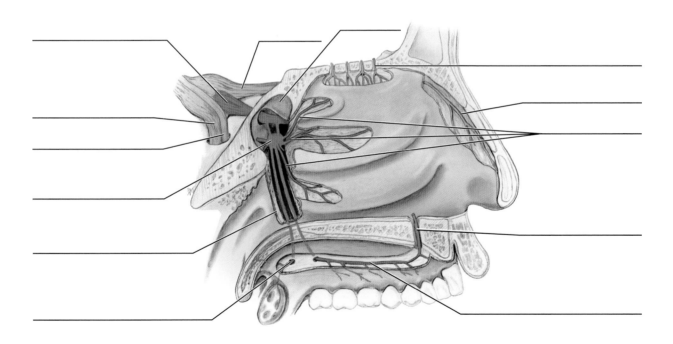

7. (Figure 8-18, *A*)

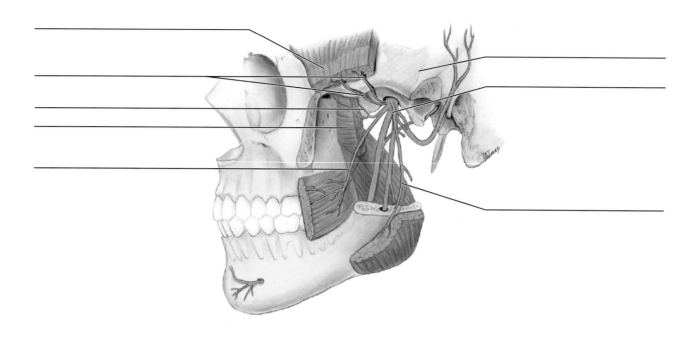

8. (Figure 8-19, *A*)

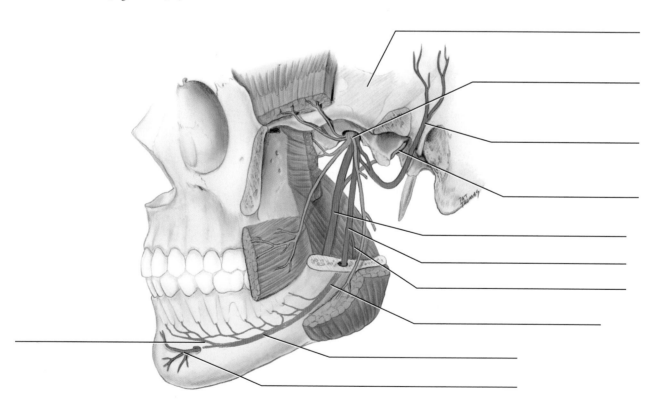

9. (Figure 8-20)

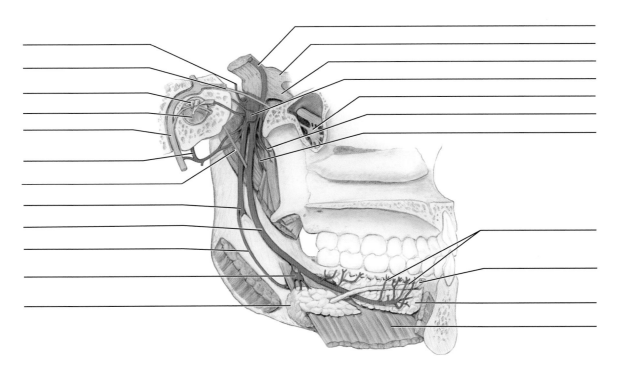

10. (Figure 8-21)

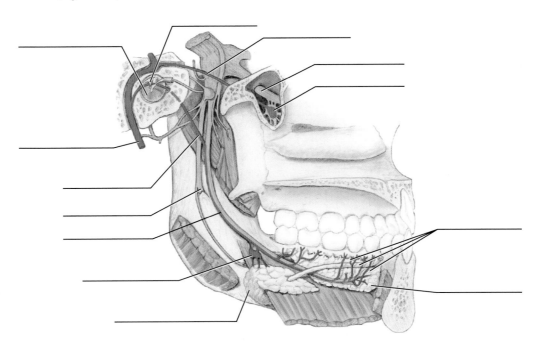

CHAPTER 9

Anatomy of Local Anesthesia

●●● LEARNING OBJECTIVES

1. Define and pronounce the **key terms** and **anatomic terms** in this chapter.
2. List the tissue and structures anesthetized by each type of local anesthetic injection and describe the related target areas.
3. Locate and identify the anatomic structures used to determine injection site for the needle for each type of local anesthetic injection on a skull and a patient.
4. Demonstrate the correct placement for the needle for each type of local anesthetic injection on a skull and a patient.
5. Identify the tissue involved during the insertion of the needle for each type of local anesthetic injection.
6. Discuss the indications of clinically effective anesthesia and possible complications associated with anatomic considerations for each type of injection.
7. Correctly complete the review questions and activities for this chapter.
8. Integrate an understanding of the anatomy of the trigeminal nerve and associated tissue into the administration of local anesthesia in clinical dental practice.

●●● KEY TERMS

Nerve block Injection that anesthetizes larger area than supraperiosteal injection because local anesthetic agent is deposited near larger nerve trunks.

Paresthesia (pare-es-**thee**-zhuh) Abnormal sensation of burning or prickling from an area.

Supraperiosteal injection (**soo**-pruh-**pare**-e-os-te-uhl) Injection that anesthetizes small area because local anesthetic agent is deposited near terminal nerve endings.

ANATOMIC CONSIDERATIONS FOR LOCAL ANESTHESIA

The management of pain through local anesthesia by dental professionals requires a thorough understanding of the anatomy of the skull, trigeminal nerve, and related structures. This chapter discusses the anatomic considerations for local anesthesia. Dental professionals will also want to refer to a current textbook on the administration of local anesthesia in dentistry for more information on actual clinical technique (see Appendix A).

The skull bones involved in local anesthetic administration are the maxilla, palatine bone, and mandible since the bones serve as hard tissue landmarks (see Chapter 3). Soft tissue structures of the face and oral cavity may serve as initial landmarks for the dental professional to visualize and palpate for local anesthesia (see Chapter 2). However, there can be variations in soft tissue anatomic topography among patients. Thus, to increase the reliability of local anesthesia procedures, the dental professional must learn to rely mainly on both visualization and palpation of hard tissue structures as landmarks when injecting patients.

The dental professional must also know the location of certain adjacent soft tissue structures, such as major blood vessels and glandular tissue, so as to avoid inadvertently injecting them (see Chapters 6 and 7, respectively). If certain soft tissue structures are accidentally injected with local anesthetic agent, complications may occur. Infections may also be spread to deeper tissue by needle tract contamination (see Chapter 12).

The trigeminal or fifth cranial nerve provides sensory information for the teeth and associated tissue (see Chapter 8). Thus the branches of the trigeminal nerve that are anesthetized before most possibly painful dental procedures include: the maxillary nerve and mandibular nerve. Understanding the location of these nerve branches in relation to the skull bones, as well as soft tissue, increases the reliability of each injection. Local anesthesia with a vasoconstrictor added to the agent can also provide hemostatic control of the area as well as prolong anesthesia during dental treatment.

Two types of local anesthetic injections are used commonly in dentistry: a supraperiosteal injection and a nerve block. The type of injection used for a given dental procedure is determined by the type and length of the procedure.

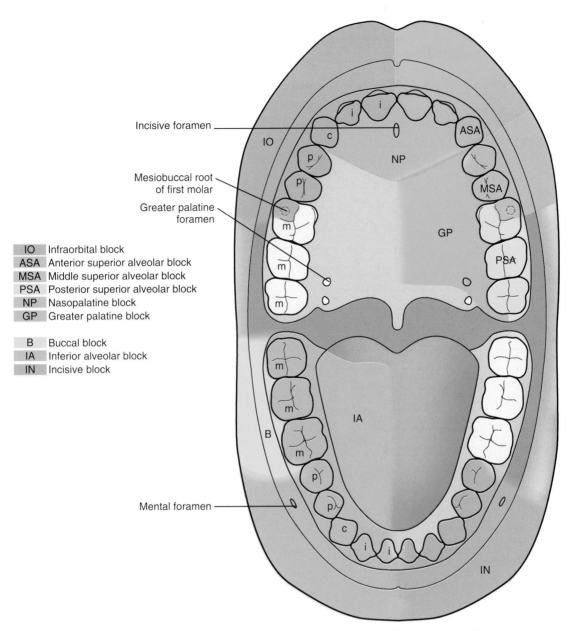

Incisive foramen

IO

i i

c

ASA

NP

p

p

MSA

Mesiobuccal root of first molar

Greater palatine foramen

m

GP

m

PSA

m

IO	Infraorbital block
ASA	Anterior superior alveolar block
MSA	Middle superior alveolar block
PSA	Posterior superior alveolar block
NP	Nasopalatine block
GP	Greater palatine block

B	Buccal block
IA	Inferior alveolar block
IN	Incisive block

m

m

IA

B

m

p

Mental foramen

p

c

i i

IN

FIGURE 9-1 Local anesthetic nerve blocks with the related structures that are anesthetized. Note that the anterior middle superior alveolar, the mental, and the Gow-Gates or Vazirani-Akinosi mandibular blocks are not included; see associated figures for clarification of these nerve blocks.

Supraperiosteal injection or *local infiltration* in dentistry anesthetizes a small area, usually one or two teeth and associated structures, by injection near the apices of the teeth. For this type of local anesthetic injection, the local anesthetic agent is deposited near terminal nerve endings. This localized deposition has varying degrees of clinical effectiveness depending on the anatomy of the region and the nearby presence of localized inflammation or infection. Additional injections and larger amounts of agent would need to be administered for anesthesia of the teeth and associated structures within a quadrant.

Nerve block in dentistry usually affects a larger area of anesthesia than a supraperiosteal injection and thus additional teeth. With the nerve block, the local anesthetic agent is deposited near larger nerve trunks. This generalized deposition has an increased level of clinical effectiveness when compared to a supraperiosteal injection and it can

be administered a distance away from localized inflammation or infection. Fewer injections and lesser amounts of agent can be used for anesthesia of the teeth and associated structures within a quadrant. This chapter mainly discusses this type of injection with its more complex anatomic basis (Figure 9-1 and Tables 9-1 to 9-3).

The proper amount of local anesthetic agent should always be used because there will be a possible lack of clinical effectiveness of the anesthesia if too little agent is used. This is commonly noted in the patient who may have large teeth with unusually long roots. The bone of the alveolar process surrounding the roots may also be excessively thick in a patient, resulting in a need for an increased volume of agent.

It is important to not start the dental treatment before the local anesthetic agent can take effect. This is a particular consideration with injections for the mandibular arch due to the anatomy of the nerve

Text continued on p. 210

TABLE 9-1	Summary of Local Anesthesia of the Maxillary Teeth and Associated Structures*						
MAXILLARY TOOTH AND TISSUE ANESTHETIZED	**ASA BLOCK**	**MSA BLOCK**	**PSA BLOCK**	**IO BLOCK**	**NP BLOCK**	**GP BLOCK**	**AMSA BLOCK**
Central Incisor							
Pulp with labial periodontium and gingiva	X			X			X
Palatal periodontium and gingiva					X		X
Lateral Incisor							
Pulp with labial periodontium and gingiva	X			X			X
Palatal periodontium and gingiva					X		X
Canine							
Pulp with labial periodontium and gingiva	X			X			X
Palatal periodontium and gingiva					X		X
First Premolar							
Pulp with buccal periodontium and gingiva		X		X			X
Palatal periodontium and gingiva						X	X
Second Premolar							
Pulp with buccal periodontium and gingiva		X		X			X
Palatal periodontium and gingiva						X	X
First Molar							
Pulp with buccal periodontium and gingiva			X				
Palatal periodontium and gingiva						X	
Second Molar							
Pulp with buccal periodontium and gingiva			X				
Palatal periodontium and gingiva						X	
Third Molar							
Pulp with buccal periodontium and gingiva			X				
Palatal periodontium and gingiva						X	

*The anesthesia for anatomic variants such as the absence of the middle superior alveolar nerve and the resultant variance of the mesiobuccal root of the maxillary first molar is not included.
AMSA, Anterior middle superior alveolar; *ASA,* anterior superior alveolar; *GP,* greater palatine; *IO,* infraorbital; *MSA,* middle superior alveolar; *NP,* nasopalatine; *PSA,* posterior superior alveolar.

TABLE 9-2	Summary of Local Anesthesia of the Mandibular Teeth and Associated Tissue*			
MANDIBULAR TOOTH AND TISSUE ANESTHETIZED	**IA BLOCK**	**BUCCAL BLOCK**	**MENTAL BLOCK**	**INCISIVE BLOCK**
Central Incisor				
Pulpal	X			X
Labial periodontium and gingiva	X		X	X
Lingual periodontium and gingiva	X			
Lateral Incisor				
Pulpal	X			X
Labial periodontium and gingiva	X		X	X
Lingual periodontium and gingiva	X			
Canine				
Pulpal	X			X
Labial periodontium and gingiva	X		X	X
Lingual periodontium and gingiva	X			

TABLE 9-2	Summary of Local Anesthesia of the Mandibular Teeth and Associated Tissue—cont'd			
MANDIBULAR TOOTH AND TISSUE ANESTHETIZED	**IA BLOCK**	**BUCCAL BLOCK**	**MENTAL BLOCK**	**INCISIVE BLOCK**
First Premolar				
Pulpal	X			X
Buccal periodontium and gingiva	X		X	X
Lingual periodontium and gingiva	X			
Second Premolar				
Pulpal	X			X
Buccal periodontium and gingiva	X		X	X
Lingual periodontium and gingiva	X			
First Molar				
Pulpal with lingual periodontium and gingiva	X			
Buccal periodontium and gingiva		X		
Second Molar				
Pulpal with lingual periodontium and gingiva	X			
Buccal periodontium and gingiva		X		
Third Molar				
Pulpal with lingual periodontium and gingiva	X			
Buccal periodontium and gingiva		X		

*The anesthesia for anatomic variants and coverage of the Gow-Gates or Vazirani-Akinosi mandibular blocks are not included since many branches of the mandibular nerve are anesthetized.
IA, Inferior alveolar.

TABLE 9-3	Review of Local Anesthesia of the Dentition and Related Structures		
	MAXILLARY ANESTHESIA		
NERVES, TEETH, AND RELATED STRUCTURES ANESTHETIZED	**LANDMARKS**	**TARGET AREA**	**INJECTION SITE**
PSA Block			
Nerves Posterior superior alveolar **Teeth** Maxillary molars in most cases; mesiobuccal root not anesthetized in approximately 28% of cases **Other Structures** Buccal periodontium and gingiva of anesthetized teeth and buccal mucosa and upper lip	Maxillary tuberosity, posterior superior alveolar foramina, maxillary mucobuccal fold, maxillary second molar, zygomatic process of maxilla, maxillary occlusal plane	Posterior superior alveolar nerve branches entering posterior superior alveolar foramina on infratemporal surface of maxilla; posterosuperior on maxillary tuberosity	Height of maxillary mucobuccal fold superior to apex of maxillary second molar, distal to zygomatic process of maxilla, with correct angulations to maxillary occlusal plane and long axis of tooth
MSA Block			
Nerves Middle superior alveolar (if present) **Teeth** Maxillary premolars and mesiobuccal root of maxillary first molar in approximately 28% of cases **Other Structures** Buccal periodontium and gingiva of anesthetized teeth and buccal mucosa and upper lip	Maxillary mucobuccal fold, maxillary second premolar	Middle superior alveolar nerve as part of superior dental plexus superior to apex of maxillary second premolar	Height of maxillary mucobuccal fold superior to apex of maxillary second premolar

Continued

TABLE 9-3	Review of Local Anesthesia of the Dentition and Related Structures—cont'd		
MAXILLARY ANESTHESIA			
NERVES, TEETH, AND RELATED STRUCTURES ANESTHETIZED	LANDMARKS	TARGET AREA	INJECTION SITE
ASA Block			
Nerves Anterior superior alveolar **Teeth** Maxillary anterior teeth **Other Structures** Labial periodontium and gingiva of anesthetized teeth and labial mucosa and upper lip	Maxillary mucobuccal fold, canine eminence, maxillary canine	Anterior superior alveolar nerve as part of superior dental plexus superior to apex of maxillary canine	Height of maxillary mucobuccal fold superior to apex of maxillary canine, just medial to and parallel with canine eminence
IO Block			
Nerves Infraorbital nerve Anterior superior alveolar Middle superior alveolar (if present) Inferior palpebral nerve Lateral nasal nerve Superior labial nerve **Teeth** Maxillary anterior teeth and premolars, as well as the mesiobuccal root of maxillary first molar in approximately 28% of cases **Other Structures** Facial periodontium and gingiva of anesthetized teeth; upper lip to midline; medial part of cheek; side of nose; lower eyelid	**Extraoral:** infraorbital rim, zygomaticomaxillary suture, infraorbital foramen **Intraoral:** maxillary mucobuccal fold, maxillary first premolar	Infraorbital nerve after entering infraorbital foramen that is slightly inferior to midpoint of infraorbital rim with zygomaticomaxillary suture	Height of maxillary mucobuccal fold superior to apex of maxillary first premolar
GP Block			
Nerves Greater palatine **Teeth** None **Other Structures** Posterior hard palate and palatal periodontium and gingiva of ipsilateral maxillary posterior teeth	Maxillary second or third molar, junction of alveolar process of maxilla and posterior hard palate, median palatine raphe overlying median palatine suture, palatal gingival margin, greater palatine foramen	Greater palatine nerve entering greater palatine foramen at junction of alveolar process of maxilla and hard palate as well as superior to apex of maxillary second or third molar; also approximately midway between median palatine raphe overlying median palatine suture and palatal gingival margin of maxillary molar	Palatal tissue anterior to greater palatine foramen
NP Block			
Nerves Nasopalatine **Teeth** None **Other Structures** Anterior hard palate and palatal periodontium and gingiva of maxillary anterior teeth bilaterally	Maxillary central incisors, anterior hard palate of maxilla, incisive papilla, incisive foramen	Right and left nerves entering incisive foramen on anterior hard palate of maxilla deep to incisive papilla and palatal to maxillary central incisors	Palatal tissue lateral to incisive papilla and palatal to maxillary central incisors

TABLE 9-3	Review of Local Anesthesia of the Dentition and Related Structures—cont'd

MAXILLARY ANESTHESIA

NERVES, TEETH, AND RELATED STRUCTURES ANESTHETIZED	LANDMARKS	TARGET AREA	INJECTION SITE
AMSA Block			
Nerves Anterior superior alveolar, middle superior alveolar, nasopalatine, greater palatine **Teeth** Maxillary anterior teeth and premolars along with maxillary first molar mesiobuccal root **Other Structures** Facial periodontium and gingiva of anesthetized teeth to midline; hard palate and palatal periodontium and gingiva of ipsilateral maxillary posterior teeth and maxillary anterior teeth bilaterally; no regional soft tissue anesthesia of upper lip and face	Maxillary premolars, palatal gingival margin, median palatine overlying median palatine suture	Small pores within maxilla of hard palate	Area on palate superior to apices of maxillary premolars and approximately midway between palatal gingival margin and median palatal raphe overlying median palatine suture

MANDIBULAR ANESTHESIA

TEETH AND RELATED STRUCTURES ANESTHETIZED	LANDMARKS	TARGET AREA	INJECTION SITE
IA Block			
Nerves Inferior alveolar, mental, incisive nerve, lingual **Teeth** Mandibular teeth to midline **Other Structures** Lingual periodontium and gingiva to midline; facial periodontium and gingiva of mandibular anterior teeth and premolars to midline; lower lip, anterior two-thirds of tongue, and floor of the mouth to midline	Medial surface of mandibular ramus, mandibular foramen, lingula, coronoid notch, pterygomandibular fold overlying raphe, pterygomandibular space, mandibular occlusal plane	Inferior alveolar nerve exiting mandibular foramen on medial surface of mandibular ramus overhung anteriorly by lingula (lingual nerve by diffusion)	Mandibular tissue on medial border of mandibular ramus within pterygomandibular space, lateral to pterygomandibular fold overlying raphe; two-thirds distance from coronoid notch to pterygomandibular fold demarcating posterior border of ramus; at approximately 6 to 10 mm superior to mandibular occlusal plane
Buccal Block			
Nerves (Long) buccal **Teeth** None **Other Structures** Buccal periodontium and gingiva of mandibular molars	Most distal mandibular molar, anterior border of mandibular ramus, retromolar pad overlying triangle	(Long) buccal nerve on anterior border of mandibular ramus in area of retromolar pad overlying triangle	Buccal mucosa distal and buccal to most distal mandibular molar
Mental Block			
Nerves Mental **Teeth** None **Other Structures** Facial periodontium and gingiva of mandibular anterior teeth and premolars to midline; lower lip and skin of chin to midline	Mandibular premolars, mental foramen, mandibular mucobuccal fold	Mental nerve entering mental foramen inferior to apices of mandibular premolars or location determined by radiographs and/or palpation	Anterior to mental foramen at depth of mandibular mucobuccal fold

Continued

TABLE 9-3	Review of Local Anesthesia of the Dentition and Related Structures—cont'd

MANDIBULAR ANESTHESIA

TEETH AND RELATED STRUCTURES ANESTHETIZED	LANDMARKS	TARGET AREA	INJECTION SITE
Incisive Block			
Nerves Mental, incisive **Teeth** Mandibular anterior teeth and premolars to the midline **Other Structures** Facial periodontium and gingiva of anesthetized teeth to midline; lower lip and skin of chin to midline	Mandibular premolars, mental foramen, mandibular mucobuccal fold	Incisive nerve merging with mental nerve within mental foramen inferior to apices of mandibular premolars or location determined by radiographs and/or palpation	Anterior to mental foramen at depth of mandibular mucobuccal fold
Gow-Gates Mandibular Block			
Nerves Inferior alveolar, lingual, (long) buccal, mental, incisive, mylohyoid, auriculotemporal **Teeth** Mandibular teeth to midline **Other Structures** Facial and lingual periodontium and gingiva of anesthetized teeth to midline; lower lip, anterior two-thirds of tongue and floor of the mouth to midline and probably buccal periodontium and gingiva of mandibular molars; skin over zygomatic bone and posterior part of buccal and temporal regions; additional innervation by way of mylohyoid nerve to muscles and also can serve as afferent nerve for mandibular first molar	**Extraoral:** Intertragic notch at lower border of the tragus, ipsilateral labial commissure **Intraoral:** Mesiolingual cusp of maxillary second molar, buccal mucosa just distal to maxillary second molar	Anteromedial border of neck of mandibular condyle	Buccal mucosa on medial surface of mandibular ramus, just distal to height of mesiolingual cusp of maxillary second molar
Vazirani-Akinosi Mandibular Block			
Nerves Inferior alveolar, lingual, mental, incisive, mylohyoid **Teeth** Mandibular teeth to midline **Other Structures** Lingual periodontium and gingiva to midline; facial periodontium and gingiva of mandibular anterior teeth and premolars to midline and probably buccal periodontium and gingiva of mandibular molars; lower lip, anterior two-thirds of tongue, and floor of the mouth to midline; additional innervation by way of mylohyoid nerve to muscles that can also serve as afferent nerve for mandibular first molar	Coronoid process, medial surface of mandibular ramus, pterygomandibular space, maxillary tuberosity, mucogingival junction of maxillary third or second molar, maxillary occlusal plane	Medial surface of mandibular ramus within pterygomandibular space adjacent to maxillary tuberosity	Medially past coronoid process and parallel to maxillary occlusal plane; then buccal mucosa at height of mucogingival junction of maxillary third or second molar

pathway as well as the mandible. In addition, when working within the confines of quadrant dentistry, the injections should be administered from posterior to anterior, with the dental treatment commencing in the same directions again due to the anatomy of the nerve pathway.

As noted earlier, there must never be an injection directly through an area with an abscess, cellulitis, or osteomyelitis so as to prevent the spread of dental (or odontogenic) infection (see Chapter 12). Also, the effectiveness of local anesthetic agents is greatly reduced when administered adjacent to areas of infection. Additional amounts may

be needed in this situation, but at the same time it is always important to keep in mind the maximal recommended dosage for each patient.

MAXILLARY NERVE ANESTHESIA

The maxillary nerve and its branches can be anesthetized in various ways depending on the extent of the procedure anticipated and the structures requiring local anesthesia (see Figure 9-1; see Tables 9-1 and 9-3). Most local anesthesia of the maxillae is more clinically effective than that of the mandible because the facial cortical plate of the maxillae is less dense and more porous than that of the mandible over similar teeth, and anesthesia from the palatal surface is also possible. This decrease in density of the maxillae compared to the mandible can be demonstrated with a panoramic radiograph (see Figure 3-46).

In addition, there is less anatomic variation of both the maxillae and palatine bones as well as associated nerves with respect to local anesthetic landmarks when compared with similar mandibular structures, making the maxillary injections more routine, and usually without the need for any troubleshooting if there is lack of clinical effectiveness of local anesthetic agent administered (see Chapter 3). However, this does not mean that maxillary injections do not have any complications that can occur. But unlike mandibular arch anesthesia, the entire maxillary arch can usually undergo anesthesia without complications.

Maxillary facial anesthesia has a high level of clinical effectiveness when administered correctly as it anesthetizes both the pulp and various parts of the associated periodontium and gingiva. Pulpal anesthesia is achieved through anesthesia of each tooth's dental branches as they extend into the pulp by way of the apical foramen from the superior dental plexus. Both the hard and soft tissue of the associated periodontium and gingiva are anesthetized by way of the interdental and interradicular branches for each tooth.

The posterior superior alveolar block is recommended in most cases for anesthesia of the maxillary molars and associated buccal periodontium and gingiva within one maxillary quadrant. The middle superior alveolar block in most cases is recommended for anesthesia of the maxillary premolars and associated buccal periodontium and gingiva within one maxillary quadrant. The anterior superior alveolar block is recommended for anesthesia of the maxillary anterior teeth and associated labial periodontium and gingiva to the midline within one maxillary quadrant. The infraorbital block is recommended for anesthesia of the maxillary anterior teeth and premolars and associated facial periodontium and gingiva within one maxillary quadrant since it anesthetizes both regions covered by the middle and anterior superior alveolar blocks.

Palatal anesthesia usually involves anesthesia of the associated palatal periodontium and gingiva. However, palatal anesthesia alone usually does not provide any pulpal anesthesia to the maxillary teeth nor anesthesia of the associated facial periodontium and gingiva. Additional administration of maxillary facial anesthesia would usually be needed for complete coverage of either a sextant or quadrant when planning treatment. The greater palatine block is recommended for anesthesia of the associated palatal periodontium and gingiva of the maxillary posterior teeth within one maxillary posterior sextant. The nasopalatine block is recommended for anesthesia of the associated palatal periodontium and gingiva of the maxillary anterior teeth bilaterally from maxillary canine to canine within the maxillary anterior sextant.

Separate from these two palatal blocks, which only provide anesthesia of the associated palatal periodontium and gingiva, is the anterior middle superior alveolar block since it also provides pulpal anesthesia. This block is recommended for anesthesia of the maxillary teeth and associated facial and palatal periodontium and gingiva to the midline within one maxillary quadrant, except for those structures innervated by the posterior superior alveolar nerve. The posterior superior alveolar block can be additionally administered to allow complete maxillary quadrant anesthesia.

POSTERIOR SUPERIOR ALVEOLAR BLOCK

The **posterior superior alveolar block** (al-**vee**-uh-luhr) or *PSA block* in most cases anesthetizes the maxillary molars and associated buccal periodontium and gingiva within one maxillary quadrant if the middle superior alveolar nerve is not present, which occurs in approximately 72% of the cases. However, in some cases the mesiobuccal root of the maxillary first molar is not innervated by the posterior superior alveolar nerve, but rather by the middle superior alveolar nerve when present, which occurs in approximately 28% of the cases. Therefore a second injection to anesthetize the middle superior alveolar nerve by the block of the same name is recommended to ensure pulpal anesthesia of all the roots of the maxillary first molar. If anesthesia of the associated palatal periodontium and gingiva of these teeth is necessary, administration of the greater palatine block also may be indicated.

Target Area and Injection Site for Posterior Superior Alveolar Block. The target area for the PSA block is the posterior superior alveolar nerve branches entering the posterior superior alveolar foramina on the infratemporal surface of the maxilla (Figures 9-2 and 9-3, see Figures 3-47 and 8-13). The posterior superior alveolar foramina are posterosuperior on the maxillary

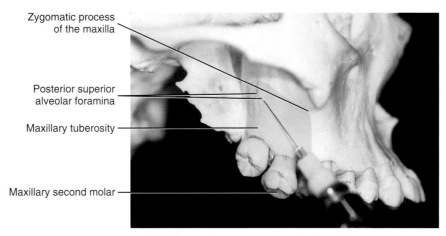

Zygomatic process of the maxilla

Posterior superior alveolar foramina

Maxillary tuberosity

Maxillary second molar

FIGURE 9-2 Target area for the posterior superior alveolar block is the posterior superior alveolar nerve branches entering the posterior superior alveolar foramina on the infratemporal surface of the maxilla. The posterior superior alveolar foramina are located posterosuperior on the maxillary tuberosity as well as superior to the apex of the maxillary second molar. Distribution of anesthesia is highlighted.

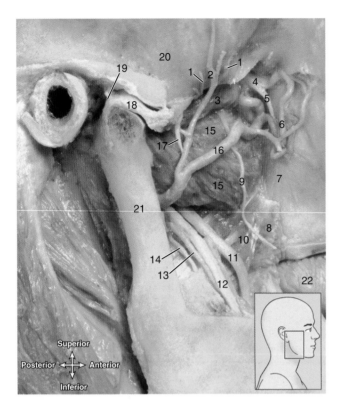

FIGURE 9-3 Dissection of the right infratemporal fossa at the target area for the posterior superior alveolar block (*see inset*; note removal of the lateral pterygoid muscle, zygomatic arch, and part of the mandible). The target area for the inferior alveolar block is also shown (see Figure 9-31). *1*, Deep temporal nerve; *2*, deep temporal artery; *3*, lateral pterygoid muscle; *4*, maxillary nerve; *5*, posterior superior alveolar nerve; *6*, posterior superior alveolar artery; *7*, infratemporal surface of maxilla; *8*, buccinator muscle; *9*, buccal nerve; *10*, medial pterygoid muscle; *11*, lingual nerve; *12*, inferior alveolar nerve; *13*, inferior alveolar artery; *14*, mylohyoid nerve; *15*, lateral pterygoid muscle; *16*, maxillary artery; *17*, masseteric nerve; *18*, joint disc of the temporomandibular joint and mandibular condyle; *19*, joint capsule; *20*, temporal bone; *21*, mandibular ramus; *22*, tongue. *(From Logan BM, Reynold PA, Hutching RT: McMinn's color atlas of head and neck anatomy, ed 4, London, 2010, Elsevier.)*

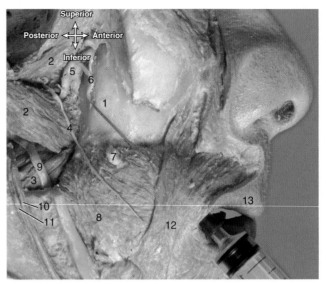

FIGURE 9-4 Dissection with needle at the injection site for a posterior superior alveolar block. The target area for the inferior alveolar block is also shown (see similar Figure 9-34). *1*, Posterior surface of maxilla; *2*, lateral pterygoid muscle; *3*, medial pterygoid muscle; *4*, buccal nerve; *5*, maxillary artery; *6*, posterior superior alveolar nerve and vessels; *7*, parotid duct; *8*, buccinator muscle; *9*, lingual nerve; *10*, inferior alveolar nerve; *11*, inferior alveolar artery; *12*, labial commissure; *13*, upper lip. *(From Logan BM, Reynold PA, Hutching RT: McMinn's color atlas of head and neck anatomy, ed 4, London, 2010, Elsevier.)*

tuberosity as well as superior to the apex of the maxillary second molar.

The injection site for the PSA block is at the height of the maxillary mucobuccal fold superior to the apex of the maxillary second molar, as well as distal to the zygomatic process of the maxilla (Figures 9-4 and 9-5). The needle is inserted into the height of the maxillary mucobuccal fold in a distal and medial direction superior to the tooth apex without contacting the maxilla in order to reduce trauma, and then the injection is administered (Figure 9-6).

In addition, the correct needle and syringe barrel angulation to the injection site must be maintained throughout using three different orientations but only one movement (Figure 9-7). This angulation should be superiorly at a 45° angle to the maxillary occlusal plane, medially at a 45° angle to the maxillary occlusal plane, and posteriorly at a 45° angle to the long axis of the maxillary second molar. To help accomplish this, the syringe barrel should be extended from the ipsilateral labial commissure. This complex orientation can be practiced using a topical anesthetic-laced long cotton tip applicator to palpate the injection site as if it were the needle and syringe, as can all the injections. A conservative

insertion technique concerning the depth of the needle should be used so as to reduce possible complications and still ensure an effective clinical outcome (discussed next).

Indications of Clinically Effective Posterior Superior Alveolar Block and Possible Complications. Usually there are no overt indications of a clinically effective PSA block since there is mainly hard tissue anesthesia with limited soft tissue anesthesia. Thus the patient frequently has difficulty determining the extent of anesthesia because the lip or tongue does not feel numb as occurs with the more commonly used inferior alveolar block or *mandibular block*. Instead, the patient will state that the teeth in the area feel dull when gently tapped, and there will be an absence of discomfort during dental procedures. It may be necessary to inform the patient of this before starting the procedure so as to reduce fears that the local anesthetic agent has not worked.

As discussed, the maxilla should not be contacted at any time during the PSA injection. If bone is contacted immediately after the needle penetrates the soft tissue, the medial angulation of the syringe barrel toward the maxillary occlusal plane at more than 45° is too great. Instead, the syringe barrel needs to be closer to the maxillary occlusal plane, thereby reducing the angle to less than 45°.

This injection has a high risk of positive aspiration due to the proximity of the posterior superior alveolar blood vessels (see Chapter 6). Inadvertent and harmless anesthesia of other branches of the mandibular nerve may occur with a PSA block because they are located lateral to the posterior superior alveolar nerve. This may result in varying degrees of mandibular lingual anesthesia and anesthesia of the lower lip in some patients; thus avoid depositing lateral to posterior superior alveolar nerve.

However, a more serious complication can occur if the needle is advanced too deep into the tissue during a PSA block (see

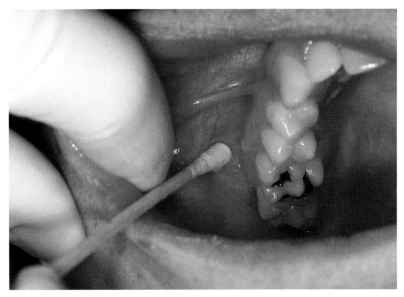

FIGURE 9-5 Injection site for the posterior superior alveolar block is palpated at the height of the maxillary mucobuccal fold superior to the apex of the maxillary second molar and distal to the zygomatic process of the maxilla.

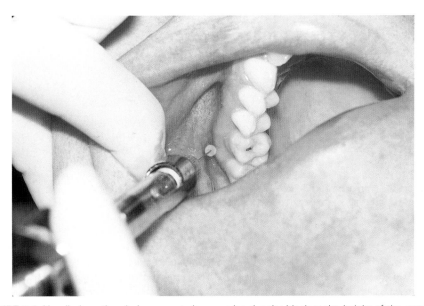

FIGURE 9-6 Needle insertion during a posterior superior alveolar block at the height of the maxillary mucobuccal fold superior to the apex of the maxillary second molar. The needle is in a distal and medial direction superior to the tooth apex without contacting the maxilla. Injection site is highlighted. *(Courtesy of Margaret J. Fehrenbach, RDH, MS.)*

Figure 9-7 and see Figure 6-13). The needle may pierce the deeper pterygoid plexus of veins and the maxillary artery if overinserted. This results in a bluish-reddish extraoral swelling of hemorrhaging blood in the tissue within the infratemporal fossa on the affected side of the face a few minutes after the injection, progressing over time inferiorly and anteriorly toward the lower anterior region of the cheek, ending in an extraoral hematoma (see Figures 3-61 and 6-19).

In addition, if the needle is contaminated, there may be a spread of a needle tract infection from the infratemporal space to the cavernous sinus (see Chapter 12). Aspiration should always be attempted in all injections before administration in order to avoid injection into blood vessels, and strict standard precautions of infection control should be observed.

MIDDLE SUPERIOR ALVEOLAR BLOCK

The **middle superior alveolar block** or *MSA block* anesthetizes maxillary premolars and possibly the mesiobuccal root of the maxillary first molar as well as the associated buccal periodontium and gingiva

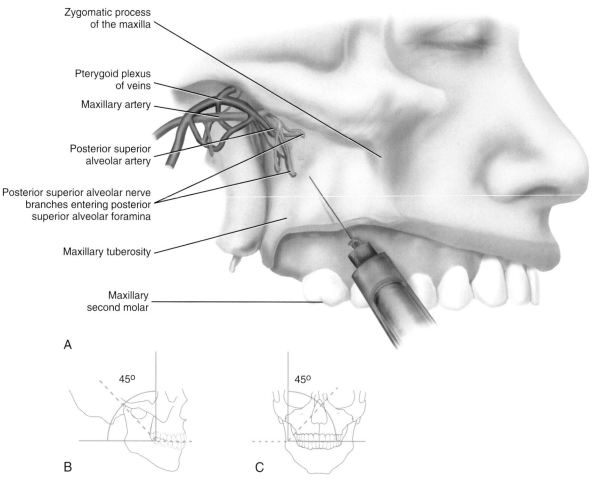

FIGURE 9-7 Correct insertion of the needle during a posterior superior alveolar block superior to the apex of the maxillary second molar without contacting the maxilla **(A).** However, if the needle is overinserted, it can pierce the pterygoid plexus of the veins and maxillary artery, which may lead to complications such as a hematoma. To prevent this complication, the needle and syringe barrel angulation should be **(B)** superiorly (*or upward*) at a 45° angle to the maxillary occlusal plane, and **(C)** medially (*or inward*) at a 45° angle to the maxillary occlusal plane, as well as posteriorly (*or backward*) at a 45° angle to the long axis of the maxillary second molar.

within one maxillary quadrant if the middle superior alveolar nerve is present to be anesthetized, which occurs in approximately 28% of the cases. To ensure complete maxillary quadrant anesthesia, most clinicians administer this block even though the middle superior alveolar nerve may not be present or when only having procedures involving the maxillary premolars.

When the middle superior alveolar nerve is absent, as occurs in approximately 72% of the cases, the region is innervated instead by both the posterior superior alveolar and the anterior superior alveolar nerves as part of the superior dental plexus, but mainly by the anterior superior alveolar nerve. If anesthesia of associated palatal periodontium and gingiva of these teeth is necessary, administration of the greater palatine block may also be indicated.

Target Area and Injection Site for Middle Superior Alveolar Block. The target area for the MSA block is the middle superior alveolar nerve if present as part of the superior dental plexus that is located superior to the apex of the maxillary second premolar (Figures 9-8 and 9-9 and see Figure 8-13). Thus the injection site is at the height of the maxillary mucobuccal fold superior to the apex of the maxillary second premolar (Figure 9-10). The needle is inserted

into the height of the maxillary mucobuccal fold until its tip is located superior to the apex of the maxillary second premolar without contacting the maxilla in order to reduce trauma, and then the injection is administered (Figure 9-11).

Indications of Clinically Effective Middle Superior Alveolar Block and Possible Complications. Indications of a clinically effective MSA block include harmless tingling and numbness of the upper lip and an absence of discomfort during dental procedures. This injection has a low risk of positive aspiration and overinsertion with complications such as a hematoma rare with the MSA block.

ANTERIOR SUPERIOR ALVEOLAR BLOCK

The **anterior superior alveolar block** or *ASA block* anesthetizes the anterior superior alveolar nerve and thus anesthetizes the maxillary anterior teeth and associated labial periodontium and gingiva to the midline within one maxillary quadrant. It is commonly used in conjunction with an MSA block instead of using an infraorbital block alone to anesthetize these teeth. Communication occurs between the middle superior alveolar nerve and both the anterior superior alveolar and posterior superior alveolar nerves as part of the superior dental plexus. Some clinicians consider the ASA block to be only a supraperiosteal injection but since it has a larger area of anesthesia and the local anesthetic agent is deposited near the larger nerve trunk of the ASA nerve, it can be considered a nerve block.

In addition, in many cases the anterior superior alveolar nerve can also involve crossover-innervation to the contralateral side in a patient; this may need to be taken into account when using local anesthesia in this area. Crossover-innervation is the overlap of terminal nerve fibers from the contralateral side of the dental arch (see Chapter 8). Thus bilateral injections of the ASA block or a supraperiosteal injection superior to the apex of the contralateral maxillary central incisor may be indicated if the patient is still feeling discomfort during treatment. If anesthesia of associated palatal periodontium and gingiva of these teeth is necessary, administration of the nasopalatine block may also be indicated.

With the expanding use of the computer-controlled local anesthesia delivery device, it was discovered that clinicians could also deliver a similar injection for anesthesia of a maxillary anterior sextant from a palatal approach using the palatal-anterior superior alveolar (P-ASA) block that combines both the ASA and the nasopalatine blocks from a deeper incisive canal injection. Thus, the anterior branches of the

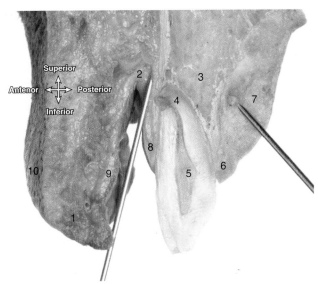

FIGURE 9-9 Dissection of a frontal section of maxilla through the maxillary first premolar. With one needle (*left*) at the injection site for middle superior alveolar block and the other needle (*right*) at the injection site for the anterior middle superior alveolar block. *1,* Upper lip; *2,* height of maxillary mucobuccal fold; *3,* alveolar process of maxilla; *4,* apex of tooth; *5,* pulp cavity; *6,* palatal gingival margin; *7,* mucoperiosteum of anterior hard palate; *8,* buccal gingival margin; *9,* labial mucosa; *10,* bucccal mucosa. *(From Logan BM, Reynold PA, Hutching RT: McMinn's color atlas of head and neck anatomy, ed 4, London, 2010, Elsevier.)*

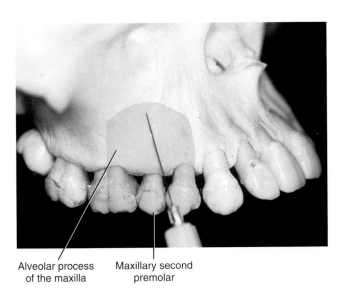

FIGURE 9-8 Target area for the middle superior alveolar block is the middle superior alveolar nerve as part of the superior dental plexus that is superior to the apex of the maxillary second premolar. Distribution of anesthesia is highlighted.

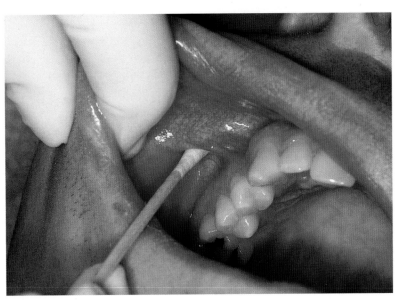

FIGURE 9-10 Injection site for the middle superior alveolar block is palpated at the height of the maxillary mucobuccal fold superior to the apex of the maxillary second premolar.

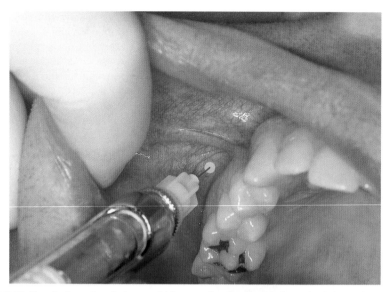

FIGURE 9-11 Needle insertion during a middle superior alveolar block at the height of the maxillary mucobuccal fold superior to the apex of the maxillary second premolar without contacting the maxilla. Injection site is highlighted. *(Courtesy of Margaret J. Fehrenbach, RDH, MS.)*

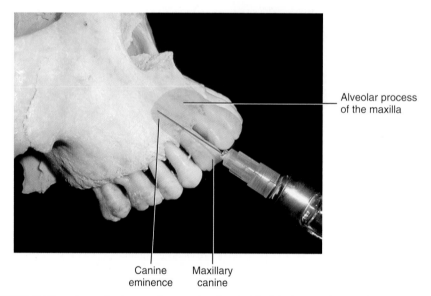

Alveolar process
of the maxilla

Canine
eminence

Maxillary
canine

FIGURE 9-12 Target area for the anterior superior alveolar block is the anterior superior alveolar nerve as part of the superior dental plexus that is superior to the apex of the maxillary canine. Distribution of anesthesia is highlighted.

anterior superior alveolar nerve as well as the nasopalatine nerve are anesthetized. This results in anesthesia of the maxillary anterior teeth and associated labial periodontium and gingiva bilaterally with the additional anesthesia of the associated palatal periodontium and gingiva bilaterally, but without causing the usual collateral anesthesia of the upper lip and muscles of facial expression. This injection can then be used when performing cosmetic dentistry procedures because after the procedures are completed, the clinician can immediately and accurately assess the patient's smile line. However, this block may be variable in anesthesia depth and duration.

Target Area and Injection Site for Anterior Superior Alveolar Block. The target area for the ASA block is the anterior superior alveolar nerve as part of the superior dental plexus that is superior to the apex of the maxillary canine (Figure 9-12 and see Figures 3-47 and 8-13).

The injection site is at the height of the maxillary mucobuccal fold superior to the apex of the maxillary canine, just medial to and parallel with the canine eminence (Figures 9-13). The needle is angled at approximately 10° off an imaginary line drawn parallel to the long axis of the maxillary canine (Figure 9-14). The needle is inserted into the height of the maxillary mucobuccal fold until its tip is superior to the apex of the maxillary canine without contacting the maxilla so as to reduce trauma, and then the injection is administered.

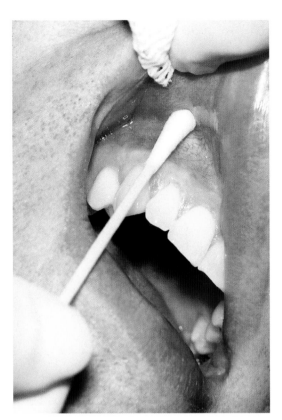

FIGURE 9-13 Injection site for the anterior superior alveolar block is palpated at the height of the maxillary mucobuccal fold superior to the apex of the maxillary canine, just medial to and parallel with the canine eminence.

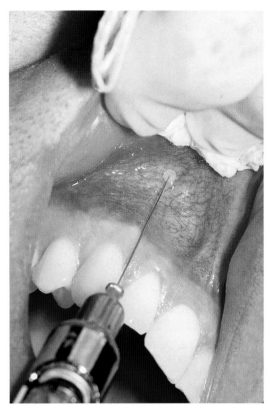

FIGURE 9-14 Needle insertion during an anterior superior alveolar block at the height of the maxillary mucobuccal fold superior to the apex of the maxillary canine without contacting the maxilla. The needle is angled at approximately 10° off an imaginary line drawn parallel to the long axis of the maxillary canine. Injection site is highlighted. *(Courtesy of Margaret J. Fehrenbach, RDH, MS.)*

Indications of Clinically Effective Anterior Superior Alveolar Block and Possible Complications. Indications of a clinically effective ASA block include harmless tingling and numbness of the upper lip and an absence of discomfort during dental procedures. This injection has a low risk of positive aspiration, and overinsertion with complications such as hematoma is rare with the ASA block.

INFRAORBITAL BLOCK

The **infraorbital block** (in-fruh-**or**-bi-tuhl) or *IO block* anesthetizes the infraorbital nerve and also both the anterior superior alveolar and middle superior alveolar nerves so as to cover the regions of both the MSA and ASA blocks with one injection. Thus the IO block anesthetizes the maxillary anterior teeth and premolars, as well as the associated facial periodontium and gingiva to the midline within one maxillary quadrant. Some clinicians believe that this block should be referred to as the *anterior superior alveolar block* to reflect the one region of the anesthetized tissue, but the more useful name comes from the infraorbital nerve anesthetized. If anesthesia of the associated palatal periodontium and gingiva of these teeth is necessary, administration of both the nasopalatine block and greater palatine block may also be indicated; additional administration of the PSA block completes maxillary quadrant anesthesia.

In addition, in many cases the anterior superior alveolar nerve involves crossover innervation to the contralateral side, so bilateral injections of the IO block (or ASA block, depending on extent of procedures) or a supraperiosteal injection superior to the apex of the

contralateral maxillary central incisor may be indicated if the patient is still feeling discomfort during treatment. Branches of the infraorbital nerve to the ipsilateral upper lip, side of the nose, and lower eyelid are also inadvertently anesthetized.

Target Area and Injection Site for Infraorbital Block. The target area for the IO block is the infraorbital nerve after entering the infraorbital foramen (Figure 9-15 and see Figures 3-47 and 8-13). Within the infraorbital foramen, the anterior superior alveolar and middle superior alveolar nerves move superiorly to join the infraorbital nerve after it enters.

To locate the infraorbital foramen, extraorally palpate the midpoint of the patient's infraorbital rim and then move slightly inferior approximately 10 mm while applying pressure until the depression created by the infraorbital foramen is felt, surrounded by smoother bone (Figure 9-16). Clinicians can palpate a "notch" or depression in the midpoint of the infraorbital rim created by the more vertical zygomaticomaxillary suture located between the zygomatic process of the maxilla (medial part) and that of the maxillary process of the zygomatic bone (lateral part) that both form the infraorbital rim (see Chapter 3).

The patient may feel soreness when pressure is applied to the infraorbital foramen due to the presence of the nearby nerve. There is also a linear relationship noted on the face that can assist with the IO block. This linear relationship is between the ipsilateral supraorbital notch, pupil of the eye looking forward, midpoint of the infraorbital rim with its zygomaticomaxillary suture, infraorbital foramen, and labial commissure (see Figure 9-16).

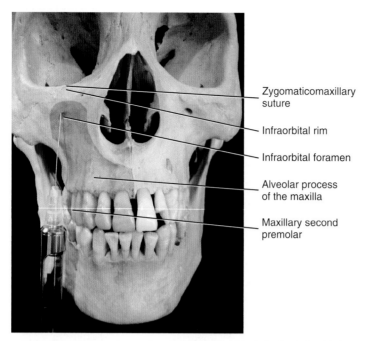

FIGURE 9-15 Target area for the infraorbital block is the infraorbital nerve after entering the infraorbital foramen. The infraorbital foramen is located slightly inferior to the midpoint of the infraorbital rim with its zygomaticomaxillary suture. Distribution of anesthesia is highlighted.

Zygomaticomaxillary suture

Infraorbital rim

Infraorbital foramen

Alveolar process of the maxilla

Maxillary second premolar

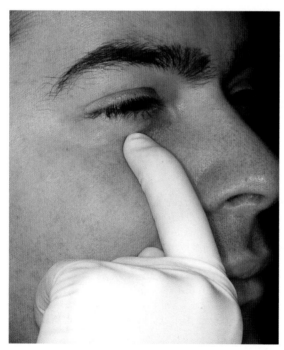

FIGURE 9-16 Demonstration of the palpation of the depression created by the infraorbital foramen for the infraorbital block by moving approximately 1 to 2 mm slightly inferior on the face from the infraorbital rim. There is also a linear relationship on the ipsilateral side of the face between the supraorbital notch, pupil of the eye looking forward, midpoint of the infraorbital rim with the zygomaticomaxillary suture, and the infraorbital foramen.

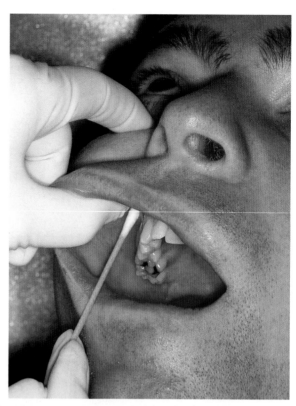

FIGURE 9-17 Injection site for the infraorbital block is palpated at the height of the maxillary mucobuccal fold superior to the apex of the maxillary first premolar. A preinjection approximation of the depth of needle insertion for the block can be made by placing one finger on the infraorbital foramen and the other finger on the proposed injection site, and then estimating the distance between the two fingers.

The injection site for the IO block is at the height of the maxillary mucobuccal fold superior to the apex of the maxillary first premolar. A preinjection approximation of the depth of needle insertion can be made by placing one finger on the infraorbital foramen and the other finger on the proposed injection site, and then estimating the distance between the two fingers (Figure 9-17).

The approximate depth of needle insertion for the IO block may vary; in a patient with a higher or deeper maxillary mucobuccal fold or more inferior infraorbital foramen, less tissue insertion will be required than in a patient with a lower or shallower maxillary mucobuccal fold or more superior infraorbital foramen.

The needle is inserted into the height of the maxillary mucobuccal fold superior to the apex of the maxillary first premolar while keeping pressure with the finger of the other hand on the infraorbital foramen during the injection (Figure 9-18). The needle is advanced while keeping it parallel with the long axis of the tooth to avoid premature contact with the maxilla. The point of gentle contact of the needle with the maxilla should be at the superior rim of the infraorbital foramen, and then the injection is administered. Maintaining the needle in contact with the bone during the injection prevents overinsertion and possible puncture of the orbit. Additional pressure is applied to the infraorbital foramen after administration to enhance local anesthetic agent diffusion.

Indications of Clinically Effective Infraorbital Block and Possible Complications. Indications of a clinically effective IO block include harmless tingling and numbness of the ipsilateral upper lip, medial part of the cheek, side of the nose, and lower eyelid because there is inadvertent anesthesia of the branches of the infraorbital

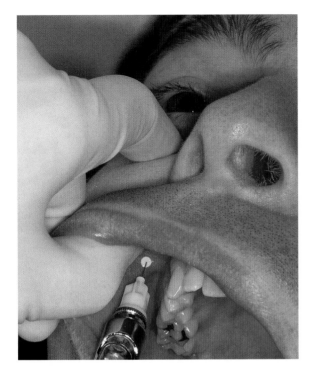

FIGURE 9-18 Needle insertion during an infraorbital block at the height of the maxillary mucobuccal fold superior to the apex of the maxillary first premolar. Injection site is highlighted. The needle is advanced while keeping it parallel with the long axis of the tooth to avoid premature contact with the maxilla. The point of contact of the needle with the maxilla should be at the superior rim of the infraorbital foramen. Pressure over the infraorbital foramen and contact with the maxilla are maintained throughout the injection. *(Courtesy of Margaret J. Fehrenbach, RDH, MS.)*

nerve. Additionally, there is numbness of the teeth and associated tissue along the distribution of both the anterior and middle superior alveolar nerves and absence of discomfort during dental procedures. Rarely the complication of a hematoma may develop across the lower eyelid and the tissue between it and the infraorbital foramen due to proximity of the area blood vessels.

GREATER PALATINE BLOCK

The **greater palatine block** (**pal**-uh-tine) or *GP block* anesthetizes the greater palatine nerve and thus anesthetizes the posterior hard palate and the associated palatal periodontium and gingiva of the ipsilateral maxillary posterior teeth within a maxillary posterior sextant.

Because the GP block does not provide anesthesia of the pulp or associated facial periodontal and gingiva of the area teeth, the administration of the MSA and PSA blocks or the IO block may also be indicated. In addition, anesthesia of the associated palatal periodontium and gingiva of the maxillary first premolar may prove inadequate because of overlapping nerve fibers from the anteriorly placed nasopalatine nerve. This lack of anesthesia may be corrected by additional administration of the nasopalatine block if the patient is still feeling discomfort during treatment.

Because the overlying palatal tissue is dense and adheres firmly to the underlying palatal bone, the use of pressure anesthesia over the depression of the greater palatine foramen posterior to the injection site to blanch the tissue throughout the injection will reduce patient discomfort. This pressure anesthesia of the tissue produces a dull ache that blocks pain impulses that arise from needle insertion and local anesthetic agent deposition.

Target Area and Injection Site for Greater Palatine Block. The target area for the GP block is the greater palatine nerve entering the greater palatine foramen from its location between the

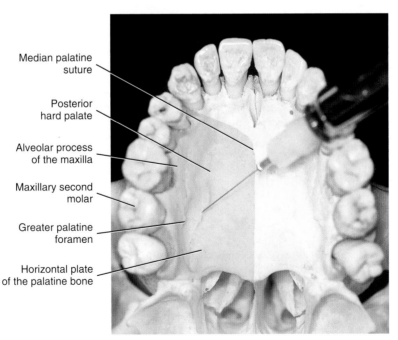

Median palatine suture
Posterior hard palate
Alveolar process of the maxilla
Maxillary second molar
Greater palatine foramen
Horizontal plate of the palatine bone

FIGURE 9-19 Target area for the greater palatine block is the greater palatine nerve entering the greater palatine foramen in the horizontal plate of the palatine bone. The greater palatine foramen is usually located at the junction of the alveolar process of the maxilla and the posterior hard palate as well as superior to the apex of the maxillary second or third molar. Distribution of anesthesia is highlighted.

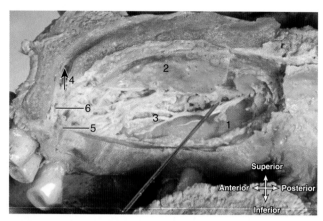

FIGURE 9-20 Dissection of the hard palate with a needle at the injection site for the greater palatine block. The injection site for the nasopalatine block is also shown (see Figure 9-25). *1,* Greater palatine foramen; *2,* mucoperiosteum of hard palate; *3,* greater palatine nerve traveling horizontally; *4,* incisive canal (*with arrow*); *5,* incisive foramen; *6,* nasopalatine nerve. *(From Logan BM, Reynold PA, Hutching RT: McMinn's color atlas of head and neck anatomy, ed 4, London, 2010, Elsevier.)*

mucoperiosteum and horizontal plate of palatine bone of the posterior hard palate (Figures 9-19 and 9-20 and see Figures 3-44 and 8-14).

The greater palatine foramen is noted as a depression on the palatal surface, usually at the junction of the alveolar process of the maxilla and posterior hard palate, as well as superior to the apex of the maxillary second (in children) or third molar (in adults), which is approximately 10 mm medial and directly superior to the palatal gingival margin. Thus this depression can be palpated approximately midway between the median palatine raphe overlying the median palatine suture and the palatal gingival margin of the maxillary molar, starting near to the most distal maxillary molar and moving inward. This landmark of the greater palatine foramen is where pressure anesthesia is applied throughout the injection.

In patients who have a vaulted palate, the greater palatine foramen will appear closer to the dentition. Conversely, in patients with a more shallow palate, the foramen will appear closer to the midline. In patients lacking a visible depression for the greater palatine foramen, the other surface landmarks are useful and palpation of the area may help to emphasize the depression of the foramen.

The site of injection for the GP block is the palatal tissue anterior to the greater palatine foramen (Figure 9-21). The needle is inserted into the previously blanched palatal tissue at a 90° angle to the palate, with the needle bowing slightly (Figure 9-22). The needle is advanced until the palatine bone is gently contacted, and then the injection is administered.

There is no need to enter the greater palatine canal when administering the injection. Although such an entrance is not potentially hazardous, it is not necessary for this block and would prove difficult with the angulation of the needle as recommended.

Indications of Clinically Effective Greater Palatine Block and Possible Complications. Indications of a clinically effective GP block are numbness of the posterior hard palate and an absence of discomfort during dental procedures. Some patients may become uncomfortable and may gag if the soft palate becomes inadvertently and harmlessly anesthetized, a distinct possibility given the proximity of the lesser palatine nerve and its foramen.

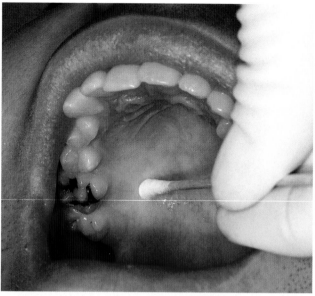

FIGURE 9-21 Palpation of the depression created by the greater palatine foramen, which is the site for pressure anesthesia during the greater palatine block. The greater palatine foramen is usually at the junction of the alveolar process of the maxilla and the posterior hard palate as well as superior to the apex of the maxillary second or third molar. Injection site for the greater palatine block is the palatal tissue anterior to the greater palatine foramen (see Figure 9-22). The surrounding palatal tissue is blanched due to the pressure on the greater palatine foramen throughout the injection for the greater palatine block to ensure pressure anesthesia.

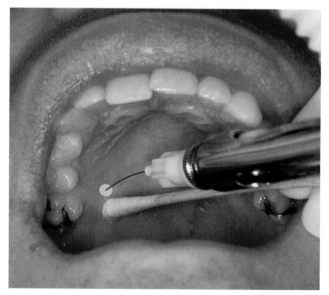

FIGURE 9-22 Needle insertion during a greater palatine block of the palatal tissue anterior to the greater palatine foramen until contact is made with bone of the palate. The greater palatine foramen is usually at the junction of the alveolar process of the maxilla and the posterior hard palate, superior to the apex of the maxillary second or third molar, and approximately midway between the median palatine raphe overlying the median palatine suture and the palatal gingival margin of the maxillary molar. Injection site is highlighted. The needle is at a 90° angle to the palate. Needle may bow slightly, and the blanching of surrounding palatal tissue due to pressure on the greater palatine foramen is maintained throughout the injection to ensure pressure anesthesia. *(Courtesy Margaret J. Fehrenbach, RDH, MS.)*

NASOPALATINE BLOCK

The **nasopalatine block** (nay-zo-**pal**-uh-tine) or *NP block* anesthetizes the anterior hard palate and the associated palatal periodontium and gingiva for the maxillary anterior teeth bilaterally from maxillary canine to canine within the maxillary anterior sextant. Thus both the right and the left nasopalatine nerves are anesthetized by this one block.

However, the NP block does not anesthetize the pulp nor associated facial periodontal and gingiva of the area teeth, so additional anesthesia by the administration of the ASA block or the IO block may be indicated. In addition, anesthesia of the associated palatal periodontium and gingiva of the maxillary canines may prove inadequate because of overlapping nerve fibers from the posteriorly placed greater palatine nerves. This lack of anesthesia may be corrected by additional administration of the GP block if the patient is still feeling discomfort during treatment.

Because the dense overlying palatal tissue adheres firmly to the underlying maxilla, the use of pressure anesthesia on the contralateral side of the injection site of the incisive papilla to blanch the tissue throughout the injection will reduce patient discomfort. This pressure anesthesia to the tissue produces a dull ache to block pain impulses that arise from needle insertion and local anesthetic agent deposition.

Target Area and Injection Site for Nasopalatine Block. The target area for the NP block is both the right and left nasopalatine nerves entering the incisive foramen of the maxillae from the mucosa of the anterior hard palate, deep to the incisive papilla, and palatal to the maxillary central incisors (Figures 9-23 and 9-24; see Figures 3-44, 8-14, and 9-20). The incisive foramen is located at the midline between the articulating palatine processes of the maxillae.

However, the injection site for the NP block is the palatal tissue lateral to the incisive papilla, which is usually located at the midline approximately 10 mm palatal to the maxillary central incisors in case there is no telltale bulge of the structure of the incisive papilla (Figure 9-25). Never insert the needle directly into the incisive papilla since this can be extremely painful to the patient. Pressure anesthesia is administered on the palatal tissue on the contralateral side of the incisive papilla throughout the injection.

The needle is inserted for the NP block into the previously blanched palatal tissue at a 45° angle to the anterior hard palate (Figure 9-26). The needle is advanced into the tissue until the maxilla is gently contacted, and then the injection is administered. There is no need to enter the incisive canal by way of the incisive foramen; in fact the needle cannot enter the foramen with the recommended position of the needle.

Indications of Clinically Effective Nasopalatine Block and Possible Complications. Indications of a clinically effective NP block include numbness of the anterior hard palate and an absence of discomfort during dental procedures. Complications such as hematoma are extremely rare.

ANTERIOR MIDDLE SUPERIOR ALVEOLAR BLOCK

The **anterior middle superior alveolar block** or *AMSA block* anesthetizes a large area innervated by the anterior and middle superior alveolar nerves as well as the nasopalatine and greater palatine nerves within the maxillary arch. Thus the single-site palatal injection of the AMSA block can anesthetize the maxillary anterior teeth and premolars along with the mesiobuccal root of the maxillary first molar, as well as associated facial periodontium and gingiva of anesthetized teeth to the midline, hard palate, and associated palatal periodontium and gingiva of the ipsilateral maxillary posterior teeth and maxillary anterior teeth bilaterally. This anesthesia is without the usual collateral anesthesia of the upper lip and muscles of facial expression. However the ipsilateral maxillary molars may have anesthesia of the associated palatal periodontium and gingiva, but do not have pulpal anesthesia nor anesthesia of the associated buccal periodontium and gingiva. Additional administration of the PSA block will add this necessary anesthesia coverage to complete maxillary quadrant anesthesia.

This injection is commonly used in cosmetic dentistry because after the procedures are completed, the clinician can immediately and accurately assess the patient's smile line. Studies show that this injection is best accomplished with a computer-controlled local anesthetic

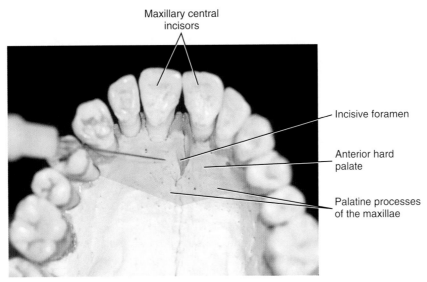

FIGURE 9-23 Target area for the nasopalatine block is both the right and left nasopalatine nerves entering the incisive foramen of the maxillae. The incisive foramen is located on the anterior hard palate, deep to the incisive papilla, and palatal to maxillary central incisors. The foramen is in the midline between the articulating palatine processes of the maxillae. Distribution of anesthesia is highlighted.

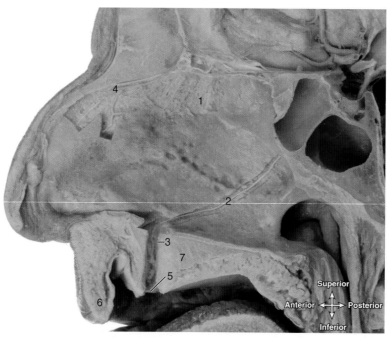

FIGURE 9-24 Dissection of a sagittal section of the left side of the nasal septum near the target area for the nasopalatine block. *1,* Olfactory nerve; *2,* nasopalatine nerve; *3,* incisive canal; *4,* anterior ethmoidal nerve; *5,* incisive foramen; *6,* upper lip; *7,* anterior hard palate. However, parts of the mucous membranes of the nasal septum have also been removed to show the principal nerves of the nasal septum. *(From Logan BM, Reynold PA, Hutching RT:* McMinn's color atlas of head and neck anatomy, *ed 4, London, 2010, Elsevier.)*

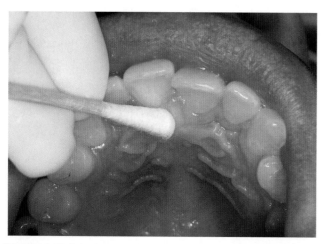

FIGURE 9-25 Injection site for the nasopalatine block is palpated at the palatal tissue lateral to the incisive papilla on the anterior hard palate and palatal to maxillary central incisors. Blanching of the palatal tissue on the contralateral side of the incisive papilla is continued during the injection to ensure pressure anesthesia.

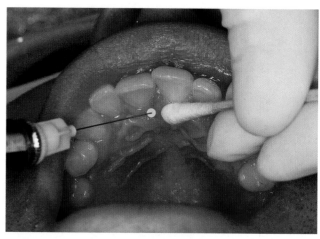

FIGURE 9-26 Needle insertion during a nasopalatine block of the palatal tissue lateral to the incisive papilla and palatal to maxillary central incisors until contact is made with the maxilla. The needle is at a 45° angle to the palate. Injection site highlighted. Blanching of the palatal tissue on the contralateral side of the incisive papilla is continued during the injection to ensure pressure anesthesia. *(Courtesy of Margaret J. Fehrenbach, RDH, MS.)*

delivery device because it regulates the pressure and volume ratio of agent delivered, which is not readily attained with a manual syringe. In addition, more recent studies show that due to the extensive anatomy involved, this block may be variable in the depth and duration of anesthesia, and does not provide a high level of hemostatic control. Due to this variability, it may not be adequate for dental procedures that need a longer and deeper level of anesthesia, as well as clinically effective hemostatic control.

Target Area and Injection Site for Anterior Middle Superior Alveolar Block. The target area for the AMSA block is the small pores within the maxilla of the hard palate (Figure 9-27 and see Figure 9-9). As the local anesthetic agent penetrates the pores, it has access from the anterior to middle part of the superior dental plexus, which then anesthetizes the teeth as well as the associated facial and palatal periodontium and gingiva as indicated earlier.

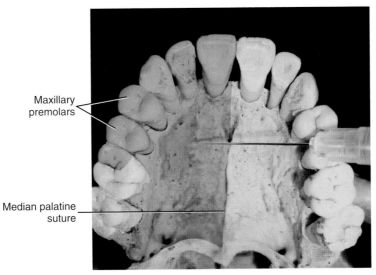

FIGURE 9-27 Target area for the anterior middle superior alveolar block is the pores within the maxillae of the hard palate. Distribution of anesthesia is highlighted.

Maxillary premolars

Median palatine suture

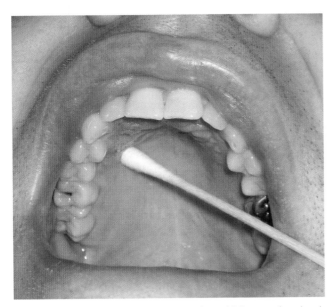

FIGURE 9-28 Injection site for the anterior middle superior alveolar block is palpated at an area on the palate superior to the apices of the maxillary premolars as well as approximately midway between the palatal gingival margin and the median palatine raphe overlying the median palatine suture.

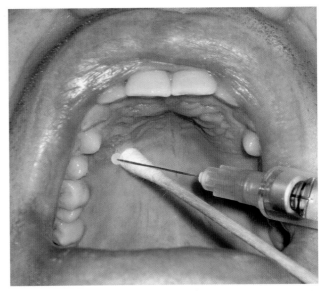

FIGURE 9-29 Needle insertion during an anterior middle superior alveolar block of the palatal tissue using a computer-controlled local anesthetic delivery device until contact is made with the maxilla at an area on the palate superior to the apices of the maxillary premolars as well as approximately midway between the palatal gingival margin and the median palatine raphe overlying the median palatine suture. The needle is at a 45° angle to the hard palate with the syringe barrel coming from the contralateral premolars. Injection site is highlighted. Blanching of the nearby palatal tissue is continued throughout the injection to ensure pressure anesthesia. *(Courtesy of Margaret J. Fehrenbach, RDH, MS.)*

The injection site for the AMSA block is an area on the hard palate superior to the apices of the maxillary premolars, and approximately midway between the palatal gingival margin and the median palatal raphe overlying the median palatine suture (Figure 9-28 and see Figure 3-48).

The use of pressure anesthesia throughout this injection near the injection site to blanch the tissue throughout the injection will reduce patient discomfort. This pressure anesthesia to the tissue produces a dull ache to block pain impulses that arise from needle insertion and local anesthetic agent deposition.

The previously blanched tissue is inserted with the needle at a 45° angle to the hard palate with the handpiece of the delivery device syringe coming from the contralateral premolars. The needle is

advanced until the maxilla is gently contacted, and then the injection is administered (Figure 9-29).

Some clinicians use a bidirectional rotation needle insertion technique with the handpiece of the delivery device syringe instead of the usual linear insertion technique to allow the needle to more easily enter the firmer tissue of the palate. In addition, a prepuncture technique that acts as a type of topical anesthesia can also be utilized by placing the bevel of the needle toward the palatal tissue with a cotton applicator on top of the needle tip. The clinician then applies light pressure on the cotton applicator to slightly puncture the tissue while administering a small amount of the agent from the delivery device without leakage and while still maintaining pressure anesthesia. The rest of the agent is then administered with less discomfort and no need for pressure anesthesia to continue.

Indications of Clinically Effective Anterior Middle Superior Alveolar Block and Possible Complications. Indications of a clinically effective AMSA block include variable numbness of the large area that is usually innervated by the anterior and middle superior alveolar nerves as well as the nasopalatine and greater palatine nerves. Blanching also remains present on the palatal tissue after the AMSA block due to the increased local anesthetic agent dispensed. However, if excessive, it may cause postoperative tissue ischemia and sloughing. Thus if excessive blanching is noted, slowing or stopping the delivery device for a few seconds to allow the local anesthetic agent to dissipate will diminish the chance of this postoperative event as well as control the overall amount of agent used. Other complications are extremely rare.

MANDIBULAR NERVE ANESTHESIA

The mandibular nerve and its branches can be anesthetized in various ways depending on the tissue and structures requiring anesthesia (see Figure 9-1; see Tables 9-2 and 9-3). However, a supraperiosteal injection of the mandible is not as clinically effective as that of the maxillae because overall the mandible is denser and less porous than the maxillae over similar teeth, especially within the mandibular posterior sextant. This increase in density of the mandible compared to the maxillae can be demonstrated with a panoramic radiograph (see Figure 3-50). For this reason, nerve blocks are preferred to supraperiosteal injections in most parts of the mandible, unlike the maxillae.

Substantial variation also exists in the anatomy of local anesthetic landmarks of the mandible and its nerves, compared with similar structures in the maxillae, complicating mandibular anesthesia. Thus the need for troubleshooting of cases may arise with a lack of clinical effectiveness of anesthetic administered for the mandible. This text covers some of the most common variations of the mandible (see Chapter 3).

Any pulpal anesthesia for these blocks is achieved through anesthesia of each nerve's dental branches as they extend into the pulp by way of each tooth's apical foramen from the inferior dental plexus. Both the hard and soft tissue anesthesia of the associated periodontium and gingiva is by way of the interdental and interradicular branches for each tooth.

The inferior alveolar block is recommended for anesthesia of the mandibular teeth and associated lingual periodontium and gingiva to the midline, as well as the associated facial periodontium and gingiva of the mandibular anterior teeth and premolars to the midline within one mandibular quadrant. The buccal block is recommended for anesthesia of the associated buccal periodontium and gingiva of the mandibular molars within one mandibular quadrant.

The mental block is recommended for anesthesia of the associated facial periodontium and gingiva of the mandibular anterior teeth and premolars to the midline within one mandibular quadrant. The incisive block is recommended for anesthesia of the mandibular anterior teeth and premolars, as well as the associated facial periodontium and gingiva to the midline within one mandibular quadrant.

The more encompassing Gow-Gates mandibular block anesthetizes the entire mandibular nerve within one mandibular quadrant and thus is highly recommended for quadrant dentistry or with lack of clinical effectiveness of an administered inferior alveolar block.

The Vazirani-Akinosi mandibular block has a large area of coverage of the mandibular nerve within one mandibular quadrant similar to the inferior alveolar block. The Vazirani-Akinosi mandibular block is recommended in a patient with severe trismus or when there is difficulty in administering the inferior alveolar block as well as when the patient is too fearful to open for anesthesia. These two mandibular blocks can also both be used when the patient has a history of IA block failure owing to anatomic variability or accessory innervation.

INFERIOR ALVEOLAR BLOCK

The **inferior alveolar block** or *IA block* is also known as the *mandibular block* and is the most commonly used injection in dentistry. The IA block anesthetizes the mandibular teeth to the midline and associated lingual periodontium and gingiva to the midline, as well as the associated facial periodontium and gingiva of the mandibular anterior teeth and premolars to the midline within one mandibular quadrant. Thus the IA block anesthetizes the inferior alveolar nerve and its nerve branches as well as the lingual nerve. However, since not all of the nerve branches of the mandibular nerve are anesthetized with an IA block it is not considered a *true* mandibular block; in contrast, the Gow-Gates mandibular block is considered a *true* mandibular block since the entire mandibular nerve is anesthetized within one mandibular quadrant (discussed later in this chapter).

Additional use of the buccal block may be indicated if anesthesia of the associated buccal periodontium and gingiva of the mandibular molars is also necessary to complete the mandibular quadrant anesthesia. In some cases there is crossover-innervation between the left and right incisive nerves, similar to what occurs with the ASA block in the maxillae (see Chapter 8). The incisive nerve is a branch of the mandibular nerve that serves the mandibular anterior teeth. If this is the case, a bilateral IA block can be used, but it is not recommended due to the increased risk of complications.

Therefore, bilateral IA blocks are usually avoided unless absolutely necessary. This is because bilateral injections of this block produce anesthesia of the entire body of the tongue and floor of the mouth. This numbness can cause difficulty with swallowing and speech, especially in patients with full or partial removable mandibular dentures, until the effects of the local anesthetic agent wear off. Comprehensive dental treatment planning can usually prevent the need for bilateral IA blocks by treating the mandible in quadrants or even sextants.

More often, the use of a contralateral incisive block or a facially or lingually placed supraperiosteal injection in the tissue inferior to the apices of the mandibular teeth that fail to achieve initial pulpal anesthesia may be indicated during treatment. This would include when the patient feels discomfort during treatment or when a larger scope of anesthesia is necessary such as the entire mandibular arch. However, supraperiosteal injections on the facial surface of the mandibular anterior sextant are more clinically effective than those on the facial surface of the mandibular posterior sextant but less effective overall than injections over the maxillae in similar locations. Again, these differences in clinical effectiveness are due to increased density of the facial cortical plate of the mandible as compared to that of the maxillae and even these differences can even vary along the length of the mandible from anterior to posterior (see Figure 3-50).

Target Area and Injection Site for Inferior Alveolar Block. The target area for the IA block is the inferior alveolar nerve exiting the mandibular foramen on the medial surface of the mandibular ramus, overhung anteriorly by the lingula as can be noted on a panoramic radiograph (Figures 9-30, 9-31, and 9-32; see Figures 9-3, 3-50, 3-52, and 3-53). The adjacent anteriorly placed lingual

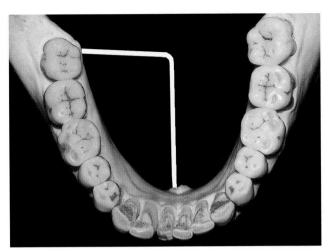

FIGURE 9-30 Distribution of anesthesia by the inferior alveolar block is highlighted.

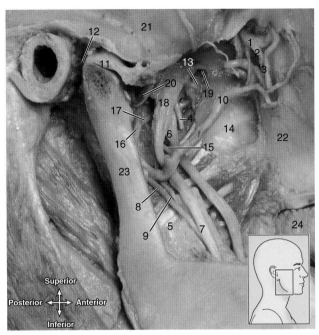

FIGURE 9-31 Dissection of the right infratemporal fossa at the target area for the inferior alveolar block (*see inset*; note removal of the lateral pterygoid muscle, zygomatic arch, and part of the mandible). The target area for the posterior superior alveolar block is also shown (see Figure 9-3). *1*, Maxillary nerve; *2*, posterior superior alveolar nerve; *3*, posterior superior alveolar artery; *4*, buccal nerve; *5*, medial pterygoid muscle; *6*, lingual nerve; *7*, inferior alveolar nerve; *8*, inferior alveolar artery; *9*, mylohyoid nerve; *10*, maxillary artery; *11*, joint disc of temporomandibular joint and mandibular condyle; *12*, joint capsule; *13*, medial pterygoid nerve; *14*, lateral pterygoid plate; *15*, chorda tympani nerve; *16*, middle meningeal artery; *17*, accessory meningeal artery; *18*, mandibular nerve; *19*, lateral pterygoid nerve; *20*, auriculotemporal nerve; *21*, temporal bone; *22*, maxilla; *23*, mandibular ramus; *24*, tongue. (*From Logan BM, Reynold PA, Hutching RT: McMinn's color atlas of head and neck anatomy, ed 4, London, 2010, Elsevier.*)

nerve will also be anesthetized as the local anesthetic agent diffuses, so there is no need for a separate injection to this nerve (see Figures 8-19 and 8-20). However, the agent must be accurately deposited within 1 mm of the target area to achieve clinically effective anesthesia, which may prove difficult because most of the deeper target anatomy is not visible to the clinician since it is at an approximate depth of 16 mm. Instead, surface landmarks must be relied upon.

The injection site for the IA block is at the depth of the pterygomandibular space on the medial border of the mandibular ramus at the correct height and anteroposterior direction determined for the injection (Figures 9-33 and 9-34). Hard tissue landmarks are mainly used to locate the injection site, such as the coronoid notch and the mandibular occlusal plane, to reduce errors caused by patient soft tissue variance.

The height of the injection for the IA block is determined by palpating the coronoid notch, the greatest depression on the anterior border of the ramus (see Figures 3-52 and 3-53). To determine the injection height, it helps to visualize an imaginary horizontal line that extends posteriorly from the coronoid notch to the pterygomandibular fold as it turns upward toward the soft palate, demarcating the posterior border of the mandibular ramus (Figure 9-35). Clinicians can palpate extraorally the posterior border of the mandibular ramus, but with this intraoral technique that is not usually necessary.

The pterygomandibular fold overlies the deeper pterygomandibular raphe, which is located between the buccinator and superior pharyngeal constrictor muscles. This fold extends from behind the most distal mandibular molar and retromolar pad and runs horizontally to the posterior border of the mandible and then turns superior to the junction of hard and soft palates, separating the buccal mucosa from the pharynx (see Figure 2-21). This fold stretches to become accentuated as the patient opens the mouth comfortably wider, which is an important instruction to relate to the patient when administering this block.

This imaginary horizontal line denoting the injection height of the IA block is also parallel to and approximately 6 to 10 mm superior to the mandibular occlusal plane in the majority of adults. However, in children and small adults, this imaginary horizontal line for the injection height should be more inferiorly positioned than the usual height and thus closer to the mandibular occlusal plane (see Figure 9-35). In regard to children this is because the mandible has not reached its full mature size. In contrast, in partially edentulous patients with only the

mandibular premolars and/or anterior teeth present, the location of the mandibular foramen may appear to be more superior because the occlusal plane of the molars is not present as a guide as when a full dentition is present.

The anteroposterior direction of the IA block injection is determined at the same time as the determination of the correct height of the injection. To determine this anteroposterior direction, it helps to visualize an imaginary vertical line that is approximately two-thirds of the distance between the coronoid notch and the pterygomandibular fold as it turns upward toward the soft palate, demarcating the posterior border of the mandibular ramus (see Figure 9-35). Clinicians can again palpate extraorally the posterior border of the mandibular ramus but with this intraoral technique that is not usually necessary. Although older sources give the location of the mandibular foramen as three-fourths along the ramus, most recent studies on skulls show its position as approximately two-thirds the distance from the coronoid notch to the posterior border of the mandibular ramus; all these recent studies show that it is slightly posterior to the middle of the mandibular ramus.

Thus, the injection site of the IA block is determined by the intersection of these two imaginary lines, one horizontal and one vertical, which meet at the deepest part of the pterygomandibular space, lateral to both the pterygomandibular fold and the sphenomandibular

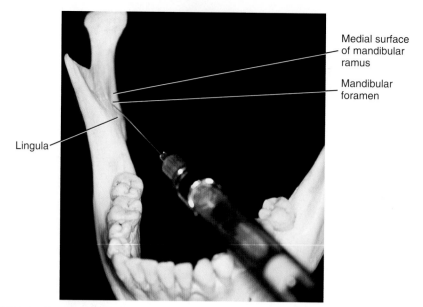

FIGURE 9-32 Target area for the inferior alveolar block is the inferior alveolar nerve exiting the mandibular foramen. The mandibular foramen is located on the medial surface of the mandibular ramus, overhung anteriorly by lingula. The adjacent anteriorly placed lingual nerve will also be anesthetized as the local anesthetic agent diffuses.

Labels on figure: Medial surface of mandibular ramus; Mandibular foramen; Lingula

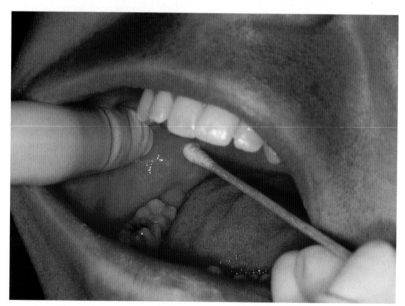

FIGURE 9-33 Injection site for the inferior alveolar block is palpated at the depth of the pterygomandibular space on the medial surface of the mandibular ramus.

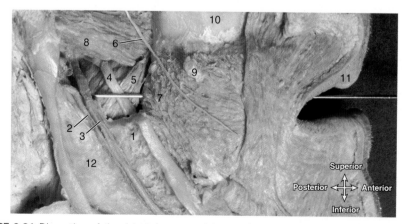

FIGURE 9-34 Dissection of the right infratemporal fossa with a needle at the injection site for the inferior alveolar block. Note how "lingual shock" could occur as the needle passes by the lingual nerve during administration of the block. *1,* Lingula; *2,* inferior alveolar artery; *3,* inferior alveolar nerve; *4,* lingual nerve; *5,* medial pterygoid muscle; *6,* buccal nerve; *7,* buccinator muscle; *8,* lateral pterygoid muscle; *9,* parotid duct; *10,* maxilla; *11,* upper lip; *12,* mandibular ramus. *(From Logan BM, Reynold PA, Hutching RT: McMinn's color atlas of head and neck anatomy, ed 4, London, 2010, Elsevier.)*

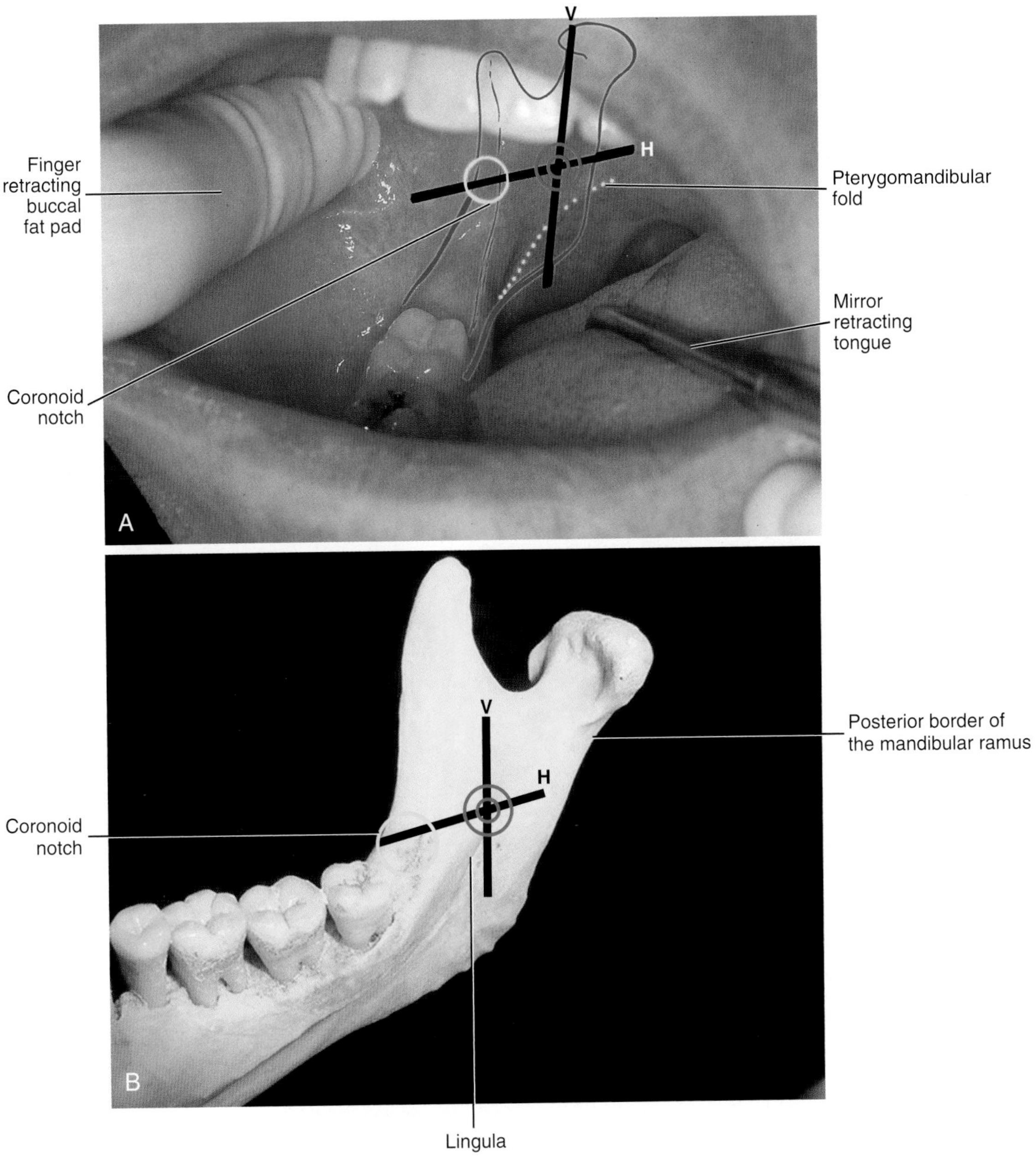

FIGURE 9-35 A, Injection site for inferior alveolar block *(bullseye)* is determined from the intersection of an imaginary horizontal line *(H)* noting the correct injection height with a vertical line *(V)* noting the correct anteroposterior direction so it is approximately two-thirds the distance from the coronoid notch to the posterior border of the mandibular ramus. Using this determination, the injection site is within the depth of the pterygomandibular space, lateral to the pterygomandibular fold *(dashed line)*, and at the same height as the coronoid notch *(yellow circle).* **B,** Medial surface of the mandibular ramus with the bony landmarks and imaginary lines for the inferior alveolar block noted again. **(A,** *courtesy of Margaret J. Fehrenbach, RDH, MS.)*

ligament (Figure 9-36; see Figures 9-35 and 11-8). To accomplish this, the syringe barrel is usually superior to the contralateral mandibular second premolar and at the contralateral labial commissure.

For the IA block, the needle is inserted into the soft tissue and advanced within the pterygomandibular space until gentle contact with the bony medial surface of the mandibular ramus, and then the injection is administered (Figures 9-37 and 9-38). It is not necessary to deposit small amounts of local anesthetic agent to anesthetize the adjacent anteriorly and laterally placed lingual nerve at approximately 16 m after the needle enters the tissue for the IA block because

anesthesia will occur through diffusion of the agent. These small amounts injected will also not reduce any tissue discomfort for the patient. Nor is it necessary to save any agent from the target area to deposit upon leaving the soft tissue for the same reason.

Inferior Alveolar Block Troubleshooting Paradigm. Even though the IA block is the most commonly used dental injection, it is not always initially clinically effective; the level for a lack of clinical effectiveness is approximately 15% to 20%. This may mean that the patient must be reinjected to achieve the necessary anesthesia of the tissue. However, the careful clinician will use a troubleshooting

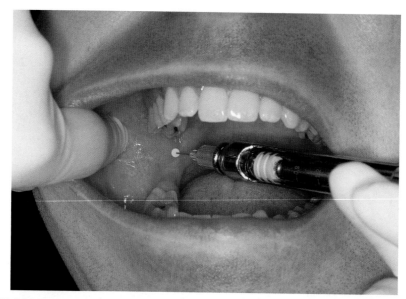

FIGURE 9-36 Needle insertion during an inferior alveolar block of the mandibular tissue. The needle is advanced within the pterygomandibular space until contact with the medial surface of the mandibular ramus. Injection site is highlighted. Note that the syringe barrel is usually superior to the contralateral mandibular second premolar and mandibular occlusal plane as well as at the contralateral labial commissure. *(Courtesy of Margaret J. Fehrenbach, RDH, MS.)*

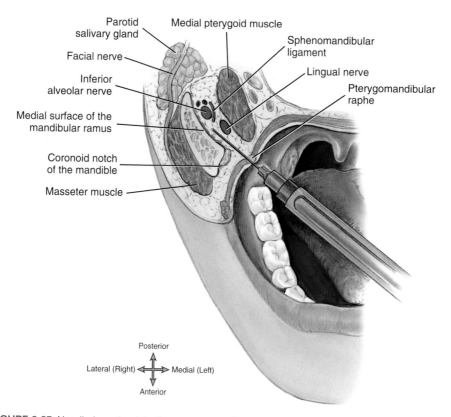

FIGURE 9-37 Needle insertion into the pterygomandibular space *(dashed line)* for an inferior alveolar block until contact with the medial surface of the mandibular ramus. However, if the needle is inserted too far posteriorly, it may enter the parotid salivary gland containing the seventh cranial or facial nerve, causing the complication of transient facial paralysis.

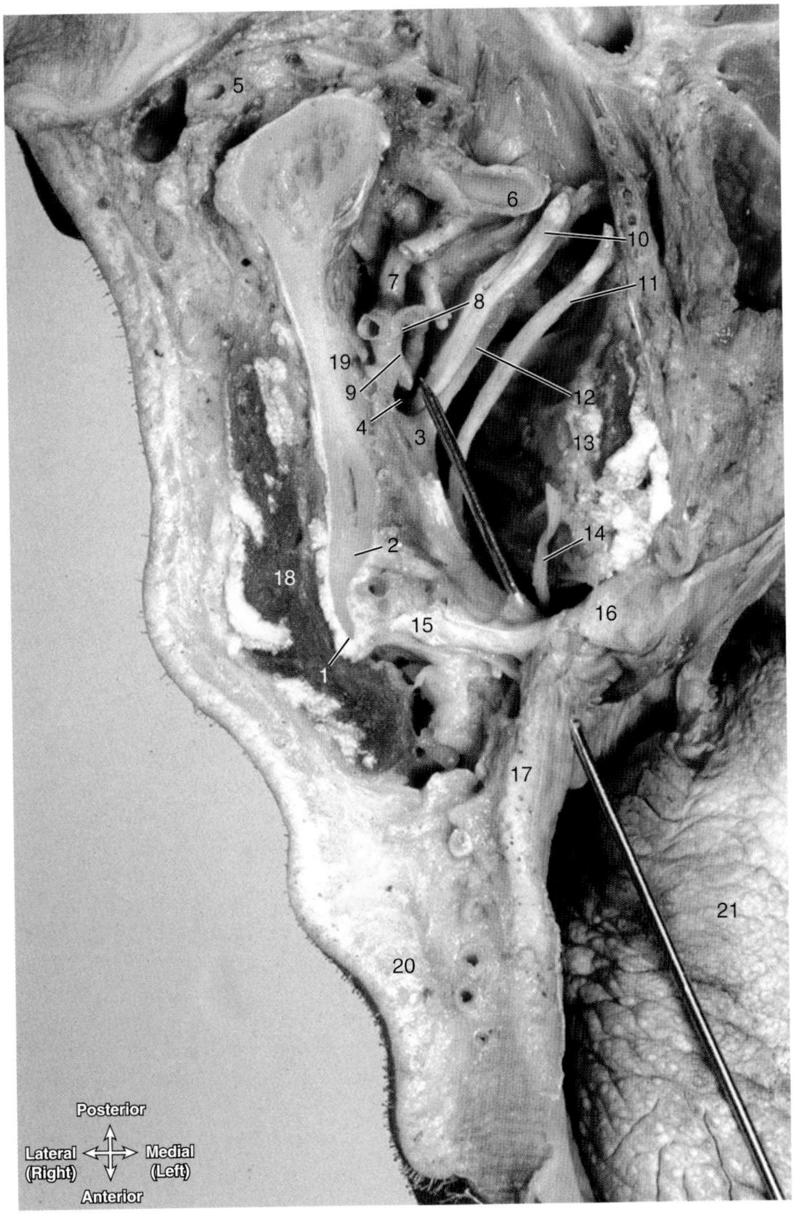

FIGURE 9-38 Dissection of a transverse section of the right infratemporal fossa with a needle at the injection site for the inferior alveolar block. *1,* Coronoid notch superior to external oblique ridge; *2,* mylohyoid line; *3,* lingula; *4,* mandibular foramen; *5,* parotid salivary gland; *6,* styloid process; *7,* maxillary artery; *8,* inferior alveolar vein; *9,* inferior alveolar artery; *10,* inferior alveolar nerve; *11,* lingual nerve; *12,* sphenomandibular ligament; *13,* medial pterygoid muscle; *14,* buccal nerve; *15,* temporalis muscle insertion; *16,* pterygomandibular raphe; *17,* buccinator muscle; *18,* masseter muscle; *19,* medial surface of mandibular ramus; *20,* buccal fat pad; *21,* tongue. *(From Logan BM, Reynold PA, Hutching RT: McMinn's color atlas of head and neck anatomy, ed 4, London, 2010, Elsevier.)*

injection paradigm in order to achieve clinical effectiveness every time the IA block is used.

First, the clinician should reassess a panoramic film of the patient if available, and from this note the mandibular foramen (see Figure 3-50). Second, the clinician should reassess the target area visually and by palpation of the landmarks. In addition, consideration should be made to the height of the insertion point, needle and syringe barrel angulations, and depth of insertion. This complex orientation can be practiced using a topical anesthetic-laced long cotton tip applicator to palpate the injection site as if it were the needle and syringe, as can all the injections. Lack of consistent clinical effectiveness is due in part to anatomic variation in the height of the mandibular foramen on the medial side of the mandibular ramus

and the great depth of soft tissue insertion required to achieve pulpal anesthesia.

To further complicate matters, not many patients are symmetric in their anatomic positioning of related mandibular structures so the paradigm for the IA block can be different on each side of the patient's oral cavity. Documenting these anatomic variations as well as any technique adjustments that were implemented in the patient's chart will assist the clinician during subsequent appointments. Other techniques to achieve mandibular anesthesia, such as the Gow-Gates or Vazirani-Akinosi mandibular blocks, may also be used when the IA block lacks clinical effectiveness (discussed later).

If bone is contacted immediately after the needle is inserted into the soft tissue when trying to administer an IA block, it is possible that the insertion point was too inferior and/or too far lateral from the pterygomandibular fold overlying the raphe, thus leaving the needle tip too far anterior on the medial surface of the mandibular ramus (see Figures 9-37 and 9-38). The needle tip may have entered either the temporalis muscle insertion, which may cause discomfort, or may have come into contact with the mylohyoid line (internal oblique ridge) of the mandible. The correction is made after withdrawing the needle by having the syringe barrel more anterior or closely superior to the mandibular anterior teeth when it is reinserted; with this correction the needle tip is more posterior.

In contrast, if bone is not contacted when trying to administer an IA block even with the correct depth of insertion by the needle, the needle tip is located too far posterior on the medial surface of the mandibular ramus (see Figures 9-37 and 9-38). The needle tip may enter the medial pterygoid muscle and be medial to the sphenomandibular ligament instead of lateral to it. The correction is made after withdrawing the needle by having the syringe barrel more posterior or closely superior to the mandibular molars when it is reinserted; with this correction the needle tip is more anterior. In addition, if the insertion and deposition are too shallow as discussed and bone is not contacted but the local anesthetic agent is administered, the medially located sphenomandibular ligament can become an outer physical barrier. This ligament can prevent the agent coming into contact with the deeper mandibular foramen and inferior alveolar nerve, thus preventing the more profound pulpal anesthesia and allowing only the more superficial lingual nerve to be anesthetized. In addition, the needle within the medial pterygoid muscle may cause trismus.

At all times, it is important not to deposit the local anesthetic agent if bone is not contacted on an insertion of the needle for an IA block. The needle tip may be too posterior and thus rest within the parotid salivary gland carrying the facial or seventh cranial nerve, resulting in serious complications (discussed later; see Figures 9-37 and 9-38).

If there is still lack of clinical effectiveness and it is mainly noted on the mandibular first molar even after proceeding with the troubleshooting injection paradigm, there may be accessory innervation present for this tooth. Current thinking supports the mylohyoid nerve as the nerve that may be involved in the accessory mandibular innervation of the mandibular first molar.

To correct this situation of accessory innervation, local anesthesia of the mylohyoid nerve using a supraperiosteal injection in the lingual tissue on the medial border of the mandible inferior to the apex of the tooth is indicated. This additional anesthetic technique is discussed in most current dental local anesthesia texts (see Appendix A). The clinician may instead attempt an additional block that may have an increased level of clinical effectiveness compared to the IA block, such as the Gow-Gates or Vazirani-Akinosi mandibular blocks, possibly due to providing additional anesthesia for the mylohyoid nerve (both discussed later in this chapter).

Another reason for incomplete anesthesia following an IA block is a bifid inferior alveolar nerve, which can be detected by noting a second mandibular canal on an intraoral radiograph (see Chapters 3 and 8). In such cases a second mandibular foramen, more inferiorly placed, exists; however, studies show that it occurs in less than approximately 1% of the cases. To work with this anatomic anomaly, the local anesthetic agent is deposited more inferiorly to the usual anatomic landmarks for the target area of the IA block or the Gow-Gates mandibular block is administered instead.

Indications of Clinically Effective Inferior Alveolar Block and Possible Complications. Indications of a clinically effective IA block include harmless numbness and tingling of the lower lip to the midline because the mental nerve, a branch of the inferior alveolar nerve, is anesthetized. This is a good indication that the inferior alveolar nerve

has been initially anesthetized, but it is not a reliable indicator of the depth of anesthesia, especially concerning pulpal anesthesia.

Another indication is harmless numbness and tingling of the body of the tongue and floor of the mouth to the midline, which indicates that the lingual nerve, a branch of the mandibular nerve, is anesthetized. Important to note is that this anesthesia of the tongue may occur without anesthesia of the inferior alveolar nerve due to the outer barrier presented by the more shallow sphenomandibular ligament (see earlier discussion). Possibly the needle was not advanced deeply enough into the tissue to anesthetize the deeper inferior alveolar nerve. The most reliable indicator of a clinically effective IA block is an absence of discomfort during dental procedures.

In addition, "lingual shock" as the needle passes by the lingual nerve may occur during administration. The patient may make an involuntary movement, varying from a slight opening of the eyes to jumping up in the chair. This reaction is only momentary, and anesthesia will quickly occur.

One complication with an IA block is transient facial paralysis if the seventh cranial or facial nerve is mistakenly anesthetized. This can occur because of an incorrect administration of local anesthetic agent into the parotid salivary gland that carries the facial or seventh cranial nerve or because the medial surface of the mandibular ramus was not contacted, as was discussed earlier (see Figures 9-37 and 9-38). This causes temporary unilateral loss of motor function to the facial expression muscles. The patient will experience the inability to close the eyelid and drooping of the ipsilateral labial commissure on the affected side as the muscles of facial expression become anesthetized. The loss of motor function is temporary and fades within a few hours once the action of the agent resolves (see Chapter 4).

This injection has a high risk of positive aspiration due to the proximity of the inferior alveolar blood vessels to the target nerves. Another related complication such as a hematoma can also occur due to these blood vessels being pierced by the needle even when the block is administered correctly (see Figure 6-18). Muscle soreness or limited movement of the mandible is rarely noted with this block when administered correctly. However, self-inflicted trauma such as lower lip biting and resulting swelling can occur due to anesthesia of the lower lip especially with children or those with physical or developmental disabilities.

Trauma can occur during an administration of the IA block, possibly to the lingual nerve, causing paresthesia of the nerve (see Chapter 8). Paresthesia is an abnormal sensation from an area such as burning or prickling, like a "pins-and-needles" feeling. Some studies demonstrate that paresthesia may be due to lack of adequate fascia around the lingual nerve or possibly neurotoxicity from the local anesthetic agent, especially in patients that receive multiple injections to the area. Other studies do not reach any set conclusions but state that nerve trauma can occur during nerve blocks. Paresthesia can also occur with the spread of dental infection (see Chapter 12), but it mainly occurs due to problematic surgical extraction of impacted third molars as well as mandibular posterior implant placement. Avoidance of further local anesthesia in the area is recommended to allow for resolution of any nerve damage. Finally, if the needle is contaminated, there may be a needle tract infection within the pterygomandibular space, which can spread to the cervical spaces.

BUCCAL BLOCK

The **buccal block** (or *long buccal block*) (**buk**-uhl) anesthetizes the (long) buccal nerve and thus the associated buccal periodontium and gingiva of the mandibular molars within one mandibular quadrant. Many times this block is not necessary if the buccal tissue is not impacted by the dental procedures provided. However, the buccal block, together with an IA block, will complete the mandibular quadrant anesthesia.

Target Area and Injection Site for Buccal Block. The target area for the buccal block is the (long) buccal nerve on the anterior border of the mandibular ramus in the area of the retromolar pad overlying the retromolar triangle (Figure 9-39 and see Figure 2-21 and 8-18). This catches the buccal nerve as it passes anteriorly to the anterior border of the mandibular ramus, crossing the external oblique ridge, and through the buccinator muscle before it enters the buccal region. Thus the injection site is the buccal mucosa that is distal and buccal to the most distal mandibular molar (Figure 9-40). The syringe barrel is parallel and directly superior to the mandibular occlusal plane on the side of injection. The needle is advanced until it gently contacts the mandible, and then the injection is administered (Figure 9-41).

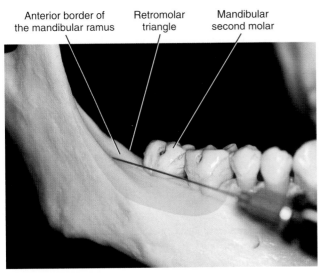

FIGURE 9-39 Target area for the buccal block is the buccal nerve on the anterior border of the mandibular ramus in the area of the retromolar pad overlying the retromolar triangle. Distribution of anesthesia is highlighted.

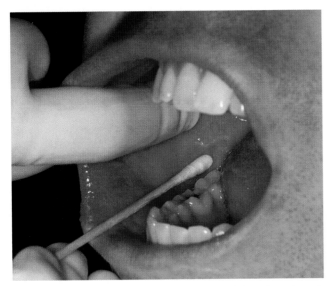

FIGURE 9-40 Injection site for the buccal block is palpated at the buccal mucosa that is distal and buccal to the most distal mandibular molar.

Indications of Clinically Effective Buccal Block and Possible Complications. Usually there are no overt indications of a clinically effective buccal block because of the location and small size of the anesthetized region. There is usually only an absence of discomfort with dental procedures. In some cases self-inflicted trauma such as a cheek bite occurs. This injection has a low risk of positive aspiration and the complication of a hematoma rarely occurs.

MENTAL BLOCK

The **mental block (men**-tuhl) anesthetizes the mental nerve and thus the associated facial periodontium and gingiva of the mandibular anterior teeth and premolars to the midline within one mandibular quadrant. If pulpal anesthesia is necessary on the mandibular anterior teeth and premolars, administration of an incisive block (discussed later) or use of the IA block, Gow-Gates, or Vazirani-Akinosi mandibular blocks may be considered instead. This block also does not provide any anesthesia of the associated lingual periodontium and gingiva of the involved teeth so additional use of a supraperiosteal injection in the lingual tissue on the medial border of the mandible inferior to the apices of these teeth may also be used.

Target Area and Injection Site for Mental Block. The target area for the mental block is the mental nerve entering the mental foramen. This block catches the mental nerve before it merges with the incisive nerve within the mandibular canal to form the inferior alveolar nerve (Figures 9-42 and 9-43 and see Figures 3-52 and 8-19).

The mental foramen is usually located on the lateral surface of the mandible inferior to the apices of the mandibular premolars. The mental foramen can be located on a radiograph before administering the injection to allow for a better determination of its position during palpation. However, studies show that the mental foramen can be as far posterior as the apex of the mandibular first molar or as far anterior as the apex of the mandibular canine. The mental foramen in adults faces posterosuperiorly (see Chapter 3 for more discussion).

To locate the mental foramen for the mental block, palpate intraorally the depth of the mandibular mucobuccal fold starting out inferior to the apex of the mandibular first molar and moving to the apex

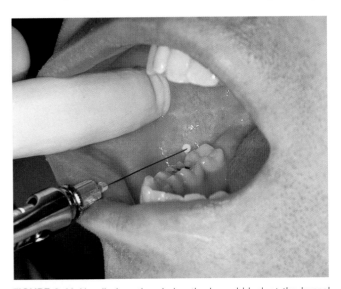

FIGURE 9-41 Needle insertion during the buccal block at the buccal mucosa that is distal and buccal to the most distal mandibular molar. The syringe barrel is parallel to the mandibular occlusal plane on the side of injection. The needle is advanced until contact with the mandible. Injection site is highlighted. *(Courtesy of Margaret J. Fehrenbach, RDH, MS.)*

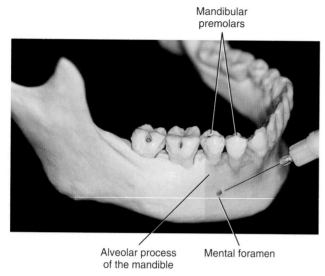

Mandibular premolars

Alveolar process of the mandible

Mental foramen

FIGURE 9-42 Target area for the mental block is the mental nerve entering the mental foramen. The mental foramen is usually located on the lateral surface of the mandible inferior to the apices of the mandibular premolars. Distribution of anesthesia is highlighted.

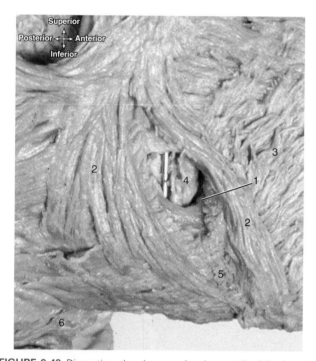

Superior
Posterior ←→ Anterior
Inferior

FIGURE 9-43 Dissection showing a probe deep at the injection site for either the mental block or incisive block. *1,* mental foramen; *2,* depressor anguli oris muscle; *3,* depressor labii inferioris muscle; *4,* mental nerve and vessels; *5,* lower chin; *6,* neck. *(From Logan BM, Reynold PA, Hutching RT: McMinn's color atlas of head and neck anatomy, ed 4, London, 2010, Elsevier.)*

of the mandibular canine or at a site indicated by a radiograph until a depression is felt on the lateral surface of the mandible, surrounded by smoother bone (Figure 9-44). The patient will comment that pressure in this area produces soreness due to the presence of the nearby nerve.

The injection site for a mental block is anterior to the mental foramen on the lateral surface of the mandible at the depth of the mandibular mucobuccal fold with the needle in the now recommended horizontal position, the syringe barrel resting on the lower

lip. The needle is advanced without contacting the mandible, and then the injection is administered (Figure 9-45). There is no need to enter the mental foramen to achieve anesthesia; in fact the needle cannot enter the foramen with the now recommended use of a horizontal position for the syringe.

Indications of Clinically Effective Mental Block and Possible Complications. Indications of a clinically effective mental block are harmless tingling and numbness of the lower lip and an absence of discomfort during dental procedures. This injection has a high risk of positive aspiration due to the proximity of the mental blood vessels. However, the complication of a hematoma rarely occurs.

INCISIVE BLOCK

The **incisive block** (in-**sy**-siv) anesthetizes the mental and incisive nerves and thus the mandibular anterior teeth and premolars, as well as associated facial periodontium and gingiva to the midline within one mandibular quadrant. However, if anesthesia of the associated lingual periodontium and gingiva of these teeth is necessary, the additional use of a supraperiosteal injection in the lingual tissue on the medial border of the mandible inferior to the apices of these teeth may also be used, or an IA block would be administered instead. The incisive block is also used when there is crossover-innervation from the contralateral incisive nerve and there is still discomfort during treatment on the mandibular anterior teeth after administering an IA block.

Target Area and Injection Site for Incisive Block. The target area for the incisive block is the incisive nerve within the mental foramen. This block catches the incisive nerve as it merges with the mental nerve and before it continues on in the mandibular canal to form the inferior alveolar nerve (Figure 9-46; see Figures 9-43, 3-52, and 8-19).

The mental foramen is usually located on the lateral surface of the mandible inferior to the apices of the mandibular premolars. The mental foramen in adults faces posterosuperiorly (see Chapter 3 for more discussion). The mental foramen can be located on a radiograph before administering the injection to allow for a better determination of its position. However, studies show that the mental foramen can be as far posterior as the apex of the mandibular first molar or as far anterior as the apex of the mandibular canine.

To locate the mental foramen for the incisive block, palpate intraorally the depth of the mandibular mucobuccal fold starting out inferior to the apex of the mandibular first molar and moving to the apex of the mandibular canine or at a site indicated by a radiograph until a depression is felt on the lateral surface of the mandible, surrounded by smoother bone (see Figure 9-44). The patient will comment that pressure in this area produces soreness due to the presence of the nearby nerve.

The injection site for an incisive block is anterior to the mental foramen at the depth of the mandibular mucobuccal fold with the needle in the now recommended horizontal position, the syringe barrel resting on the lower lip. The needle is advanced without contacting the mandible, and then the injection is administered (see Figure 9-45). It is important to note that it is not necessary to have the needle enter the mental foramen to achieve a clinically effective block; in fact, the needle cannot enter the foramen with the now recommended use of a horizontal position for the syringe.

More local anesthetic agent is deposited within the tissue for the incisive block than for the mental block, and pressure is applied to the injection site after the injection to enhance agent diffusion. Thus this pressure forces more of the agent into the mental foramen, anesthetizing first the shallow mental nerve and then the deeper incisive

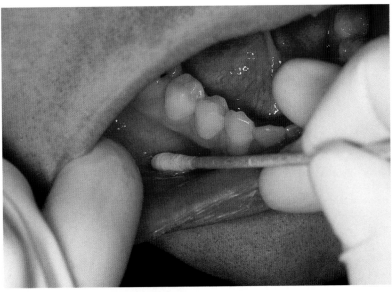

FIGURE 9-44 Palpation for either the mental block or incisive block of the depression created by the mental foramen on the lateral surface of the mandible, usually located in the depth of the mandibular mucobuccal fold inferior to the apices of the mandibular premolars. The injection site for either the mental block or incisive block is anterior to the mental foramen.

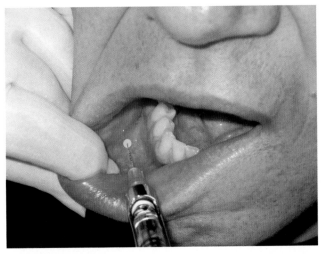

FIGURE 9-45 Needle insertion during either a mental block or incisive block at the depth of the mandibular mucobuccal fold anterior to the mental foramen on the lateral surface of the mandible, without contacting the mandible. The mental foramen is usually inferior to the apices of the mandibular premolars. Injection site is highlighted. Note that the syringe barrel is resting on the lower lip. *(Courtesy of Margaret J. Fehrenbach, RDH, MS.)*

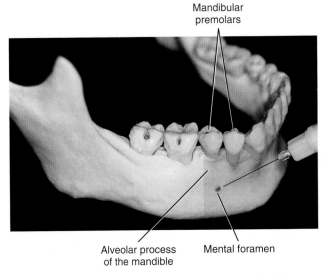

FIGURE 9-46 Target area for the incisive block is the incisive nerve merging with the mental nerve within the mental foramen. The mental foramen is usually located on the lateral surface of the mandible inferior to the apices of the mandibular premolars. Distribution of anesthesia is highlighted.

nerve. Thus anesthesia of the tissue innervated by the mental nerve will precede that of the deeper incisive nerve's tissue, with soft tissue anesthesia preceding pulpal anesthesia.

Indications of Clinically Effective Incisive Block and Possible Complications. Indications of a clinically effective incisive block are the same as the mental block with harmless tingling and numbness of the lower lip, except that there is pulpal anesthesia as well as anesthesia of the associated facial periodontium and gingiva of the involved teeth, and there is an absence of discomfort during more invasive dental procedures. This injection, similar to the mental block, has a high risk of positive aspiration due to the proximity of the incisive blood vessels. However, as with a mental block, a hematoma rarely occurs.

GOW-GATES MANDIBULAR BLOCK

The nerves anesthetized with the **Gow-Gates mandibular block** or *G-G block* include the inferior alveolar, lingual, mental, incisive, mylohyoid, and auriculotemporal nerves as well as the (long) buccal nerve approximately 75% of the time (Figure 9-47 and see Figures 8-16 and 8-17). The G-G block is considered a *true* mandibular block because it anesthetizes the entire mandibular nerve or third division and its branches. Therefore the G-G block will anesthetize the mandibular teeth to the midline and associated lingual periodontium and gingiva, as well as the associated facial periodontium and gingiva of the mandibular anterior teeth and premolars to the midline and probably the buccal periodontium and gingiva of the mandibular molars within one mandibular quadrant.

The G-G block is usually recommended for mandibular quadrant dentistry and in cases when the IA block is not clinically effective. One of the major advantages of the block is that it has an increased level of clinical effectiveness compared to that of an IA block, even taking into account a slightly more complicated procedure. Studies show that its higher level of clinical effectiveness may be related to the block being able to provide additional anesthesia to the mylohyoid nerve that has been shown to be involved in the lack of clinical effectiveness of the IA block due to accessory innervation (see earlier discussion). Thus it can be used when the patient has a history of IA block failure owing to anatomic variability or accessory innervation. Additional administration of the buccal block to anesthetize the associated buccal periodontium and gingiva of the mandibular molars may also be indicated to complete the mandibular quadrant anesthesia similar to the IA block.

Target Area and Injection Site for Gow-Gates Mandibular Block. The target area for the G-G block is the anteromedial border of the neck of the mandibular condyle, just inferior to the insertion of the lateral pterygoid muscle and lateral to the medial pterygoid muscle as well as medial to the mandibular ramus (Figure 9-48 and see Figures 4-23, 8-18, and 8-20).

The extraoral landmarks for the G-G block include the ipsilateral intertragic notch of the ear and the labial commissure (Figure 9-49 and see Figures 2-4 and 2-10). The pathway of the needle parallels the imaginary extraoral line connecting the ipsilateral intertragic notch and the labial commissure.

The injection site is located intraorally on the buccal mucosa of the medial surface of the mandibular ramus, just distal to the height of the mesiolingual cusp of the maxillary second molar (Figure 9-50). Initially the needle is used to determine the height for the injection by placing the needle just inferior to the mesiolingual cusp of the maxillary second molar (Figure 9-51). The injection height of the G-G block is more superior to the mandibular occlusal plane than that of an IA block, approximately 10 to 25 mm, depending on the patient's size. When a maxillary third molar is present, the injection site will be just distal to that tooth.

The needle is inserted into the buccal mucosa distal to the maxillary second molar at the established height. The needle is advanced while maintaining the needle pathway and injection height until the neck of the mandibular condyle is gently contacted; the injection is then administered (Figure 9-52). The syringe barrel is maintained superior to the

contralateral mandibular canine-to-premolar region and aligned parallel to the determined needle pathway. By contacting the bone of the neck of the mandibular condyle, the needle avoids causing traumatic injury to the area blood vessels, temporomandibular capsule, and otic ganglion.

It is also recommended that the patient open the mouth as comfortably wide as possible during the entire injection. The condyle assumes a more frontal position with the mouth open, and the injection site

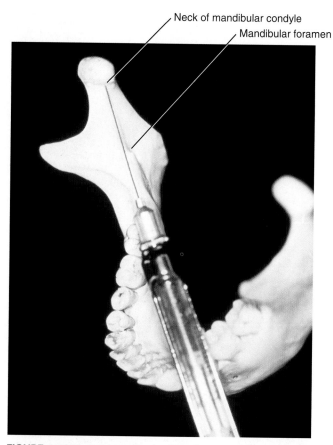

FIGURE 9-48 Target area for the Gow-Gates mandibular block is at the anteromedial border of the neck of the mandibular condyle.

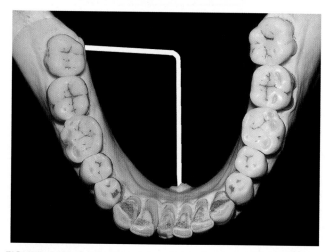

FIGURE 9-47 Distribution of anesthesia by Gow-Gates mandibular block is highlighted and includes structures innervated by the mandibular nerve. This is also the same intraoral area anesthetized by the Vazirani-Akinosi mandibular block with the additional anesthesia of the auriculotemporal nerve; and the buccal peridontium and gingiva of the mandibular molars are probably anesthetized (shown).

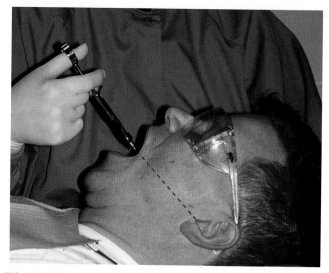

FIGURE 9-49 Imaginary extraoral line *(dashed line)* for determining the pathway of the needle for the Gow-Gates mandibular block. This extraoral line connects the ipsilateral intertragic notch of the ear and the labial commissure.

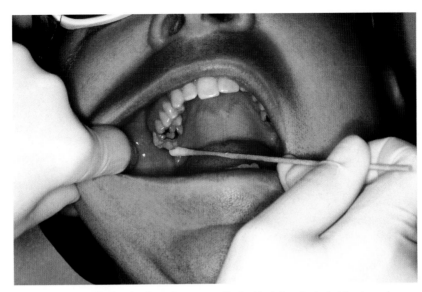

FIGURE 9-50 Injection site for the Gow-Gates mandibular block is palpated at the buccal mucosa just distal to the height of the mesiolingual cusp of the maxillary second molar, with its needle pathway determined by following a line extraorally connecting the intertragic notch of the ear and the ipsilateral labial commissure.

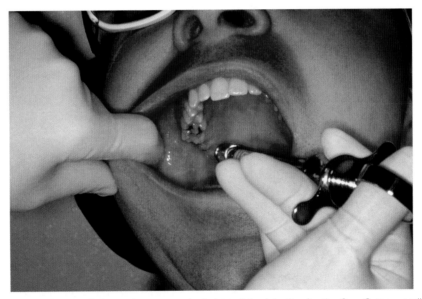

FIGURE 9-51 The needle is used to assess the height of the injection for the Gow-Gates mandibular block by initially placing the needle just inferior to the mesiolingual cusp of the maxillary second molar.

becomes closer to the mandibular nerve trunk, which is preferred during this injection (see Chapter 5). In contrast, with a more closed mouth the condyle will move out of the injection site and the soft tissue will become thicker. In addition, leaving the mouth open after administration will allow complete diffusion of the local anesthetic agent to the inferior alveolar nerve since it places the nerve closer to the injection site at the neck of the mandibular condyle; using a bite block may be helpful.

Gow-Gates Mandibular Block Troubleshooting Paradigm. Similar to the IA block (and also the V-A block), a troubleshooting paradigm may be used to achieve clinical effectiveness with the G-G block. Even before the injection is administered, the placement of the tragus in regard to facial surface needs to be considered since the angle of injection varies according to the degree to which the tragus diverges from the ear. As a rule, the flatter the tragus lies in relation to

the facial surface, the more anterior the syringe barrel position should be or more closely superior to the contralateral mandibular canine. In contrast, the closer the tragus is to a 90° angle to the facial surface, the more posterior the syringe barrel position should be or more closely superior to the contralateral mandibular second premolar.

If bone is not contacted on the neck of the mandibular condyle even with the usual depth of insertion, a greater depth may be required for larger patients or those with a markedly flaring mandibular ramus. If this is not the case with the patient, it can be due to deflection of the needle in a mesial direction. The correction is to withdraw the needle completely and instead bring the syringe barrel more posterior or more closely superior to the contralateral mandibular second molar. This correction moves the needle tip more anterior when it is reinserted or more closely superior to the mandibular canine, which should ensure contact with the bone of the neck.

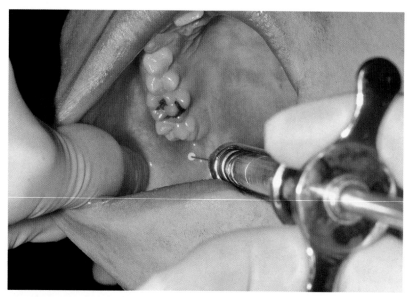

FIGURE 9-52 Needle insertion during a Gow-Gates mandibular block at the buccal mucosa just distal to the maxillary second molar at the established height. The needle is advanced while maintaining the needle pathway and the injection height until the neck of the mandibular condyle is contacted. The syringe barrel is maintained superior to the contralateral mandibular canine-to-premolar region. Injection site is highlighted. *(Courtesy of Margaret J. Fehrenbach, RDH, MS.)*

Indications of Clinically Effective Gow-Gates Mandibular Block and Possible Complications. Indications of a clinically effective G-G block are numbness of the mandibular teeth and numbness of the associated facial and lingual periodontium and gingiva. Inadvertently, the anterior two-thirds of the tongue, the floor of the mouth, and the body of the mandible and inferior mandibular ramus, as well as the skin over the zygomatic bone and the posterior buccal and temporal regions to the midline, will undergo numbness.

If the buccal periodontium and gingiva of the mandibular molars do not have an adequate level of anesthesia, the buccal block can be additionally administered. As the buccal nerve is approximately 23 mm from the injection site at the condyle, there is a significant reduction in the concentration of the anesthetic solution consequently affecting the block.

The two main disadvantages of the G-G block are the numbness of the lower lip, as well as the temporal and buccal regions as discussed, and the longer time necessary for the local anesthetic agent to take effect. The increased time is due to the larger size of the nerve trunk being anesthetized and the distance of the trunk from the site of deposition, which is approximately 5 to 10 mm. Thus this block may be contraindicated for certain patients who do not like the feeling of numbness to last too long as well as children or those with physical or developmental disabilities.

Another advantage other than the large area anesthetized and its clinical effectiveness is that the injection has a longer duration than the IA block because the area of the injection is less vascular and a larger volume of local anesthetic agent is usually administered. This injection is contraindicated in cases with limited ability to open the mouth, but trismus is rarely a complication; instead a Vazirani-Akinosi mandibular block would be indicated. The risk of positive aspiration is low for the G-G block since the inferior alveolar blood vessels are further away from the target site than they are with the IA block; thus hematoma is also rare.

VAZIRANI-AKINOSI MANDIBULAR BLOCK

The nerves anesthetized with the **Vazirani-Akinosi mandibular block** (vaz-i-ron-ee **ak**-ee-no-see) or *V-A block* include the inferior alveolar,

lingual, mental, incisive, and mylohyoid nerves within the pterygomandibular space as well as the (long) buccal nerve approximately 75% of the time (see Figures 8-16, 17 and 9-47). Thus it is not considered a *true* mandibular block because it does not anesthetize the entire mandibular nerve and its branches as does the G-G block. Instead the V-A block is more similar to the IA block in anesthetic coverage. Therefore, the V-A block will anesthetize the mandibular teeth to the midline and associated lingual periodontium and gingiva, as well as the associated facial periodontium and gingiva of the mandibular anterior teeth and premolars to the midline and probably the buccal periodontium and gingiva of the mandibular molars within one mandibular quadrant.

In contrast to these other mandibular quadrant blocks, the V-A block is a closed-mouth mandibular block. Thus this block has a major advantage over these other mandibular blocks since it allows clinically adequate anesthesia of a patient that has severe trismus, which is a limited mandibular opening as a result of infection, trauma, or postinjection complication (see Chapters 7 and 12). The V-A block is also useful when soft tissue structures such as the tongue or buccal fat pad persistently obstruct the view of the intraoral landmarks used in the IA block (see earlier discussion) or for the edentulous patient without any dentition landmarks during implant surgery.

In addition, this block can be used for the fearful patient who does not want to open for anesthesia. Finally, this mandibular block can be used if the patient has a history of IA block failure owing to anatomic variability or accessory innervation. However, the V-A block is contraindicated in patients with an acute infection or inflammation within the pterygomandibular space or maxillary tuberosity region.

Additional administration of the buccal block to anesthetize the associated buccal periodontium and gingiva of the mandibular molars may also be indicated to complete the mandibular quadrant anesthesia similar to the IA block. However, it is important to consider that there is greater clinical effectiveness with the V-A block when compared to the IA block in many cases since the mylohyoid nerve is additionally anesthetized, a nerve that has been associated with accessory innervation of the mandibular first molar.

Target Area and Injection Site for Vazirani-Akinosi Mandibular Block. The target area for the V-A block is the medial

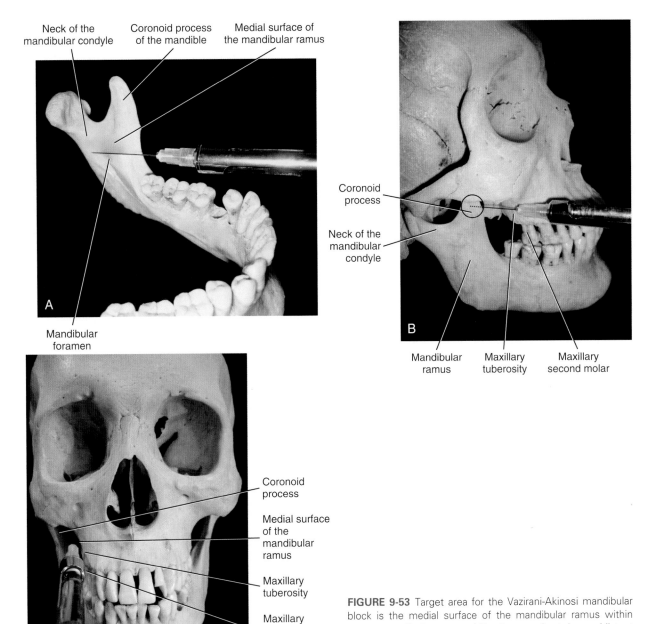

Neck of the mandibular condyle

Coronoid process of the mandible

Medial surface of the mandibular ramus

Mandibular foramen

Coronoid process

Neck of the mandibular condyle

Mandibular ramus

Maxillary tuberosity

Maxillary second molar

Coronoid process

Medial surface of the mandibular ramus

Maxillary tuberosity

Maxillary second molar

FIGURE 9-53 Target area for the Vazirani-Akinosi mandibular block is the medial surface of the mandibular ramus within pterygomandibular space (**A**) at approximately equidistant between the mandibular foramen and neck of the mandibular condyle (*dashed line in circle*) (**B**) as well as being adjacent to the maxillary tuberosity (**C**).

surface of mandibular ramus within the pterygomandibular space approximately equidistant between the mandibular foramen and the neck of the mandibular condyle as well as being adjacent to the maxillary tuberosity (Figure 9-53).

The patient is asked to gently occlude the posterior teeth, with the muscles of mastication remaining as relaxed as possible. If the muscles are clenched, the pterygomandibular space will be obliterated, which will prevent the agent from contacting the nerves within it. However, the intraoral landmarks must be visible during the injection so retraction of the check and its buccal fat pad is needed; using a retractor instrument is highly recommended. The intraoral landmarks for the V-A block are the medial surface of the mandibular ramus, maxillary tuberosity, and mucogingival junction of the maxillary third or second molar.

The injection site is the buccal mucosa between the medial surface of the mandibular ramus and the maxillary tuberosity, with the syringe barrel parallel to the maxillary occlusal plane (Figures 9-54). Thus this injection is administered at a site more inferior than the G-G block but more superior than the IA block. The injection height of the V-A block is determined by placing the needle at the same height as the mucogingival junction of the maxillary third or second molar directly across from the tooth (Figures 9-55).

The needle is directed medially past the coronoid process and then inserted into the buccal mucosa at the established height. The needle is then advanced posteriorly and slightly laterally without contacting the medial surface of the mandibular ramus, unlike the IA block, with the hub of the syringe ending up opposite the mesial aspect of the maxillary second molar (Figure 9-56). With the needle tip within the

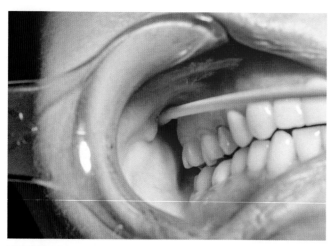

FIGURE 9-54 Injection site for the Vazirani-Akinosi mandibular block is palpated at the buccal mucosa with the injection height at the same height as the mucogingival junction of the maxillary third or second molar directly across from the tooth. *(From Fehrenbach MJ, Logothetis, DD: Mandibular anesthesia. In Logothetis DD, editor: Local anesthesia for the dental hygienist, ed 2, St Louis, 2017, Elsevier.)*

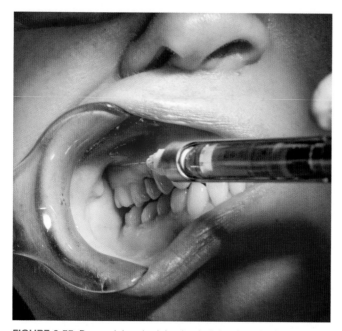

FIGURE 9-55 Determining the injection height of the Vazirani-Akinosi mandibular block by placing the needle at the same height as the mucogingival junction of the maxillary third or second molar directly across the way. Using a retractor instrument is highly recommended. *(From Fehrenbach MJ, Logothetis, DD: Mandibular anesthesia. In Logothetis DD, editor: Local anesthesia for the dental hygienist, ed 2, St Louis, 2017, Elsevier.)*

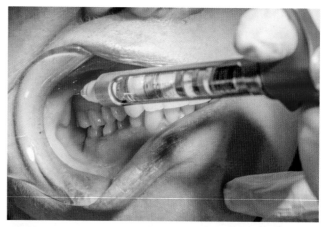

FIGURE 9-56 Needle insertion during a Vazirani-Akinosi mandibular block at the buccal mucosa between the medial surface of the mandibular ramus and the maxillary tuberosity, with the syringe barrel parallel to the maxillary occlusal plane. The needle was first directed medially past the coronoid process. The exact insertion point is hard to discern due to buccal frenum interference. The needle is advanced posteriorly and slightly laterally without contacting the medial surface of the mandibular ramus, and with the hub of the syringe ending up opposite the mesial aspect of the maxillary second molar. *(From Fehrenbach MJ, Logothetis, DD: Mandibular anesthesia. In Logothetis DD, editor: Local anesthesia for the dental hygienist, ed 2, St Louis, 2017, Elsevier.)*

maxillary tuberosity (see discussion next). The depth of insertion will vary with the anteroposterior size of the patient's mandibular ramus.

Vazirani-Akinosi Mandibular Block Troubleshooting Paradigm. Similar to the IA block, a troubleshooting paradigm may be used to achieve clinical effectiveness with the V-A block. Although no bone should be contacted with this block as discussed, if the mandibular ramus obstructs needle placement, it often occurs early. It is usually due to contact with the outer coronoid process since the insertion point is too far laterally placed; it may be corrected by reinserting the needle at a more medial position.

However, if the needle is placed too medially, it will end up resting medial to the sphenomandibular ligament and only the superficial lingual nerve will become anesthetized and not the deeper inferior alveolar nerve. And administering the agent too early and with the needle too shallow will also cause this same situation with its lack of depth to the anesthesia.

Out of a concern for the risk of complications, the clinician may also inject the agent at too inferior a position, again similar to the IA block. To correct this situation, the insertion of the needle can be at or slightly above the level of the mucogingival junction of the maxillary second or third molar across the way.

Indications of Clinically Effective Vazirani-Akinosi Mandibular Block and Possible Complications. Indication of a clinically effective V-A block is numbness of structures that are very similar in scope as that of the IA block. Also, since motor nerve paralysis develops as quickly as or quicker than sensory anesthesia, the patient with trismus begins to notice an increased ability to open the jaws shortly after the deposition of local anesthetic agent. If there is still trismus present later during the dental appointment, the V-A block can also be readministered. If trismus has subsided for the patient but there is additional discomfort noted during the dental procedures, then an IA block, G-G block, or a supraperiosteal injection can also be administered.

There is decreased risk of positive aspiration as well as hematoma formation as compared to the IA block since the inferior alveolar artery

center of the pterygomandibular space, the injection is administered (see Figure 11-8). The goal is to fill the pterygomandibular space with the agent so as to get full contact of the agent with the inferior alveolar and lingual nerves in the space.

Due to the closed-mouth situation, it may be difficult to visualize the path of the needle so the depth of the needle is always a concern and must be carefully controlled; the depth is approximately half the mesiodistal length of the mandibular ramus as measured from the

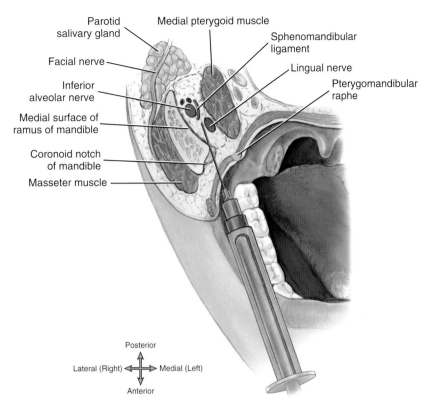

Posterior
Lateral (Right) ◄──►◄──► Medial (Left)
Anterior

FIGURE 9-57 Needle insertion into the midsection of the pterygomandibular space *(dashed line)* during a Vazirani-Akinosi mandibular block without contacting the medial surface of the mandibular ramus unlike the inferior alveolar block (see Figure 9-37). The depth of the needle is approximately half the mesiodistal length of the mandibular ramus as measured from the maxillary tuberosity. However, if the needle is inserted too far posteriorly, it may enter the parotid salivary gland containing the seventh cranial or facial nerve, causing the complication of transient facial paralysis.

and vein are further away from the injection site than they are with the IA block; it is also less traumatic than the G-G block with the mouth needing to stay open for a long time (see earlier discussions).

However, depth of the needle must be considered to avoid administration of local anesthetic agent into the parotid salivary gland containing the seventh cranial or facial nerve. This may cause the complication of transient facial paralysis; see earlier discussion related to the IA block's possible complications (see Figure 9-57).

REVIEW QUESTIONS

1. An extraoral hematoma can result from an INCORRECTLY administered posterior superior alveolar local anesthetic block because the needle was overinserted and thus penetrated which of the following?
   A. Parotid salivary gland
   B. Pterygoid plexus of veins
   C. Floor of the nasal cavity
   D. Lateral orbital wall
   E. Seventh cranial or facial nerve

2. Which of the following local anesthetic blocks has the SAME injection site as the incisive local anesthetic block?
   A. Nasopalatine block
   B. Greater palatine block
   C. Inferior alveolar block
   D. Buccal block
   E. Mental block

3. Which of the following nerves is NOT anesthetized during an inferior alveolar local anesthetic block?
   A. Buccal nerve
   B. Lingual nerve
   C. Mental nerve
   D. Incisive nerve

4. Which of the following local anesthetic blocks uses pressure anesthesia of the tissue to reduce patient discomfort?
   A. Posterior superior alveolar block
   B. Mental block
   C. Greater palatine block
   D. Inferior alveolar block
   E. Buccal block

5. Which of the following regions is usually anesthetized during an infraorbital local anesthetic block?
   A. Bilateral anterior hard palate
   B. Buccal gingiva of maxillary molars
   C. Upper lip, side of nose, and lower eyelid
   D. Palatal gingiva of maxillary anterior teeth
   E. Side of face, upper eyelid, and bridge of nose

6. If the mesiobuccal root of the maxillary first molar is NOT anesthetized by a posterior superior alveolar local anesthetic block, the dental professional should additionally administer a
   A. posterior superior alveolar block.
   B. (long) buccal block.
   C. middle superior alveolar block.
   D. nasopalatine block.

7. Which of the following is an important landmark to locate before administering an inferior alveolar local anesthetic block?
   A. Coronoid notch
   B. Tongue
   C. Buccal fat pad
   D. Mental foramen

8. The injection site for the greater palatine local anesthetic block is usually located on the palate near which of the following?
   A. Maxillary first premolar
   B. Maxillary second or third molar
   C. Incisive papilla
   D. Infraorbital foramen

9. If an extraction of a permanent maxillary lateral incisor is scheduled, which of the following local anesthetic blocks needs to be administered?
   A. Posterior superior alveolar block
   B. Middle superior alveolar block
   C. Nasopalatine block
   D. Greater palatine block

10. Transient facial paralysis can occur with which INCORRECTLY administered local anesthetic block?
    A. Posterior superior alveolar block
    B. Middle superior alveolar block
    C. Nasopalatine block
    D. Inferior alveolar block
    E. Mental block

11. Which local anesthetic block anesthetizes the largest intraoral area?
    A. Buccal block
    B. Inferior alveolar block
    C. Mental block
    D. Incisive block

12. Which of these situations can occur if bone is contacted immediately after the needle is inserted into the soft tissue when administering an inferior alveolar local anesthetic block?
    A. Needle tip is located too far anteriorly on the mandibular ramus.
    B. Needle tip is located too far posteriorly on the maxillary tuberosity.
    C. Syringe barrel is superior to the maxillary anterior teeth.
    D. Syringe barrel is superior to the mandibular anterior teeth.

13. In which of the following locations is the outcome MOST clinically effective when using a supraperiosteal injection of local anesthetic?
    A. Facial surface of maxillary anterior sextant
    B. Facial surface of maxillary posterior sextant
    C. Facial surface of mandibular anterior sextant
    D. Facial surface of mandibular posterior sextant

14. If working within the mandibular anterior sextant on the exposed roots of the teeth, which local anesthetic block is MOST clinically effective and comfortable for the patient?
    A. Unilateral posterior superior alveolar block
    B. Bilateral lingual block
    C. Bilateral inferior alveolar block
    D. Bilateral incisive block

15. Which of the following local anesthetic blocks anesthetizes the associated buccal periodontium and gingiva of the mandibular molars?
    A. Buccal block
    B. Inferior alveolar block
    C. Mental block
    D. Incisive block

16. The mental foramen is USUALLY located on the lateral surface of the mandible inferior to the apices of which of the following mandibular teeth?
    A. First and second molars
    B. Second and third molars
    C. First and second premolars
    D. First premolar and canine

17. To have complete anesthesia of the maxillary quadrant, which of the following local anesthetic blocks needs to be administered along with the anterior middle superior alveolar local anesthetic block?
    A. Middle superior alveolar block
    B. Nasopalatine block
    C. Posterior superior alveolar block
    D. Anterior superior alveolar block

18. Which of the following can serve as a landmark for the anterior middle superior alveolar local anesthetic block?
    A. Incisive papilla
    B. Premolars
    C. Lesser palatine foramen
    D. Canine eminence

19. Which of the following is considered a *true* mandibular local anesthetic block because it anesthetizes the entire mandibular nerve?
    A. Posterior superior alveolar block
    B. Vazirani-Akinosi block
    C. Inferior alveolar block
    D. Gow-Gates block
    E. Buccal block

20. Which of the following landmarks should be noted when administering a Gow-Gates local anesthetic block?
    A. Maxillary second molar
    B. Contralateral labial commissure
    C. Coronoid notch
    D. Pterygomandibular space

21. Which of the following local anesthetic blocks is USUALLY associated with self-inflicted trauma?
    A. Posterior superior alveolar block
    B. Inferior alveolar block
    C. Greater palatine block
    D. Anterior middle superior alveolar block

22. Which of the following local anesthetic blocks has a HIGH risk of positive aspiration?
    A. Mental block
    B. Buccal block
    C. Vazirani-Akinosi block
    D. Middle superior alveolar block

23. Which of the following local anesthetic blocks USUALLY anesthetizes the mylohyoid nerve?
    A. Vazirani-Akinosi block
    B. Inferior alveolar block
    C. Anterior middle superior alveolar block
    D. Infraorbital block

24. In contrast to other mandibular quadrant blocks, the Vazirani-Akinosi mandibular block is a(n)
    A. *true* mandibular block.
    B. palatally administered block.
    C. closed-mouth block.
    D. extraoral block.

25. The target area for the Gow-Gates local anesthetic block is the
    A. mandibular foramen and lingula.
    B. depth of the pterygomandibular space.
    C. medial surface of the mandibular ramus.
    D. neck of the mandibular condyle.

Identification Exercises

Identify the structures on the following diagrams by filling in each blank with the correct anatomic term. You can check your answers by looking back at the figure indicated in parentheses for each identification diagram.

1. (Figure 9-7)

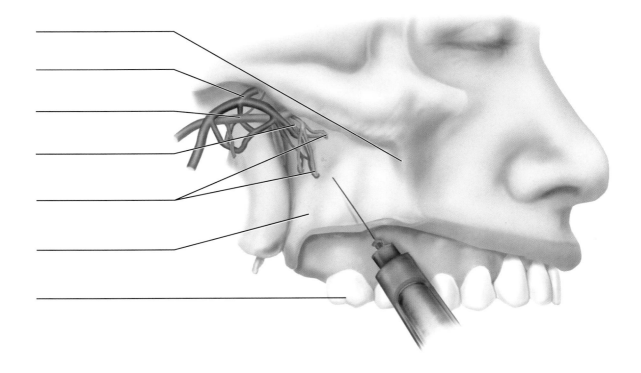

2. (Figure 9-37)

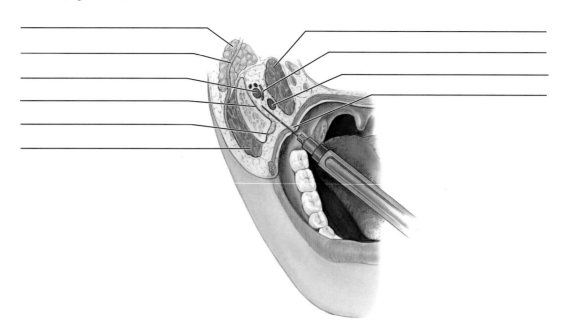

CHAPTER 10

Lymphatic System

●●● LEARNING OBJECTIVES

1. Define and pronounce the **key terms** and **anatomic terms** in this chapter.
2. List and discuss the lymphatic system and its components.
3. Locate and identify the lymph nodes of the head and neck on a diagram and patient.
4. Locate and identify the tonsils of the head and neck on a diagram and patient.
5. Identify the lymphatic drainage patterns for the head and neck.
6. Describe and discuss pathology of lymphoid tissue associated with the head and neck.
7. Correctly complete the review questions and activities for this chapter.
8. Integrate an understanding of the head and neck lymphatic system into clinical dental practice.

●●● KEY TERMS

Afferent vessel (af-uhr-uhnt) Lymphatic vessel with lymph flowing into lymph node.

Cervical lymph node levels Division of lymph nodes in neck by region using Roman numerals.

Efferent vessel (ef-uhr-uhnt) Lymphatic vessel with lymph flowing out of lymph node from node's hilus.

Hilus (hi-luhs) Depression on one side of lymph node where lymph flows out by way of efferent lymphatic vessel.

Lymph (limf) Tissue fluid draining from surrounding region and into lymphatic vessels.

Lymphadenitis (lim·fad·uh·ny·tis) Inflammation of lymph node.

Lymphadenopathy (lim-fad-uh-nop-uh-thee) Process with increase in size and change in the lymphoid tissue consistency.

Lymphatic ducts (lim-fat-ik) Larger lymphatic vessels draining smaller vessels and then emptying into venous component of vascular system.

Lymphatic system Part of immune system consisting of vessels, nodes, ducts, and tonsils.

Lymphatic vessels System of channels draining tissue fluid from surrounding regions.

Lymph nodes Organized bean-shaped lymphoid tissue filtering lymph by way of lymphocytes.

Metastasis (muh-tas-tuh-sis) Spread of cancer from primary site to secondary site.

Primary node Lymph node draining lymph from particular region.

Secondary node Lymph node draining lymph from primary node.

Tonsils (ton-sils) Masses of lymphoid tissue including palatine, lingual, pharyngeal, and tubal tonsils.

LYMPHATIC SYSTEM OVERVIEW

The lymphatic system is part of the immune system that consists of vessels, nodes, ducts, and tonsils. It helps fight disease processes such as infection and cancer and also serves other functions in the body. Although not part of the lymphatic system, the thymus gland also functions as a part of the related immune system and is discussed in Chapter 7.

LYMPHATIC VESSELS

The lymphatic vessels are a system of channels that parallel the venous blood vessels yet are more numerous in number (Figure 10-1). Tissue fluid drains from the surrounding region into the lymphatic vessels as lymph, also a clear watery fluid. Not only do the lymphatic vessels drain their region, but they also communicate with each other by way of regional lymphatic drainage, which assumes a chain-like pattern (discussed later). Lymphatic vessels are larger and thicker than the vascular system's capillaries. Unlike capillaries, lymphatic vessels have valves similar to veins. These valves ensure a one-way flow of lymph through the lymphatic vessel. Lymphatic vessels are even found within tooth pulp.

LYMPH NODES

The lymph nodes are bean-shaped bodies grouped in clusters along the connecting lymphatic vessels; they are called "glands" by patients (Figure 10-2). Positioned beside the lymphatic vessels, the lymph

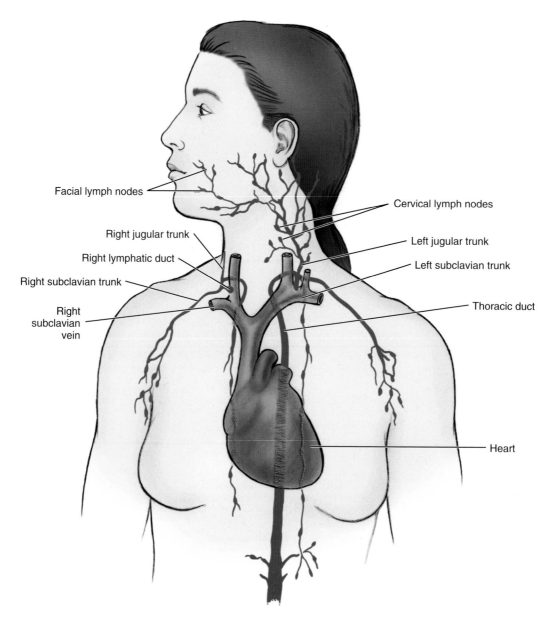

FIGURE 10-1 Lymphatic vessels and lymphatic ducts of the right and left sides of the upper body highlighted *(green)* and superimposed against the major blood vessels and heart.

nodes filter toxic products from the lymph to prevent their entry into the vascular system. The lymph nodes are composed of organized lymphoid tissue and contain lymphocytes, the white blood cells of the immune system that actively remove toxins. The removal of the toxins helps fight disease processes in the body. The nodes are also involved in the production of the lymphocytes.

Lymph nodes can be superficially located with superficial veins or located deep within the tissue with the deeper blood vessels. Lymph nodes groups are named for adjacent anatomic structures as well as their depth. In healthy patients, lymph nodes are usually small, soft, and free or mobile in the surrounding tissue. Therefore lymph nodes in a healthy patient cannot be visualized or felt when palpating their usual location during an extraoral examination of the head and neck.

REGIONAL LYMPHATIC DRAINAGE PATTERNS OF LYMPH NODES

The lymph flows into the lymph node by way of multiple afferent vessels (see Figure 10-2). On one side of the node is a depression or hilus, where the lymph flows out of the node by way of a single efferent vessel.

Since the lymph nodes are linked down a chain of lymphatic vessels, they can be classified as either primary or secondary based on their regional lymphatic drainage. Lymph from a particular region first drains into a primary node (regional node or master node). Primary nodes, in turn, drain into a secondary node (central node). In addition, lymphatic drainage from the superficial structures of the head and neck generally travel first to groups of more superficially placed lymph nodes before passing to the deeper lymph nodes.

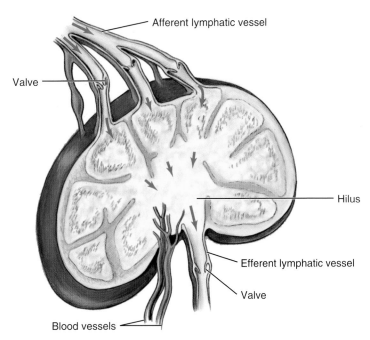

FIGURE 10-2 Lymph node with its components demonstrating the flow of lymph into and out the node; adjacent types of blood vessels are also noted *(red, artery; blue, vein)*.

TABLE 10-1	Oral Cavity Lymph Node Drainage	
STRUCTURES	**PRIMARY NODES**	**SECONDARY NODES**
Buccal mucosa	Buccal and mandibular	Submandibular
Anterior hard palate	Submandibular and retropharyngeal	Superior deep cervical
Posterior hard palate	Superior deep cervical and retropharyngeal	Inferior deep cervical
Soft palate	Superior deep cervical and retropharyngeal	Inferior deep cervical
Maxillary anterior teeth with periodontium and gingiva	Submandibular	Superior deep cervical
Maxillary first and second molars and premolars with periodontium and gingiva	Submandibular	Superior deep cervical
Maxillary third molars with periodontium and gingiva	Superior deep cervical	Inferior deep cervical
Mandibular incisors with periodontium and gingiva	Submental	Submandibular and deep cervical
Mandibular canines, premolars, and molars with periodontium and gingiva	Submandibular	Superior deep cervical
Floor of the mouth	Submental	Submandibular and deep cervical
Apex of the tongue	Submental	Submandibular and deep cervical
Body of the tongue	Submandibular	Superior deep cervical
Base of the tongue	Superior deep cervical	Inferior deep cervical
Palatine tonsils and lingual tonsil	Superior deep cervical	Inferior deep cervical

The regional lymphatic drainage pattern can be outlined for the oral cavity (Table 10-1), face and scalp (Table 10-2), and neck (Table 10-3); communication of the lymph nodes and their vessels can also be demonstrated by flow charts (see Figures 10-8, 10-11, and 10-16).

TONSILS

Tonsils consist of masses of lymphoid tissue located in the oral cavity and pharynx. Tonsils, like lymph nodes, contain lymphocytes that

remove toxins. Tonsils are located near airway and food passages to protect the body against disease processes from toxins.

LYMPHATIC DUCTS

Within the tissue located in outer regions of the body, smaller lymphatic vessels containing lymph converge into larger **lymphatic ducts** (see Figure 10-1), which empty into the venous component of the vascular system in the thorax (chest). However, the final drainage

TABLE 10-2	Head and Face Lymph Node Drainage	
STRUCTURES	**PRIMARY NODES**	**SECONDARY NODES**
Scalp	Posterior auricular, anterior auricular, superficial parotid, occipital, and accessory	Deep cervical and supraclavicular
Lacrimal gland	Superficial parotid	Superior deep cervical
External ear	Posterior auricular, anterior auricular, and superficial parotid	Superior deep cervical
Middle ear	Deep parotid	Superior deep cervical
Pharyngeal tonsil and tubal tonsil	Superior deep cervical	Inferior deep cervical
Paranasal sinuses	Retropharyngeal	Superior deep cervical
Infraorbital region and nasal cavity	Malar, nasolabial, retropharyngeal, and superior deep cervical	Submandibular and deep cervical
Cheek in buccal region	Buccal, malar, mandibular, and submandibular	Superior deep cervical
Parotid salivary gland	Deep parotid	Superior deep cervical
Temporomandibular joint	Superior deep cervical	Inferior deep cervical
Upper lip	Submandibular	Superior deep cervical
Lower lip	Submental	Submandibular and deep cervical
Chin in mental region	Submental	Submandibular and deep cervical
Sublingual salivary gland	Submandibular	Superior deep cervical
Submandibular salivary gland	Submandibular	Superior deep cervical

TABLE 10-3	Cervical Lymph Node Drainage	
STRUCTURES	**PRIMARY NODES**	**SECONDARY NODES**
Superficial anterior cervical triangle	Anterior jugular	Inferior deep cervical
Superficial lateral and posterior cervical triangles	External jugular and accessory	Deep cervical and supraclavicular
Deep posterior cervical triangle	Inferior deep cervical	Flows directly into the jugular trunk on right side or thoracic duct on left
Pharynx	Retropharyngeal	Superior deep cervical
Thyroid gland	Superior deep cervical	Inferior deep cervical
Larynx	Laryngeal	Inferior deep cervical
Esophagus	Superior deep cervical	Inferior deep cervical
Trachea	Superior deep cervical	Inferior deep cervical

endpoint of the lymphatic vessels into the lymphatic ducts depends on which side of the body is involved, which mirrors a similar concept in the vascular system (see Chapter 6).

The lymphatic system of the right side of the head and neck converge by way of the right **jugular trunk** (**jug**-u-luhr), joining the lymphatic system from the right arm and thorax (chest) to form the right lymphatic duct, which drains into the venous component of the vascular system at the junction of the right subclavian and right internal jugular veins (see Figure 6-14).

In contrast, the lymphatic vessels of the left side of the head and neck converge into the left jugular trunk, actually a short vessel, and then into the **thoracic duct** (thuh-**ras**-ik), which joins the venous component at the junction of the left subclavian and left internal jugular veins. The lymphatic system from the left arm and thorax also joins the thoracic duct. The thoracic duct is much larger than the right lymphatic duct because it drains the lymph from the entire lower half of the body for both the right and left sides.

LYMPH NODES OF HEAD

The lymph nodes of the head are paired and they usually either drain the right or left tissue, structures, or organs in each region, depending on their location. The lymph nodes of the head are also located in either a superficial or deep position relative to the surrounding tissue. The groupings of the lymph nodes of the head are based either on their location or nearby anatomic structures as well as their depth, either superficial or deep. Older terms for the lymph node groups are included for completeness.

SUPERFICIAL LYMPH NODES OF THE HEAD

Five groups of paired superficial lymph nodes are located in the head: the occipital, posterior auricular, anterior auricular, superficial parotid, and facial lymph nodes (Figure 10-3; see Figure 10-8).

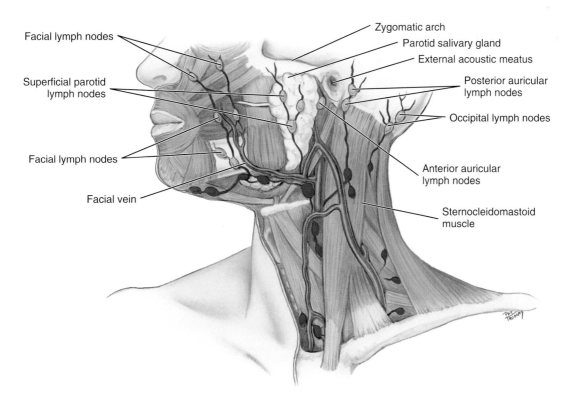

FIGURE 10-3 Superficial lymph nodes of the head and associated structures are highlighted.

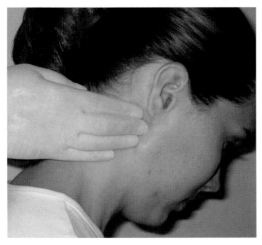

FIGURE 10-4 Demonstration of palpation of the occipital lymph nodes during an extraoral examination by tilting the patient's head forward. *(Courtesy Margaret J. Fehrenbach, RDH, MS.)*

OCCIPITAL LYMPH NODES

The **occipital lymph nodes** (ok-**sip**-i-tuhl) are approximately 1 to 3 in number. These nodes are located on the posterior base of the head in the occipital region and drain this part of the scalp (see Figure 3-21). Have the patient lean the head forward, allowing for effective bilateral palpation at the base of each side of the head during an extraoral examination for these nodes (Figure 10-4). The occipital nodes empty into the deep cervical nodes.

POSTERIOR AURICULAR, ANTERIOR AURICULAR, AND SUPERFICIAL PAROTID LYMPH NODES

The **posterior auricular nodes** (aw-**rik**-u-luhr) (or postauricular) are approximately 1 to 3 in number and are located posterior to each auricle and the external acoustic meatus, where the sternocleidomastoid (SCM) muscle inserts on the mastoid process (see Figures 2-4 and 4-1). The **anterior auricular lymph nodes** (or preauricular) are approximately 1 to 3 in number and are located immediately anterior to each tragus.

The **superficial parotid lymph nodes** (puh-**rot**-id) are up to 10 in number along with the deep parotid group and are located just superficial to each parotid salivary gland (see Figure 7-2).

The posterior auricular, anterior auricular, and superficial parotid nodes drain the external ear, lacrimal gland, and adjacent regions of the scalp and face. All of these nodes empty into the deep cervical nodes. During an extraoral examination, bilaterally palpate these nodes as well as the face and scalp anterior to and around each auricle (Figure 10-5).

FACIAL LYMPH NODES

The **facial lymph nodes** are up to 12 in number and are superficial nodes located along the facial vein with its diagonal course across the side of the face (see Figure 6-12). These nodes are usually small and variable in number. The facial nodes are further categorized into four subgroups: the malar, nasolabial, buccal, and mandibular lymph nodes.

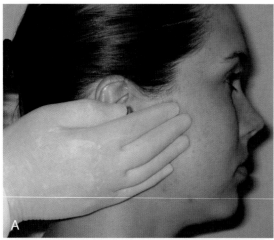

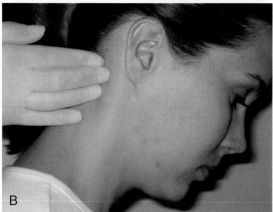

FIGURE 10-5 Demonstration of palpation of the posterior auricular, anterior auricular, and superficial parotid lymph nodes during an extraoral examination including the face **(A)** and the scalp around each ear **(B)**. *(Courtesy Margaret J. Fehrenbach, RDH, MS.)*

Nodes in the infraorbital region are the **malar lymph nodes** (**may**-luhr) (or infraorbital nodes) (see Figure 2-9). Nodes located along the nasolabial sulcus are the **nasolabial lymph nodes** (nay-zo-**lay**-be-uhl) (see Figure 2-7). Nodes around the labial commissure and just superficial to the buccinator muscle are the **buccal lymph nodes** (**buk**-uhl) (see Figure 4-11). Nodes in the tissue superior to the surface of the mandible and anterior to the masseter muscle, are the **mandibular lymph nodes** (man-**dib**-u-luhr) (see Figure 4-19).

Each facial node subgroup drains the skin and mucous membranes where the nodes are located. The facial nodes also drain from one to the other in a superior to inferior fashion, and then finally drain together into the deep cervical nodes by way of submandibular nodes. During an extraoral examination, bilaterally palpate these nodes on each side of the face, moving from the infraorbital region to the labial commissure, and then to the surface of the angle of the mandible (Figure 10-6). Infections from the teeth may spread to one of these facial nodes (see Chapter 12). When undergoing enlargement in response to the infection, these nodes can be described as being firmer and pea sized when palpated (discussed later in the chapter).

DEEP LYMPH NODES OF HEAD

The deep lymph nodes in the head region cannot be palpated during an extraoral examination due to their increased depth in the tissue. However, they still communicate with the more superficial regional nodes. The deep nodes of the head include the deep parotid and retropharyngeal lymph nodes (Figures 10-7 and 10-8). All of these deep nodes of the head drain into the deep cervical nodes.

DEEP PAROTID LYMPH NODES

The **deep parotid lymph nodes** are up to 10 in number along with the superficial parotid nodes and are located deep within the parotid salivary gland. These nodes drain the middle ear, auditory tube, and parotid salivary gland (see Figure 7-2).

RETROPHARYNGEAL LYMPH NODES

Also located near the deep parotid nodes and at the level of the atlas, which is the first cervical vertebra, are the **retropharyngeal lymph nodes** (ret-roh-far-**rin**-je-uhl), which are up to 3 in number. These nodes drain and are posterior to the palate, pharynx, paranasal sinuses, and nasal cavity (see Figure 3-62).

CERVICAL LYMPH NODES

All nodes of the neck or cervical lymph nodes are paired and they unilaterally usually either drain the right or left tissue, structures, or organs in each region, depending on their location, except for the midline submental nodes, which drain the tissue in the submental triangle bilaterally. The cervical lymph nodes are also located in either a superficial or deep position relative to the surrounding tissue. These groupings for the cervical lymph nodes are based either on their location or nearby anatomic structures as well as their depth, either superficial or deep. Older terms for the lymph node groups are included for completeness.

Clinicians can also record overall the cervical nodes, except those directly inferior to the chin, in relationship to the large SCM muscle, which defines the triangular regions of the neck (see Figure 2-23). Thus the cervical nodes can be generally discussed within three overlapping major categories: upper/middle/lower, anterior or lateral/posterior, and superficial/deep. This chapter is more specific in its discussion but recognizes this other method as workable for clinicians in a dental setting. It is important to note that the cervical lymph node groups also continue along the larynx, trachea, and thyroid gland as well as into the thorax (chest).

In addition, there is an imaging-based classification used by the medical community dividing the deep cervical lymph nodes into six cervical lymph node levels (Figure 10-9). These levels are designated by Roman numerals from I to VI, increasing in number as they become located nearer to the thorax. Other nodes not within this classification continue to be known by their anatomic name such as with the external and anterior jugular nodes and as well as the supraclavicular nodes. This text includes both the anatomic and level designations for those lymph nodes of the neck to reduce confusion for clinicians.

However, it is important to note that clinical terminology concerning the designation of cervical lymph nodes continues to evolve. This is because the designations are related to outcomes for various therapies for lymph node pathology such as the spread of squamous cell carcinoma, the most common oral cancer (see later discussion). Recent studies advocate a more precise 3-by-3 gridded system of 11 designations for more specific coverage of the neck using an overlay of both superficial and deep dissection.

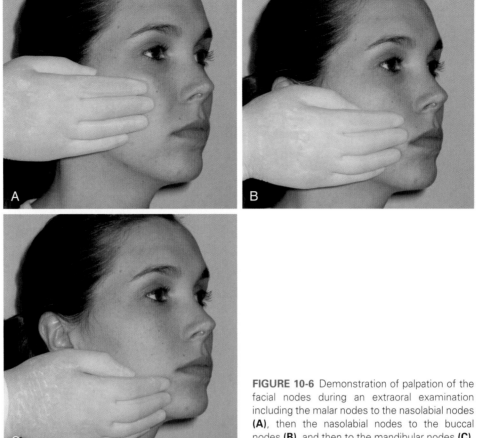

FIGURE 10-6 Demonstration of palpation of the facial nodes during an extraoral examination including the malar nodes to the nasolabial nodes **(A)**, then the nasolabial nodes to the buccal nodes **(B)**, and then to the mandibular nodes **(C)**. *(Courtesy Margaret J. Fehrenbach, RDH, MS.)*

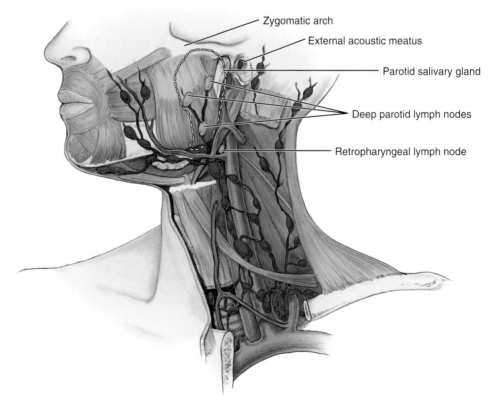

FIGURE 10-7 Deep lymph nodes of the head and associated structures are highlighted.

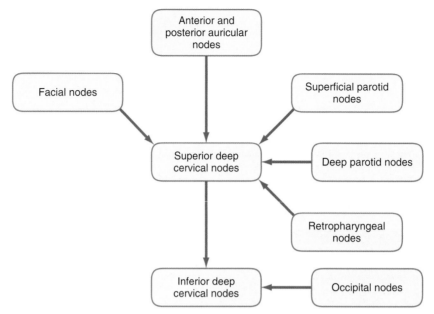

FIGURE 10-8 Lymphatic drainage of the head into the neck; note that external jugular nodes may be secondary nodes for the occipital, posterior auricular, anterior auricular, and superficial parotid nodes.

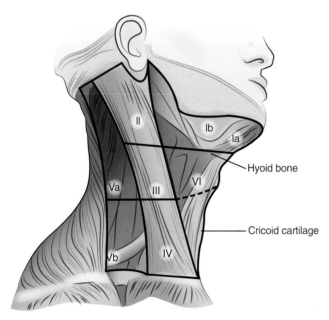

FIGURE 10-9 Levels noted for the deep cervical lymph nodes by region using Roman numerals, which increase in number as the location gets nearer to the thorax (chest).

SUPERFICIAL CERVICAL LYMPH NODES

The four groups of superficial cervical lymph nodes include: the submental, submandibular, external jugular, and anterior jugular lymph nodes (Figures 10-10 and 10-11).

SUBMENTAL LYMPH NODES

The **submental lymph nodes** (sub-**men**-tuhl) are approximately 2 to 3 in number and are located inferior to the chin within the submental fascial space, as well as the submental triangle, which is between the anterior bellies of the digastric muscles (see Figure 11-11). At this location, these nodes are near the midline inferior to the mandibular

symphysis in the suprahyoid region, and also just superficial to the mylohyoid muscle (see Figure 4-25). These cervical lymph nodes are considered to be within Level Ia (see Figure 10-9).

The submental lymph nodes bilaterally drain the lower lip, both sides of the chin, the floor of the mouth, the apex of the tongue, and the mandibular incisors with associated periodontium and gingiva. The submental nodes then empty into the submandibular nodes or directly into the deep cervical nodes.

The most common cause of nodal enlargement is from infections involving mononucleosis syndromes, Epstein-Barr virus, cytomegalovirus, toxoplasmosis, and dental infections such as periodontitis (nodal enlargement discussed later). Nodal Level Ib is also at greatest risk for involving the spread of cancers arising from the floor of the mouth, apex of the tongue, anterior sextant of the mandibular alveolar process, and lower lip (cancer is also discussed in greater detail later).

SUBMANDIBULAR LYMPH NODES

The **submandibular lymph nodes** (sub-man-**dib**-u-luhr) are approximately 3 to 6 in number and are located at the inferior border of the mandibular ramus, just superficial to the submandibular salivary gland, and within the submandibular fascial space (see Figure 11-12). They are also posterolateral to the anterior belly of the digastric muscles. These cervical lymph nodes are considered to be within Level Ib (see Figure 10-9).

The submandibular lymph nodes unilaterally drain the cheeks, upper lip, body of the tongue, anterior hard palate, and most of the teeth with associated periodontium and gingiva, except for the mandibular incisors and maxillary third molars. The submandibular nodes may be secondary nodes for the submental nodes and facial regions. The lymphatic system from both the sublingual and submandibular salivary glands also drains into these nodes. The submandibular nodes then empty into the deep cervical nodes.

The most common cause of nodal enlargement is from infections of head, neck, sinuses, ears, eyes, scalp, and pharynx (nodal enlargement discussed later). Nodal Level Ib is also at greatest risk for involving the spread of cancers arising from the oral cavity, anterior nasal

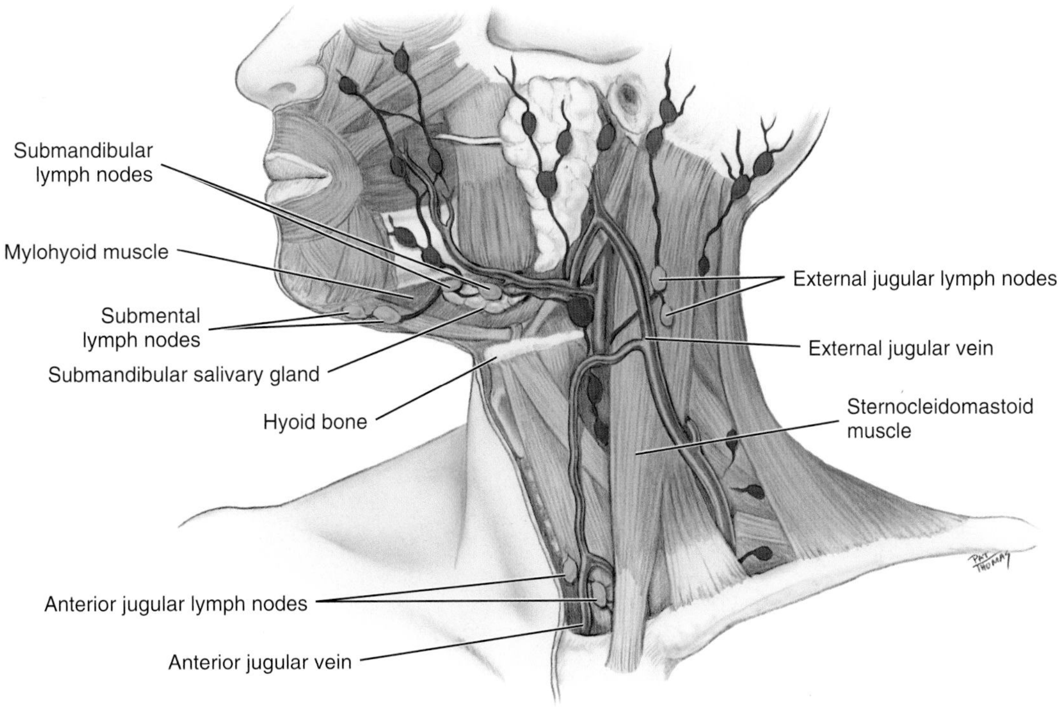

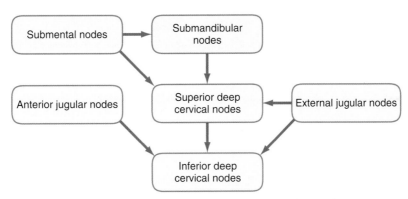

FIGURE 10-10 Superficial cervical lymph nodes and associated structures are highlighted.

FIGURE 10-11 Superficial lymphatic drainage of the neck.

cavity, soft tissue midface structures, and submandibular salivary gland (cancer is discussed in greater detail later).

During an extraoral examination, manually palpate the submental and submandibular nodes directly inferior to the chin after having the patient lower the chin (Figures 10-12 and 10-13). Then for the more laterally placed submandibular nodes, push the tissue on each side in the area over the bony inferior border of mandible, where it can be grasped and rolled. It is also recommended during additional palpation that the patient's chin be raised, the mouth slightly open, and the apex of the tongue on the hard palate to allow palpation of the nodes directly inferior to the chin against the mylohyoid muscle.

EXTERNAL JUGULAR LYMPH NODES

The **external jugular lymph nodes** (or superficial cervical nodes) are approximately 1 to 2 in number and are located on each side of the neck along the external jugular vein, superficial to the SCM

muscle (see Figure 6-13). The external jugular nodes may be secondary nodes for the occipital, posterior auricular, anterior auricular, and superficial parotid nodes. These nodes then empty into the deep cervical nodes.

ANTERIOR JUGULAR LYMPH NODES

The **anterior jugular lymph nodes** (or anterior cervical nodes) are located on each side of the neck along the length of the anterior jugular vein, anterior to the larynx, trachea, and superficial to the SCM muscle, as well as between the superficial layer of deep cervical fascia and the infrahyoid muscles. These nodes drain the infrahyoid region of the neck (Figure 6-13). The anterior jugular nodes then empty into the deep cervical nodes.

During an extraoral examination of the external and anterior jugular nodes in the middle part of the neck, have the patient turn the head to the contralateral side, which makes the important landmark of the SCM muscle more prominent (Figure 10-14). Palpate

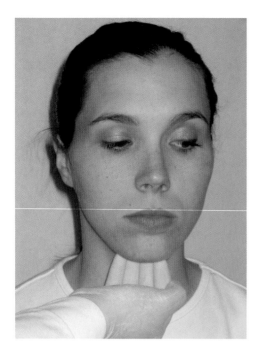

FIGURE 10-12 Demonstration of palpation of the submental and submandibular lymph nodes during an extraoral examination that are directly inferior to the chin by lowering the patient's chin. *(Courtesy Margaret J. Fehrenbach, RDH, MS.)*

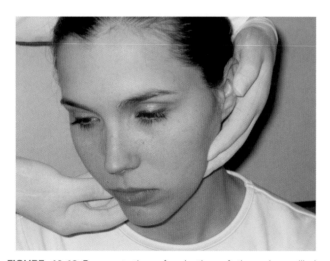

FIGURE 10-13 Demonstration of palpation of the submandibular lymph nodes that are more laterally placed during an extraoral examination by pushing the tissue in the area over the bony inferior border of the mandible on each side, where it is grasped and rolled. *(Courtesy Margaret J. Fehrenbach, RDH, MS.)*

these nodes superficially on each side of the muscle by starting at the angle of the mandible and continue the whole length of the surface of the SCM muscle to the clavicle.

DEEP CERVICAL LYMPH NODES

The **deep cervical lymph nodes** are approximately 15 to 30 in number and are located along the length of the internal jugular vein on each side of the neck, deep to the SCM muscle (Figures 10-15 and 10-16). They extend from the base of the skull to the root of the neck, adjacent to the pharynx, esophagus, and trachea.

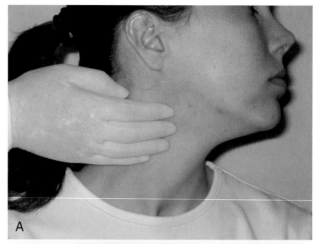

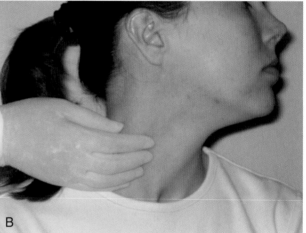

FIGURE 10-14 Demonstration of palpation of the external and anterior jugular lymph nodes during an extraoral examination using the landmark of the sternocleidomastoid muscle, starting at the angle of the mandible **(A)** and continuing down the length of the surface of the muscle to the clavicle **(B)**. *(Courtesy Margaret J. Fehrenbach, RDH, MS.)*

The deep cervical nodes can be divided into two groups based on the vertical anatomic position of the nodes relative to the point where the omohyoid muscle crosses the internal jugular vein: the superior and inferior deep cervical lymph nodes (see Figure 10-15). However, the specificity of this division is not as strong a concern in the overall drainage of the head and neck to dental professionals as it is to medical professionals. These deep cervical nodes are also considered to be within Levels II to VI (see further discussion below and see Figure 10-9).

Level II nodes include the superior one-third of the deep cervical nodes, including the jugulodigastric node. This region extends from the digastric muscle superiorly to the hyoid bone (clinical landmark) or the carotid bifurcation (surgical landmark) inferiorly. More specifically, Level IIa contains nodes in the region anterior to the accessory nerve and Level IIb is posterior to the nerve. Nodal Level II is at greatest risk for involving the spread of cancers arising from the oral cavity, nasal cavity, nasopharynx, oropharynx, laryngopharynx, larynx, and parotid salivary gland (cancer is discussed in greater detail later).

Level III includes the middle one-third of the deep cervical nodes that extends from the hyoid bone or carotid bifurcation superiorly to

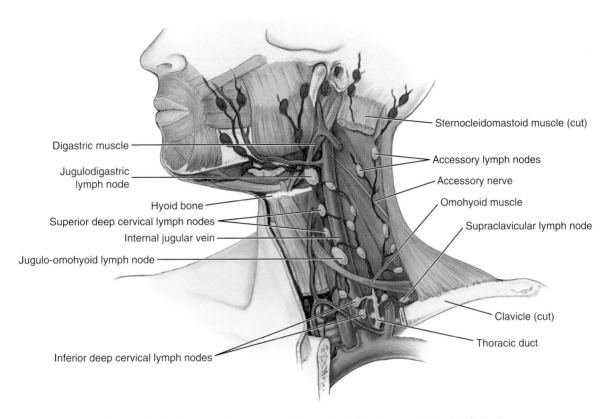

FIGURE 10-15 Deep cervical lymph nodes and associated structures are highlighted.

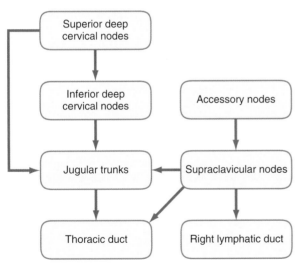

FIGURE 10-16 Lymphatic drainage of the neck.

the cricothyroid notch (clinical landmark), or inferior edge of cricoid cartilage (radiologic landmark), or omohyoid muscle (surgical landmark) inferiorly. The cricothyroid notch of the cricoid cartilage is directly inferior to the superior thyroid notch of the thyroid cartilage. Nodal Level III is at greatest risk for involving the spread of cancers arising from the oral cavity, nasopharynx, oropharynx, laryngopharynx, and larynx.

Level IV includes the inferior one-third of the deep cervical nodes that extends from the omohyoid muscle superiorly to the clavicle

inferiorly. Nodal Level IV is at greatest risk for involving the spread of cancers arising from the laryngopharynx, esophagus, and larynx.

Level V nodes extend from the skull base at the posterior border of the attachment of the SCM muscle within the posterior cervical triangle to the level of the clavicle as seen on each axial scan. More specifically, Level Va is superior to the inferior border of the cricoid cartilage and Level Vb is between inferior border of the cricoid cartilage and the superior border of the clavicle. Nodal Level V is at greatest risk for involving the spread of cancers arising from the nasopharynx and oropharynx (Level Va) as well as the thyroid gland (Level Vb).

Level VI nodes lie inferior to the lower body of the hyoid bone and between the medial margins of the left and right common carotid arteries or the internal carotid arteries within the carotid sheath. Nodal Level VI is at greatest risk for involving the spread of cancers arising from the thyroid gland, specific parts of the larynx, and esophagus.

Unlike the deep nodes of the head that cannot be palpated, the deep cervical nodes can be palpated on each side of the neck. Again, during an extraoral examination, have the patient turn the head to the contralateral side, which makes the important landmark of the SCM muscle more prominent and increases accessibility for effective palpation of these nodes (Figure 10-17 and see Figure 4-2). Palpation of the deep cervical nodes is performed on the underside of both the anterior and posterior aspects of the SCM muscle in contrast to the superficial cervical nodes that are on the muscle's surface that have already been discussed. Using bidigital palpation start at the angle of the mandible and continue down the length of the SCM muscle to the clavicle.

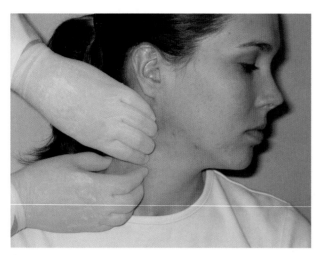

FIGURE 10-17 Demonstration of palpation of the deep cervical lymph nodes during an extraoral examination by turning the patient's head to the contralateral side and using the landmark of the sternocleidomastoid muscle with bidigital palpation on its underside from the angle of the mandible to the clavicle. *(Courtesy Margaret J. Fehrenbach, RDH, MS.)*

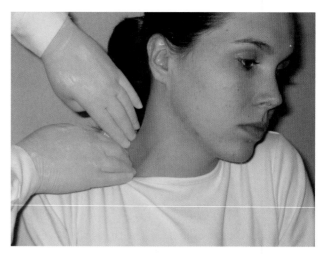

FIGURE 10-18 Demonstration of palpation of the inferior deep cervical and supraclavicular lymph nodes near the clavicle during an extraoral examination with the patient's shoulders raised up and forward. *(Courtesy Margaret J. Fehrenbach, RDH, MS.)*

SUPERIOR DEEP CERVICAL LYMPH NODES

The superior deep cervical lymph nodes are located deep underneath the SCM muscle, superior relative to the point where the omohyoid muscle crosses the internal jugular vein (see Figure 4-24). The superior deep cervical nodes are primary nodes draining the posterior nasal cavity, posterior hard palate, soft palate, base of the tongue, maxillary third molars with associated periodontium and gingiva, temporomandibular joint, esophagus, trachea, and thyroid gland. However, it is important to note that since the lymphatic drainage of the base of the tongue is bilateral in the posterior region, the contralateral node may also be affected if pathology is occurring there.

The superior deep cervical nodes may be secondary nodes for all other nodes of the head and neck, except inferior deep cervical nodes. The superior deep cervical nodes empty into the inferior deep cervical nodes or directly into the jugular trunk.

One node of the superior deep cervical nodes, the **jugulodigastric lymph node** (jug-u-lo-di-**gas**-trik) or *tonsillar node*, becomes noticeably palpable when the palatine tonsils that are drained by them undergo nodal enlargement due to infection (discussed later in the chapter). The jugulodigastric node is located inferior to the posterior belly of the digastric muscle and posterior to the mandible.

INFERIOR DEEP CERVICAL LYMPH NODES

The inferior deep cervical lymph nodes are a continuation of the superior deep cervical group. The inferior deep cervical nodes are also located deep to the SCM muscle, but inferior relative to the point where the omohyoid muscle crosses the internal jugular vein, extending into the supraclavicular fossa, superior to each clavicle (see Figure 4-24). The inferior deep cervical nodes are primary nodes draining the posterior part of the scalp and neck, the superficial pectoral region, and a part of the arm.

A possibly prominent node of the inferior deep cervical nodes, the **jugulo-omohyoid lymph node** (jug-u-lo-o-moh-**hi**-oid), is located at the angle created by the actual crossing of the omohyoid muscle and internal jugular vein. The jugulo-omohyoid node drains the tongue and submental triangle as well as associated structures and regions.

The inferior deep cervical nodes may be secondary nodes for the superficial nodes of the head and superior deep cervical nodes. Their efferent vessels form the jugular trunk, which is one of the tributaries of the right lymphatic duct on the right side and the thoracic duct on the left (see Figure 10-1). The inferior deep cervical nodes also communicate with the axillary lymph nodes that drain the breast region. Thus due to this nodal communication, the inferior deep cervical nodes are at greatest risk for involving the spread of breast cancer or adenocarcinoma (cancer is discussed in greater detail later).

ACCESSORY AND SUPRACLAVICULAR LYMPH NODES

In addition to the deep cervical lymph nodes are the accessory and supraclavicular node groups in the most inferior part of the neck (see Figure 10-15). The **accessory lymph nodes** are approximately 2 to 6 in number and are located along the eleventh cranial or accessory nerve. They drain the scalp and neck regions and then drain into the supraclavicular nodes.

The **supraclavicular lymph nodes** (soo-pruh-klah-**vik**-u-luhr) are approximately 1 to 10 in number and are located superiorly along the clavicle close to where sternum joins it. They drain the lateral cervical triangles of the neck. The supraclavicular nodes may empty into one of the jugular trunks or directly into the right lymphatic duct or thoracic duct (see Figure 10-1). These nodes are located in the final endpoint of lymphatic drainage from the entire body. Because of this location, these nodes are at greatest risk for involving the spread of cancers arising from the lungs, esophagus, and stomach (cancer is discussed in greater detail later). Therefore inspection of these nodes is important in any comprehensive patient assessment.

For those nodes near the clavicle such as the inferior deep cervical, accessory, and supraclavicular nodes, have the patient raise the shoulders up and forward, allowing for effective palpation during an extraoral examination using the trapezius muscle as a base (Figure 10-18).

TONSILS

Unlike lymph nodes, tonsils are not located along lymphatic vessels. Instead, all the tonsils drain into the superior deep cervical lymph nodes, particularly affecting the jugulodigastric lymph node if there is an infection in the region (considered the tonsillar node) (see Tables 10-1 and 10-2 and Figure 10-15). Changes in size and consistency can also occur in the tonsillar tissue similar to lymph nodes (see later discussion).

PALATINE AND LINGUAL TONSILS

The palatine tonsils, what patients call their "tonsils," are two rounded masses of variable size located in the oral cavity between the anterior and posterior faucial pillars on each side of the fauces (Figure 10-19; see Figures 2-21, 4-28, and 4-31). These two vertical folds are formed by muscles of the soft palate; the palatoglossus muscle forms the anterior faucial pillar while the palatopharyngeus muscle forms the posterior faucial pillar.

The lingual tonsil is an indistinct layer of lymphoid nodules located intraorally on the dorsal surface of the base of the tongue (Figure 10-20 and see Figure 2-17).

PHARYNGEAL AND TUBAL TONSILS

The **pharyngeal tonsil** (fuh-**rin**-je-uhl) is located on the midline of the posterior wall or roof of the nasopharynx (Figure 10-21 and see

Figure 3-66). This tonsil is also called the *adenoids* (**ad**-uh-noids) and is slightly enlarged in children but can undergo even further enlargement with infection. The **tubal tonsil** (**too**-buhl) is also located in the nasopharynx, posterior to the openings of the eustachian or auditory tube (see Figure 10-21).

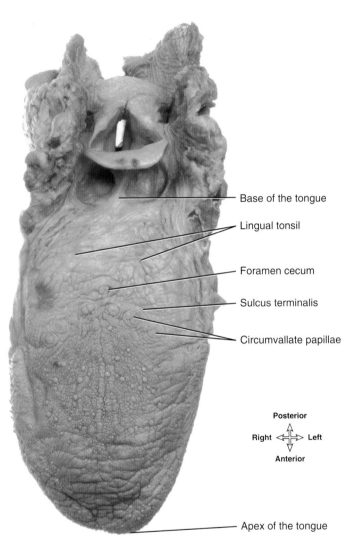

FIGURE 10-20 Dissection of the dorsal surface of the tongue, including the lingual tonsil. *(From Logan BM, Reynold PA, Hutching RT: McMinn's color atlas of head and neck anatomy, ed 4, London, 2010, Elsevier.)*

Labels: Base of the tongue; Lingual tonsil; Foramen cecum; Sulcus terminalis; Circumvallate papillae; Apex of the tongue

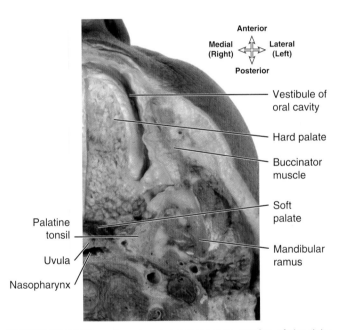

FIGURE 10-19 Dissection showing a transverse section of the right palatine tonsil, palate, and oral cavity. *(From Logan BM, Reynold PA, Hutching RT: McMinn's color atlas of head and neck anatomy, ed 4, London, 2010, Elsevier.)*

Labels: Vestibule of oral cavity; Hard palate; Buccinator muscle; Soft palate; Mandibular ramus; Palatine tonsil; Uvula; Nasopharynx

Clinical Considerations With Lymphatic System Pathology

When a patient has a disease process such as infection or cancer active in a region, the region's lymph nodes respond. The resultant dramatic increase in size and also change in consistency of the lymphoid tissue is considered **lymphadenopathy** (Figure 10-22). Lymphadenopathy results from an increase in both the size of each individual lymphocyte and the overall cell count in the lymphoid tissue. With additional larger sized lymphocytes and with increased numbers, the lymphoid tissue can better fight the disease process. When more than one group of lymph nodes is involved, it is considered *generalized lymphadenopathy*, which commonly occurs

with systemic infections such as human immunodeficiency virus (HIV) and widespread cancers such as leukemia.

The occurrence of lymphadenopathy may allow each lymph node to be visualized during an extraoral examination. More important, changes in consistency allow each involved node to be felt when palpated during the extraoral examination along the even firmer backdrop of underlying bones and muscles such as the SCM muscle or the clinician's hands. In general, the lymph nodes must be larger than approximately 10 mm in diameter to be palpable or even visualized. The involved nodes may eventually return

Continued

to their original size if the disease process subsides, or they may stay enlarged as a result of scar tissue from the lymphadenopathy and thus are still palpable, having a slightly firmer texture from the fibrosis process.

This change in lymph node consistency can range from firmer to bony hard. Nodes can remain mobile or free from the surrounding tissue during a disease. However, they can also become attached or fixed to the surrounding tissue, such as skin, bone, or muscle, as the disease process progresses to involve the regional tissue. When the nodes are involved with lymphadenopathy, the node can also feel tender to the patient when palpated. This tenderness is due to pressure on the area nerves resulting from the nodes' enlargement.

In some cases of infection, the lymph node can undergo inflammation or **lymphadenitis**. This commonly occurs with microbial infections, such as with *Staphylococcus aureus* and *Streptococcus pyogenes* infections locally with tonsillar or oral abscesses as well as systemically with mononucleosis or HIV infections. Cervical lymphadenitis or *scrofula* is still commonly seen with tuberculosis in medically compromised individuals.

A dental professional needs to examine the patient carefully for any palpable lymph nodes of the head and neck during an extraoral examination and record whether any are present (see **Appendix B**). Knowing the regional lymphatic drainage pattern may help determine the source of the infection or primary cancer site based on the findings during the examination (discussed further). In addition, a past medical history of infection or cancer could point to a recurrence if there are newly involved nodes.

The lymph nodes that are palpable due to lymphadenopathy may also help determine where a disease process such as infection or cancer is active. In addition, the examination may help determine whether the disease process has become widespread, involving a larger region and thus more secondary lymph nodes and related tissue. There is also a strong emphasis now on a multidisciplinary team management approach that includes dental professionals when treating head and neck patients with serious orofacial infections or cancer.

This documentation and history concerning palpable lymph nodes will assist in the diagnosis, treatment, and outcome of a disease process that may be present in the patient. Therefore a dental professional must understand the relationship between node location and node drainage patterns throughout the head and neck. After reading the chapter, reviewing the node location and drainage patterns in this manner will reinforce the importance of location to node function.

The dental professional needs to remember that these lymph nodes drain not only intraoral dental structures such as the teeth but also other structures of the head and neck such as the eyes, ears, nasal cavity, and deeper areas of the pharynx. A patient may need a medical referral when lymph nodes are palpable due to a disease process in these other orofacial structures.

The lymph nodes associated with the head and neck can also be involved in the spread of infection such as dental or odontogenic infection from the teeth, which is discussed in **Chapter 12**. This spread of infection can occur along the connecting lymphatic vessels of the involved lymph nodes.

Again, any palpable lymph nodes in the head and neck on a patient as well as those that are also visually noted need to be recorded, as well as any appropriate medical referrals (Figure 10-22). The changes in a node when it is involved with infection are further discussed in **Chapter 12**.

Lymphadenopathy can also occur to the tonsils, causing tissue enlargement. In most cases this enlargement of the tonsils, with the exception of the tonsils located further posterior in the tissue of the pharynx, can be visualized during an intraoral examination of the patient (see Figures 10-23 and 4-31). The intraoral tonsils may also be tender when palpated by a medical specialist and have other signs of infection such as suppuration or pus formation. Lymphadenopathy of the tonsils in both the oral cavity and pharynx may lead to more serious sequelae possibly involving airway obstruction (see **Chapter 12**). Thus a patient may need a medical referral if lymphadenopathy and other signs of infection with intraoral tonsils are noted.

Not only are lymph nodes involved with fighting disease such as infections, cancer can also start within the node as with lymphoma, which includes both Hodgkin and non-Hodgkin disease. Lymph nodes can be also involved in the spread of certain cancers (carcinomas) from epithelial tissue in the region they filter. The spread of a cancer from the original or primary site of the neoplasm to another or secondary site is considered **metastasis**. Primary nodes of the primary site then drain to the secondary site to which the cancer will later metastasize.

If the cancer is caught early enough at the primary neoplasm site or even at the secondary site of the primary lymph nodes, surgery to remove the neoplasm as well as the primary nodes often may stop metastasis. If the cancer is not stopped by the primary nodes or caught early, it will spread to secondary nodes and metastasis of the cancer will continue. Cancer cells can slowly travel, unchecked in the lymph from node to node if they are not stopped by any of the nodes along the lymphatic vessels or by removal of the involved nodes.

If the cancer metastasizes past all the connecting lymph nodes, the cancer cells of a carcinoma can enter the vascular system by way of the lymphatic ducts. The spread of cancer or metastasis by way of the blood vessels is more rapid than by way of the nodes, so the cancer in this case can quickly metastasize to the rest of the body, causing possibly fatal systemic involvement. Thus the involvement of only primary nodes in cancer may mean a better prognosis for the patient than the involvement of secondary nodes or lymphatic ducts and associated blood vessels.

When they are involved with cancer, the lymph nodes can become bony hard, and possibly fixed to surrounding tissue, structures, and organs, thus making them nonmobile as the cancer grows and spreads. The cancerous nodes are usually not as tender initially to palpation as those involved with infection; however, painful palpation can be a late finding when the cancer begins to involve surrounding nerve tissue. In summary, it is important to note that those nodes involved with only an acute infection are only slightly firmer, extremely mobile, and with increased tenderness as compared to nodes involved with cancer (see **Chapter 12**). Patients will undergo lymph node biopsy for further diagnosis of any strongly suspicious head and neck lymph nodes and possibly ultrasonography (USG) since this imaging modality is considered to be superior to others in this regard.

The vast majority of cancer patients have palpable enlarged lymph nodes. And most importantly to dental professionals, at least 80% of head and neck cancers spread to the cervical lymph nodes as part of tumor's pathogenesis. Nodal metastasis is the single most prognostic factor for the 5-year survival rate of squamous cell carcinoma of the head and neck. In general, such an occurrence of nodal metastasis decreases the overall survival by 50%. The level of nodal metastasis (see earlier discussion) and the number and size of nodes are also significant and these factors correlate with distant metastasis. However, nodal metastasis is a more complex multistep process and cannot be explained by enlargement only.

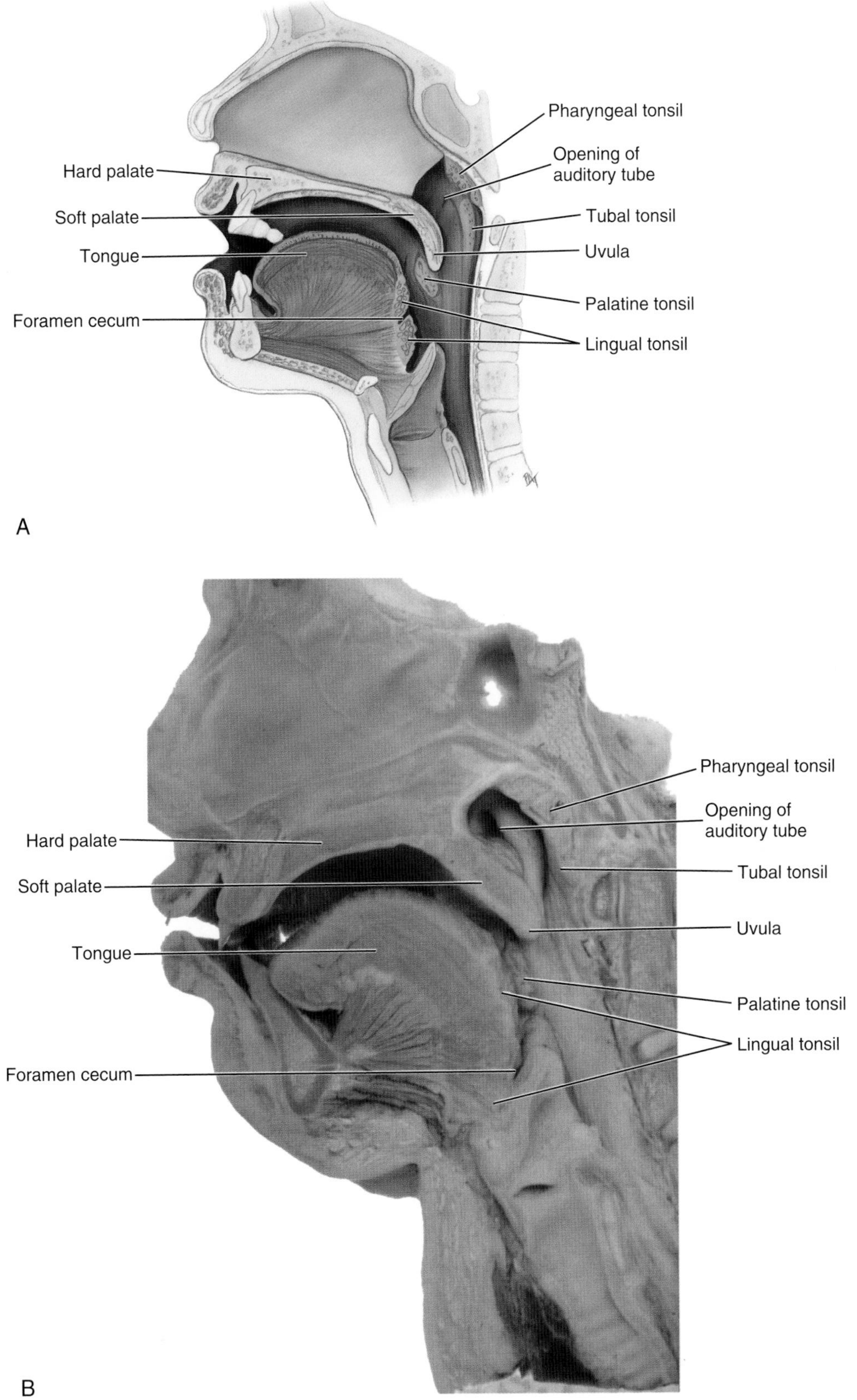

FIGURE 10-21 Pharynx with the palatine tonsil, lingual tonsil, pharyngeal tonsil, and tubal tonsil upon sagittal section **(A)**, with dissection **(B)**. (**B** *from Reynolds PA, Abrahams PH: McMinn's interactive clinical anatomy: head and neck, ed 2, London, 2001, Elsevier.*)

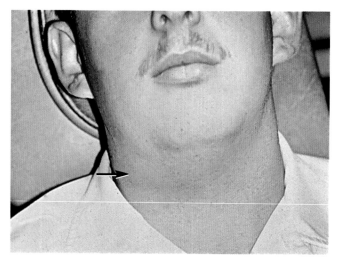

FIGURE 10-22 Unilateral lymphadenopathy of the submandibular lymph nodes on a patient that caused the dramatic nodal enlargement *(arrow)* that was both palpable as well as visually noted. There is also a loss of cervical symmetry of the neck. *(Courtesy Margaret J. Fehrenbach, RDH, MS.)*

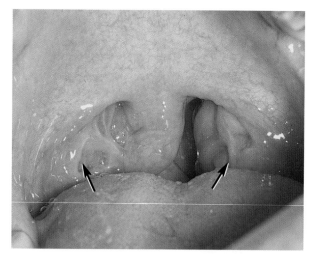

FIGURE 10-23 Bilateral lymphadenopathy of the palatine tonsils *(arrows)* on a patient. *(Courtesy Margaret J. Fehrenbach, RDH, MS.)*

REVIEW QUESTIONS

1. Which of the following lymph node groups have BOTH superficial and deep nodes?
   A. Facial nodes
   B. Buccal nodes
   C. Parotid nodes
   D. Occipital nodes
   E. Submandibular nodes

2. Which of the following structures leave each individual lymph node at the hilus?
   A. Lymphatic ducts
   B. Tonsillar tissue
   C. Efferent lymphatic vessels
   D. Afferent lymphatic vessels

3. Which of the following lymph node groups are considered subdivisions of the facial lymph nodes?
   A. Sublingual, submandibular, zygomatic, and buccal nodes
   B. Infraorbital, nasal, buccal, and submental nodes
   C. Mandibular, lingual, malar, and zygomatic nodes
   D. Malar, buccal, nasolabial, and mandibular nodes
   E. Zygomatic, nasolabial, masseteric, and submental nodes

4. Which of the following components of the lymphatic system usually have one-way valves?
   A. Arteries
   B. Veins
   C. Vessels
   D. Nodes
   E. Ducts

5. Which type of nodes drain lymph from a local region before the lymph flows to a more distant region?
   A. Primary nodes
   B. Secondary nodes
   C. Central nodes
   D. Tertiary nodes

6. The buccal lymph nodes are located superficial to which of the following structures?
   A. Sublingual gland
   B. Buccinator muscle
   C. Sternocleidomastoid muscle
   D. Parotid salivary gland
   E. Submandibular salivary gland

7. Which of the following lymph node groups extends from the base of the skull to the root of the neck?
   A. Facial nodes
   B. Deep cervical nodes
   C. Occipital nodes
   D. Jugulodigastric nodes
   E. Anterior jugular nodes

8. Where are the external jugular lymph nodes located?
   A. Anterior to the hyoid bone
   B. Along the external jugular vein
   C. Deep to the sternocleidomastoid muscle
   D. Close to the symphysis of the mandible

9. Into which area does the thoracic duct empty?
   A. Aortic arch of the body
   B. Superior vena cava of the body
   C. Junction of the right and left brachiocephalic veins
   D. Junction of the left internal jugular and subclavian veins

10. Which of the following are the primary lymph nodes draining the skin and mucous membranes of the lower face?
    A. Occipital nodes
    B. Malar nodes
    C. Submandibular nodes
    D. Superficial parotid nodes
    E. Deep parotid nodes

11. Which of the following are secondary lymph nodes for the occipital nodes?
    A. Buccal nodes
    B. Submental nodes
    C. Submandibular nodes
    D. Deep cervical nodes
    E. Supraclavicular nodes

12. Which of the following lymph node groups are BOTH considered superficial cervical lymph nodes?
    A. External and anterior jugular nodes
    B. Superficial and deep jugular nodes
    C. Medial and lateral jugular nodes
    D. Internal and external jugular nodes

13. Which of the following statements concerning the submental lymph nodes is CORRECT?
    A. They are located deep to the mylohyoid muscle.
    B. They are located between the mandibular symphysis and hyoid bone.
    C. They drain the labial commissure and base of tongue.
    D. They are secondary nodes for deep cervical nodes.

14. Which muscle needs to be made more prominent on a patient to achieve effective palpation of the region where the superior deep cervical lymph nodes are located?
    A. Masseter muscle
    B. Trapezius muscle
    C. Sternocleidomastoid muscle
    D. Epicranial muscle

15. Where is the lingual tonsil located within the head and neck?
    A. Posterior to the auditory tube's opening
    B. On the superior posterior wall of the nasopharynx
    C. At the base of the tongue
    D. Between the anterior and posterior faucial pillars

16. Which of the following lymph nodes often becomes easily palpable when the palatine tonsils are inflamed?
    A. Jugulo-omohyoid node
    B. Jugulodigastric node
    C. Submental nodes
    D. Facial nodes

17. Which of the following lymph node groups are primary nodes for the maxillary third molar if it becomes associated with caries or periodontal disease?
    A. Submental nodes
    B. Submandibular nodes
    C. Superior deep cervical nodes
    D. Inferior deep cervical nodes

18. If a patient with breast cancer has involvement with the axillary nodes, which lymph node groups in the neck primarily communicate with these nodes?
    A. Superior deep cervical nodes
    B. Inferior deep cervical nodes
    C. Submental nodes
    D. Submandibular nodes

19. At which site in the oral cavity are the palatine tonsils located?
    A. Dorsal surface of tongue
    B. Submandibular fossa
    C. Between anterior and posterior faucial pillars
    D. Surrounding the faucial arch

20. Which of the following descriptions characterizes lymph nodes when they are involved in metastasis?
    A. Always tender
    B. Usually bony hard
    C. Always mobile
    D. Usually decreased in size

21. What is the last location noted for the lymph before reentering the vascular system?
    A. Several deep lymph nodes
    B. Entry into lymphatic vessels through the walls
    C. Thoracic duct
    D. Thymus gland

22. Which of the following situations causes enlargement of the lymph nodes?
    A. Amount of intergland lymph is large.
    B. Accumulation of bacteria and viruses causes the node to expand.
    C. More protein is lost from the circulatory system and winds up in the nodes.
    D. White blood cells in the node multiply to fight an infection.

23. Which of the following are prominent lymph nodes that drain BOTH the tongue and submental triangle?
    A. Jugulo-omohyoid nodes
    B. Jugulodigastric nodes
    C. Mandibular nodes
    D. Accessory nodes

24. Which tonsil is also called the adenoids and can be slightly enlarged in children?
    A. Palatine tonsil
    B. Pharyngeal tonsil
    C. Tubal tonsil
    D. Lingual tonsil

25. Which of the following lymph node groups drain the infrahyoid region of the neck?
    A. Malar nodes
    B. External jugular nodes
    C. Anterior jugular nodes
    D. Accessory nodes

Identification Exercises

Identify the structures on the following diagrams by filling in each blank with the correct anatomic term. You can check your answers by looking back at the figure indicated in parentheses for each identification diagram.

1. (Figure 10-1)

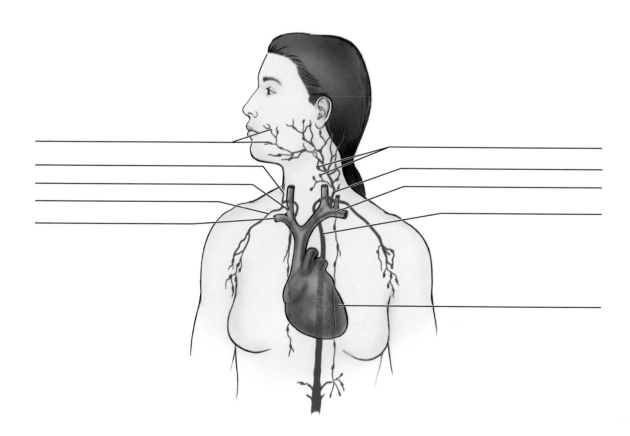

2. (Figure 10-2)

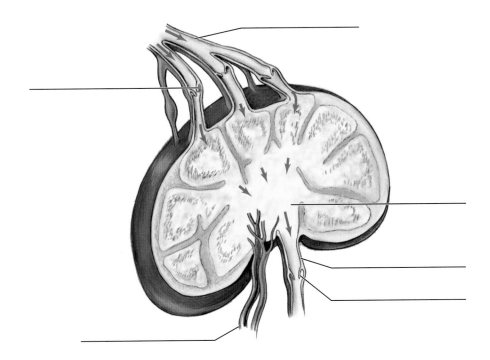

3. (Figure 10-3)

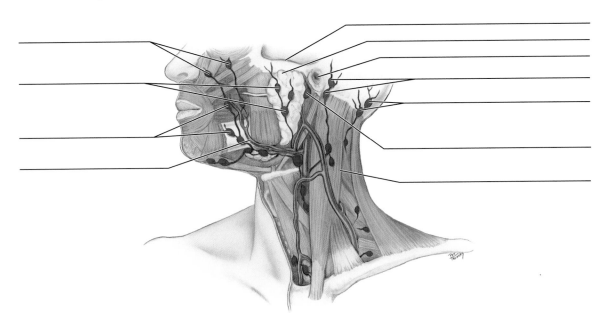

4. (Figure 10-7)

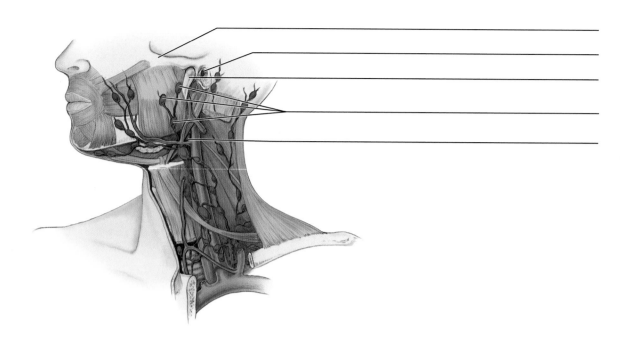

5. (Figure 10-10)

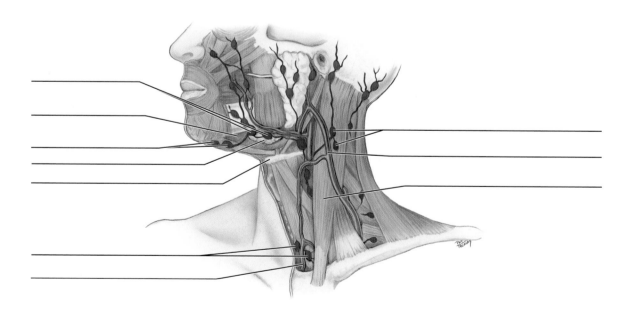

6. (Figure 10-15)

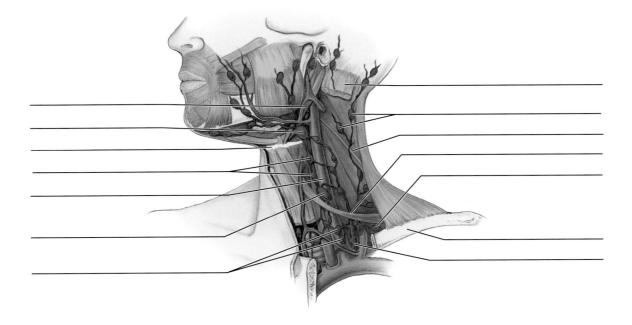

7. (Figure 10-21, *A*)

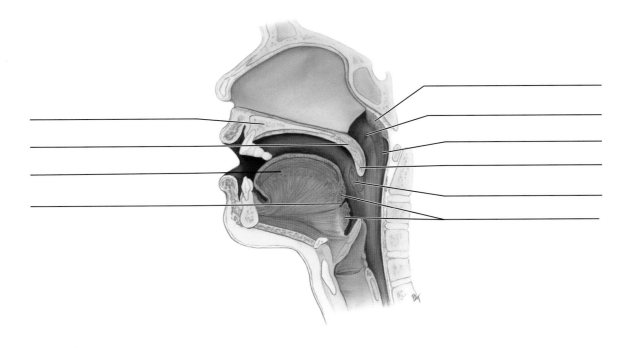

CHAPTER 11

Fasciae and Spaces

●●● LEARNING OBJECTIVES

1. Define and pronounce the **key terms** and **anatomic terms** in this chapter.
2. Locate and identify the fasciae of the head and neck on a diagram, skull, and patient.
3. Locate and identify the major spaces of the head and neck on a diagram, skull, and patient.

4. Discuss the communication between the major spaces of the head and neck.
5. Correctly complete the review questions and activities for this chapter.
6. Integrate an understanding of fasciae and spaces into the overall study of head and neck anatomy as well as a clinical dental practice.

●●● KEY TERMS

Fascia/Fasciae (fas-she-uh, **fas-**she-ee) Layers of fibrous connective tissue underlying skin and surrounding

muscles, bones, vessels, nerves, organs, other structures.

Fascial spaces (fas-she-uhl) Potential spaces between layers of fascia.

FASCIAE AND SPACES OVERVIEW

Fascia (plural, fasciae) consists of layer upon layer of fibrous connective tissue. The fascia lies just deep to and connected to the skin that surrounds the much deeper muscles, bones, vessels, nerves, organs, and other structures.

Potential spaces are created between the layers of fascia of the body because of the sheetlike nature of fasciae. These potential spaces are termed fascial spaces or *fascial planes*. It is important to remember that these fascial spaces are not actually empty spaces, as they contain structures or parts of structures moving through the space as well as loose connective tissue for more padding. Other spaces are also present in the head that are not necessarily created by fascia but by other structures such as bones and muscles; both types of spaces are considered in this chapter.

Thus this chapter discusses the fasciae of the face and neck that surround both superficial and deep structures. Potential spaces created between the body's layers of fasciae are also discussed. A three-dimensional view of the systems and structures of the head and neck is additionally presented for a more thorough understanding of these anatomic regions (see Chapter 1).

FASCIAE OF HEAD AND NECK

In areas of the body including the head and neck, the fasciae can be divided into either the superficial fasciae or the deep fasciae. Layers of superficial fascia are found just deep to and attached to the skin.

In most cases, the layers of superficial fascia separate skin from deeper structures, allowing the skin to move independently of these deeper structures. The layers of superficial fascia vary in thickness in different parts of the body and are composed of fat as well as irregularly arranged connective tissue. The blood vessels and nerves of the skin also travel in the superficial fasciae; most of these larger blood vessels and nerves have already been discussed in previous chapters.

In contrast, the layers of deep fascia cover the deeper structures of the body including the head and neck, such as the bones, muscles, nerves, and vessels. Again, most of these deeper structures have already been discussed in previous chapters. These layers of deep fascia consist of a dense and inelastic fibrous tissue forming sheaths around these deeper structures.

SUPERFICIAL FASCIAE OF FACE AND NECK

The layers of superficial fasciae of the body do not usually enclose muscles, except for the superficial fasciae of the face and neck (Figure 11-1, Table 11-1). The superficial fascia of the face encloses the muscles of facial expression (see Figure 4-5). The superficial cervical fascia of the neck contains the platysma muscle, which covers most of the anterior cervical triangle of the neck (see Figures 2-23 and 4-17).

DEEP FASCIAE OF FACE AND JAWS

The layers of deep fasciae of the face and jaws are divided into: the temporal, masseteric-parotid, and pterygoid fasciae. These layers of

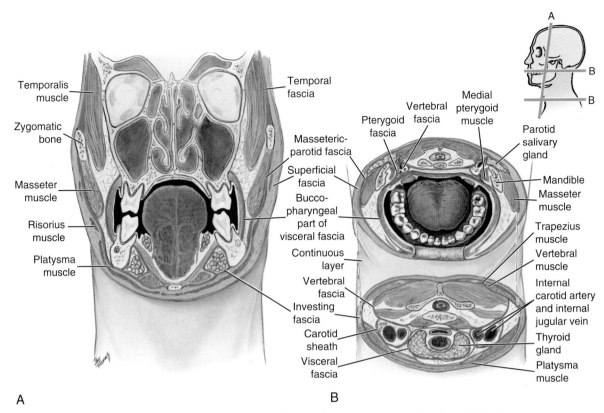

FIGURE 11-1 Frontal section of the head and neck of the head and neck *(see inset)* highlighting the fasciae of the face **(A)**. Transverse sections at the oral cavity and then at the neck *(see inset)* highlighting the continuous nature of the investing fascia **(B)**.

TABLE 11-1	Fasciae of Head and Neck
FASCIAE OF THE HEAD AND NECK	**RELATIONSHIP TO HEAD AND NECK STRUCTURES**
Superficial Fasciae of Face and Neck	
Superficial fascia of the face	Encloses muscles of facial expression
Superficial cervical fascia of the neck	Contains platysma muscle that covers anterior cervical triangle of the neck
Deep Fasciae of Face and Jaws (Continuous With Investing Layer of Deep Cervical Fascia as Well as Each Other)	
Temporal fascia	Covers temporalis muscle and structures superior to the zygomatic arch
Masseteric-parotid fascia	Covers masseter muscle and structures inferior to the zygomatic arch; surrounds parotid salivary gland
Pterygoid fascia	Located on the medial surface of the medial pterygoid muscle
Deep Cervical Fasciae (From External to Internal in Location and Continuous With Each Other)	
Investing fascia	Surrounds the neck, continuing onto the masseteric-parotid fascia; splits around and encloses two salivary glands (submandibular and parotid) and two muscles (sternocleidomastoid and trapezius); surrounds the infrahyoid muscles, running from the hyoid bone inferiorly to the sternum
Carotid sheath	Runs inferiorly along each side of the neck; contains the internal carotid and common carotid arteries and the internal jugular vein, as well as the tenth cranial or vagus nerve; borders vascular compartment of neck
Visceral fascia	Runs inferiorly along each side of the neck; contains the trachea, esophagus, and thyroid gland; borders the visceral compartment of the neck
Buccopharyngeal fascia	Encloses entire superior part of the alimentary canal; continuous with the fascia covering the buccinator muscle, where the muscle comes together with the superior pharyngeal constrictor muscle at the pterygomandibular raphe (pterygomandibular fold)
Vertebral fascia*	Covers the spinal cord, cervical vertebrae, and associated vertebral muscles; borders the vertebral compartment of the neck

*Some anatomists distinguish a separate layer of the vertebral fascia called the *alar fascia*, which runs from the base of the skull to connect with the visceral fascia inferiorly in the neck.

deep fasciae of the face and jaws are continuous with each other (see Figure 11-1).

The **temporal fascia** (**tem**-puh-ruhl) covers the temporalis muscle and structures superior to the zygomatic arch (see Figures 3-14 and 4-22). The **masseteric-parotid fascia** (mass-i-**tare**-ik-puh-**rot**-id) covers the masseter muscle and structures inferior to the zygomatic arch and surrounds the parotid salivary gland (see Figure 4-22). The **pterygoid fascia** (**ter**-i-goid) is located on the medial surface of the medial pterygoid muscle (see Figure 4-23). The deep fasciae of the face and jaws are also continuous with the investing layer of the deep cervical fascia.

DEEP CERVICAL FASCIAE

The layers of deep cervical fasciae include: the investing fascia, carotid sheath, visceral fascia, buccopharyngeal fascia, and vertebral fascia (Figures 11-2 and 11-3; see Chapter 3). Again, it is important to note that the layers of the various regions of deep cervical fasciae are continuous with each other. Later in this chapter, the compartments of the neck are discussed in relationship to the deep cervical fasciae (see Figure 11-15).

Investing Fascia. The **investing fascia** is the most external layer of deep cervical fascia. This fascia surrounds the neck, continuing onto the masseteric-parotid fascia. This fascia also splits around two salivary glands (submandibular and parotid) and two muscles

(sternocleidomastoid and trapezius), enclosing them completely. Branching laminae from this fascia also provide the deep fasciae that surround the infrahyoid muscles, running from the hyoid bone inferiorly to the sternum.

Carotid Sheath With Visceral and Buccopharyngeal Fasciae. The **carotid sheath** (kuh-**rot**-id) is a bilateral tube of deep cervical fascia deep to the investing fascia and sternocleidomastoid muscle, running inferiorly along each side of the neck from the base of the skull to the thorax (chest). The carotid sheath contains the internal carotid and common carotid arteries and the internal jugular vein, as well as the tenth cranial or vagus nerve (see Figure 6-2 and 3-19 as well as Chapters 6 and 8, respectively). All these carotid sheath contents travel between the braincase and thorax (chest). The carotid sheath also borders the vascular compartments of the neck that is discussed later in this chapter (see Figure 11-15).

Deep and parallel to each carotid sheath is the **visceral fascia** (**vis**-er-uhl) or *pretracheal fascia*, which is a single midline tube of deep cervical fascia running inferiorly along the neck. This fascia contains the trachea, esophagus, and thyroid gland. The visceral fascia also borders the visceral compartment of the neck that is discussed later in this chapter (see Figure 11-15).

Nearer to the skull, the visceral fascial layer located posterior and lateral to the pharynx is the **buccopharyngeal fascia** (buk-ko-fuh-**rin**-je-uhl). This deep cervical fascia encloses the entire superior part of the alimentary canal and is continuous with the fascia covering the

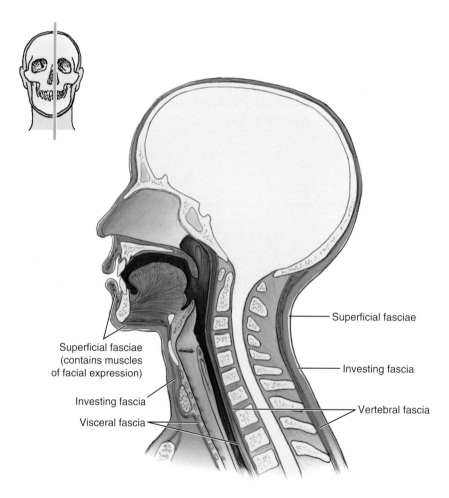

FIGURE 11-2 Midsagittal section of the head and neck *(see inset)* highlighting the deep cervical fasciae.

Labels in figure:
- Superficial fasciae (contains muscles of facial expression)
- Investing fascia
- Visceral fascia
- Superficial fasciae
- Investing fascia
- Vertebral fascia

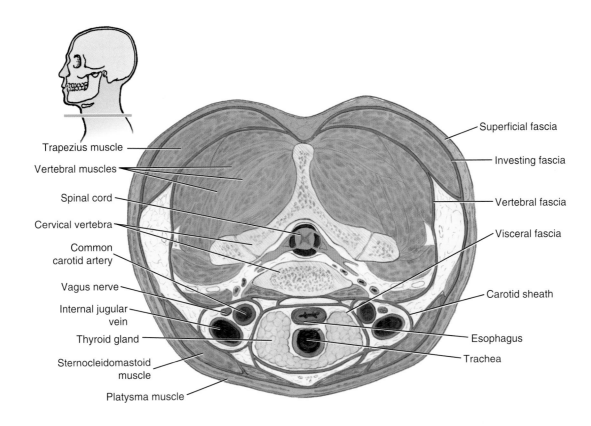

FIGURE 11-3 Transverse section of the neck *(see inset)* highlighting the deep cervical fasciae.

buccinator muscle, a location where the buccinator muscle and the superior pharyngeal constrictor muscle come together at the pterygomandibular raphe (see Figures 4-11 and 4-29), which is present in the oral cavity as the pterygomandibular fold (see Figure 4-31). The pterygomandibular raphe or fold is a landmark for the local anesthetic administration for the inferior alveolar block (see Figures 9-37 and 9-38).

Vertebral Fascia. The deepest layer of the deep cervical fascia, the **vertebral fascia** (**ver**-tuh-bruhl) or *prevertebral fascia*, covers the spinal cord, cervical vertebrae, and associated vertebral muscles. The vertebral fascia borders the vertebral compartment of the neck discussed later in this chapter (see Figure 11-15). Some anatomists distinguish a separate layer of the vertebral fascia called the *alar fascia*, which runs from the base of the skull to connect with the visceral fascia inferiorly in the neck.

SPACES OF HEAD AND NECK

A dental professional must have an understanding of the anatomic aspects of the spaces of the head and neck when examining a patient. These spaces communicate with each other directly, as well as through the associated blood and lymph vessels contained within the space. Thus communication may allow the spread of dental (or odontogenic) infection from an initial superficial area in the face and jaws to more vital deeper structures in the neck or even travel to the brain. The spread of infection by way of these spaces may have serious consequences; the role of spaces in the spread of dental (or odontogenic) infection is discussed further in Chapter 12. Again, the study of these spaces also allows the clinician to form a three-dimensional view of head and neck anatomy (see Chapter 1).

SPACES OF FACE AND JAWS

The spaces of the face and jaws or *cranial spaces* can communicate with each other and with the cervical fascial spaces. However, unlike the neck, the spaces of the face and jaws are often defined by the arrangement of muscles and bones forming borders, in addition to the surrounding fasciae. Thus many of the major spaces located in the head are not strictly considered fascial spaces. The major spaces of the face and jaws include: the vestibular space of the maxilla, vestibular space of the mandible, canine space, parotid space, buccal space, masticator space, space of the body of the mandible, submental space, submandibular space, and sublingual space (Table 11-2).

Vestibular Space of the Maxilla. The space of the upper jaw, the **vestibular space of the maxilla** (ves-**tib**-u-luhr) (mak-**sil**-uh), is located medial to the buccinator muscle and inferior to the attachment of this muscle along the alveolar process of the maxilla (Figure 11-4 and see Figures 3-45 and 4-11). Its lateral wall is the oral mucosa. This space communicates with the maxillary molars and associated periodontium and gingiva and thus can become involved with dental (or odontogenic) infections within this space.

Vestibular Space of the Mandible. The space of the lower jaw, the **vestibular space of the mandible** (**man**-di-buhl) is located between the buccinator muscle and overlying oral mucosa (see Figure 11-4 and see Figures 3-51 and 4-11). This space is bordered by the attachment of the buccinator muscle onto the alveolar process of the mandible. This important space of the lower jaw communicates with the mandibular posterior teeth and associated periodontium and gingiva, as well as the space of the body of the mandible, and thus can become involved with dental (or odontogenic) infections within this space.

TABLE 11-2	Major Spaces of Face and Jaws			
SPACE	**LOCATION**	**CONTENTS**	**COMMUNICATION PATTERN**	**SOURCE OF POSSIBLE INFECTION**
Maxillary vestibular space	Between buccinator muscle and oral mucosa of maxilla		Maxillary molars and associated periodontium and gingiva	Maxillary molars and associated periodontium and gingiva
Mandibular vestibular space	Between buccinator muscle and oral mucosa of mandible		Mandibular posterior teeth and associated periodontium and gingiva as well as body of mandible	Mandibular posterior teeth and associated periodontium and gingiva
Canine space	Within superficial fascia covering canine fossa	Angular artery and vein as well as the infraorbital nerve and vessels	Buccal space	Maxillary canine
Buccal space	Between buccinator muscle and masseter muscle	Buccal fat pad	Canine space, pterygomandibular space, and space of the body of mandible	Maxillary premolar or molar as well as mandibular molar
Parotid space	Enveloping parotid salivary gland	Parotid salivary gland, and part of facial nerve, external carotid artery, and retromandibular vein	Parapharyngeal space	Parotid salivary gland infection
Masticator space	Area of mandible and muscles of mastication	Temporal, submasseteric, and infratemporal spaces	All parts with each other and also with submandibular and parapharyngeal spaces	
Temporal space	Part of masticator space between temporal fascia and temporalis muscle	Fat tissue	Infratemporal and submasseteric spaces	Infratemporal and pterygomandibular space
Infratemporal space	Part of masticator space between lateral pterygoid plate, maxillary tuberosity, and mandibular ramus	Maxillary artery and branches, mandibular nerve and branches, and pterygoid plexus of veins	Temporal, submasseteric, submandibular, and parapharyngeal spaces	Maxillary third molar as well as needle tract infection
Pterygomandibular space	Part of infratemporal space between medial pterygoid muscle and mandibular ramus	Inferior alveolar nerve, lingual nerve, and inferior alveolar blood vessels	Submandibular and parapharyngeal spaces	Mandibular second or third molar with associated pericoronitis as well as needle tract infection
Submasseteric space	Part of masticator space between masseter muscle and external surface of mandibular ramus	Masseteric artery and vein	Temporal and infratemporal spaces	Mandibular third molar (rare)
Space of the body of mandible	Periosteum covering mandible	Mandible and inferior alveolar nerve and branches with associated blood vessels	Vestibular space of mandible, buccal, submental, submandibular, and sublingual spaces	Mandibular teeth
Submental space	Midline between mandibular symphysis and hyoid bone	Submental lymph nodes and anterior jugular vein origin	Space of the body of mandible, as well as submandibular and sublingual spaces	Mandibular anterior teeth or anterior extension from submandibular space
Submandibular space	Medial to mandible and inferior to mylohyoid muscle	Submandibular lymph nodes and salivary gland and parts of facial artery	Infratemporal, submental, sublingual, and parapharyngeal spaces	Mandibular posterior teeth as well as spread from contralateral submandibular space
Sublingual space	Medial to mandible and superior to mylohyoid muscle	Sublingual salivary gland and ducts, and parts of lingual nerve and artery and hypoglossal nerve	Space of the body of mandible, as well as submental and submandibular spaces	Mandibular first molar or premolar

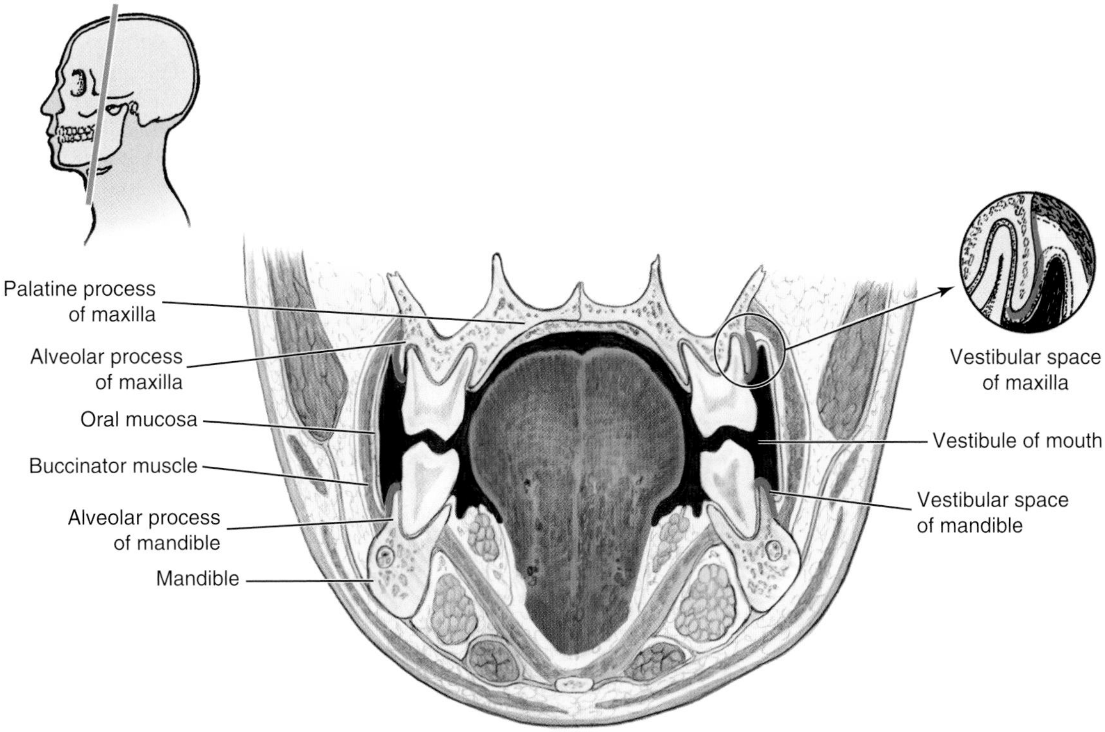

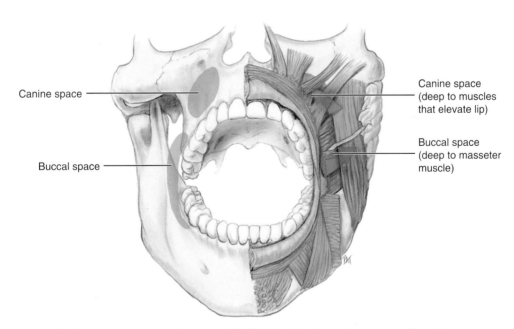

FIGURE 11-4 Frontal section of the head and neck *(see inset)* highlighting both the maxillary vestibular space and mandibular vestibular space.

Palatine process of maxilla

Alveolar process of maxilla

Oral mucosa

Buccinator muscle

Alveolar process of mandible

Mandible

Vestibular space of maxilla

Vestibule of mouth

Vestibular space of mandible

Canine space

Buccal space

Canine space (deep to muscles that elevate lip)

Buccal space (deep to masseter muscle)

FIGURE 11-5 Frontal view of the head highlighting both the canine space and buccal space.

Canine Space. The **canine space** (**kay**-nine) is located superior to the upper lip and lateral to the apex of the maxillary canine (Figure 11-5 and see Figure 3-45). This space is deep to the overlying skin and muscles of facial expression that elevate the upper lip, the levator labii superioris and zygomaticus minor muscles (see Figure 4-13). The floor of the space is the canine fossa of the maxilla, which is covered by periosteum (see Figure 3-47). This space is bordered anteriorly by the orbicularis oris muscle and posteriorly by the levator anguli

oris muscle (see Figure 4-10). The space contains the angular artery and vein as well as the infraorbital nerve and vessels (see Figure 6-6).

The canine space communicates with the buccal space. If the canine space is involved in a dental (or odontogenic) infection, the source is usually the maxillary canine and there is unilateral loss of the depth to the overlying nasolabial sulcus (see Table 12-1 and Figure 2-7).

Buccal Space. The **buccal space** (**buk**-uhl) is the fascial space formed between the buccinator muscle (actually the buccopharyngeal fascia) and masseter muscle (see Figures 4-11 and 11-10, *B*). Therefore the buccal space is inferior to the zygomatic arch, superior to the mandible, lateral to the buccinator muscle, and medial and anterior to the masseter muscle. This bilateral space is partially covered by the platysma muscle, as well as by an extension of fascia from the parotid salivary gland capsule (see Figures 4-17 and 7-2). The space contains the buccal fat pad, parotid duct, and facial artery (see Figures 2-12 and 6-6).

The buccal space communicates with the canine space, pterygomandibular space, and space of the body of the mandible. If the buccal space is involved in a dental (odontogenic) infection, the source is usually from a maxillary premolar or molar as well as a mandibular molar. The patient with this type of infection within this space appears similar to the cartoon image of toothache with a wrapped swollen cheek that extends to the ipsilateral labial commissure (see Figure 12-6 and Table 12-1).

Parotid Space. The **parotid space** (puh-**rot**-id) is a fascial space created inside the investing fascial layer of the deep cervical fascia as it envelops the parotid salivary gland (Figure 11-6 and see Figure 7-2). The space contains not only the entire parotid salivary gland but also much of the length of the seventh cranial or facial nerve as well as the external carotid artery and retromandibular vein. Usually infection is from nonodontogenic sources but instead involves the gland. Communication occurs with parapharyngeal space; thus parotid salivary gland infection can involve serious complications when it spreads to this cervical space.

Masticator Space. The **masticator space** (mass-ti-**kay**-tor) is a general term used to include the entire area of the mandible and associated muscles of mastication (see Figures 4-19 to 4-23). Thus it includes: the temporal, infratemporal, and submasseteric spaces, as well as the masseter muscle and both the mandibular ramus and body of the mandible. All parts of the masticator space communicate with each other, as well as with the submandibular space and a nearby cervical fascial space, the parapharyngeal space (discussed later).

As stated before, a part of the masticator space is the **temporal space**, which is formed by the temporal fascia anterior to the temporalis muscle; it can be divided into either the superficial or deep temporal spaces (Figure 11-7; see Figure 3-59). This space is located between the fascia and muscle. Therefore the temporal space extends from the superior temporal line inferiorly to the zygomatic arch and infratemporal crest. The space contains fat tissue and communicates with the infratemporal and submasseteric spaces.

If the temporal space is involved in infection, the source usually involves other nearby masticator fascial spaces, the infratemporal or pterygomandibular spaces. When involved in infection, the superficial temporal space will have its swelling limited by the outline of the temporalis fascia with extreme pain. The deep temporal space, in contrast, will have less swelling when infected and thus is difficult to initially diagnose; however, trismus is possible (see Chapter 5).

The **infratemporal space** (in-fruh-**tem**-puh-ruhl) is also part of the masticator space and occupies the infratemporal fossa, an area adjacent to the lateral pterygoid plate of the sphenoid bone and maxillary tuberosity of the maxilla (Figure 11-8, *A*; see Figures 11-7 and Figure 3-61). The space is bordered laterally by the medial surface of the mandible and the temporalis muscle. The roof is formed by the infratemporal surface of the greater wing of the sphenoid bone.

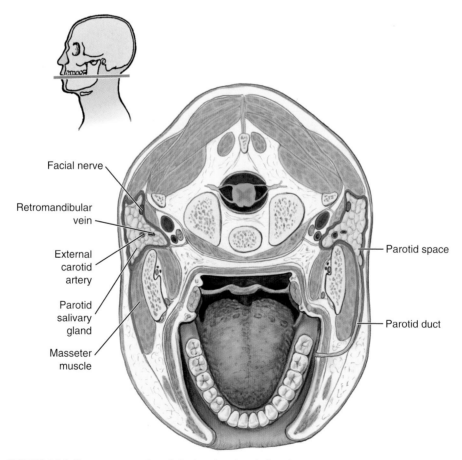

Facial nerve

Retromandibular vein

External carotid artery

Parotid salivary gland

Masseter muscle

Parotid space

Parotid duct

FIGURE 11-6 Transverse section of the head and neck *(see inset)* highlighting the parotid space.

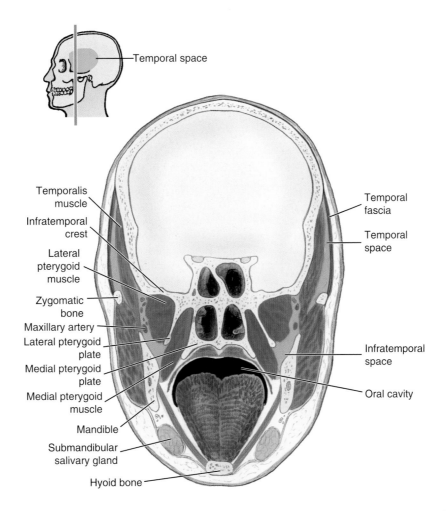

Temporal space

Temporalis muscle

Infratemporal crest

Lateral pterygoid muscle

Zygomatic bone

Maxillary artery

Lateral pterygoid plate

Medial pterygoid plate

Medial pterygoid muscle

Mandible

Submandibular salivary gland

Hyoid bone

Temporal fascia

Temporal space

Infratemporal space

Oral cavity

FIGURE 11-7 Frontal section of the head *(see inset)* highlighting both the temporal space and infratemporal space.

Medially, the space is bordered anteriorly by the lateral pterygoid plate and posteriorly by the pharynx with its visceral layer of deep fascia. There is no border inferiorly and posteriorly, instead the infratemporal space is continuous with a more inferior and deep cervical fascial space, the parapharyngeal space (discussed later).

The infratemporal space contains a part of the maxillary artery as it branches, the mandibular nerve and its branches, and the pterygoid plexus of veins. It also contains the medial and lateral pterygoid muscles. This space communicates with the temporal and submasseteric spaces, as well as with the submandibular and parapharyngeal spaces. If the infratemporal space is involved in a dental (or odontogenic) infection, the source is usually a maxillary third molar as well as needle tract infection (see Table 12-1 and see Chapter 9). With this type of infection within the space there will be extraoral swelling over the mandibular notch area and intraoral swelling in the maxillary tuberosity area, with possible trismus (see Chapter 5).

The **pterygomandibular space** (ter-i-go-man-**dib**-u-luhr) is a part of the infratemporal space and is formed by the lateral pterygoid muscle (roof), medial pterygoid muscle (medial wall), and mandibular ramus (lateral wall) (see Figure 11-8).

The pterygomandibular space is important to dental professionals because it contains the inferior alveolar nerve, lingual nerve, and inferior alveolar blood vessels. Thus the space in itself is the target

area for the inferior alveolar block as well as the Vazirani-Akinosi mandibular block (see Figures 9-37 and 9-56).

This space communicates with both the submandibular space and the parapharyngeal space of the neck (discussed later). If the pterygomandibular space is involved in a dental (or odontogenic) infection, the source is mainly a mandibular second or third molar with associated pericoronitis as well as needle tract infection (see Chapters 9 and 12). With this type of infection, there is an absence of extraoral swelling and discomfort upon swallowing or dysphagia; however, severe trismus is possible (see Table 12-1 and Chapter 5). There can also be anterior bulging of the ipsilateral part of the soft palate and faucial pillars with deviation of the uvula to the unaffected contralateral side.

Another part of the masticator space, the **submasseteric space** (sub-mas-et-**tehr**-ik), is located between the masseter muscle and the external surface of the vertical mandibular ramus (Figure 11-9). The space contains the masseteric artery and vein. This space communicates with both the temporal and infratemporal spaces. If the submasseteric space is involved in in a dental (or odontogenic) infection, which occurs rarely, the source is usually a mandibular third molar with associated pericoronitis. With this type of infection of this space there is a swelling noted at the angle of the mandible, possibly involving severe trismus and throbbing pain (see Table 12-1 and Figure 2-9 and Chapter 5).

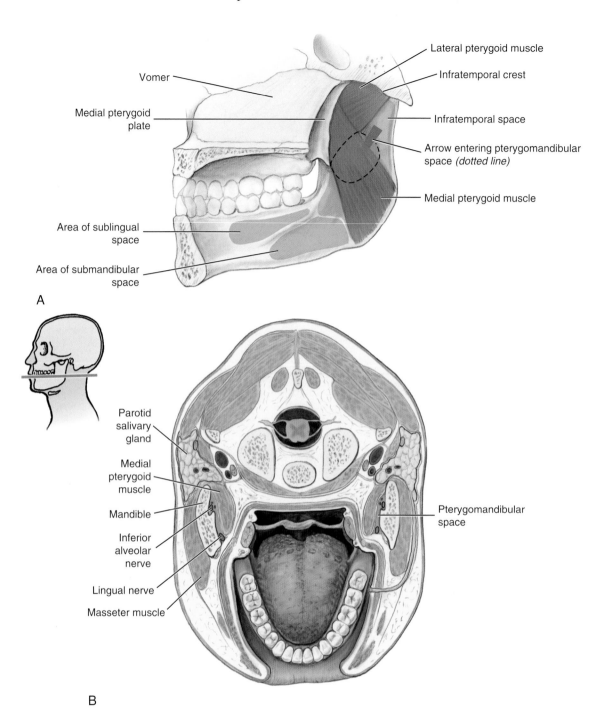

FIGURE 11-8 The skull highlighting the infratemporal space and pterygomandibular space upon mid-sagittal section **(A)**. The head and the neck highlighting the pterygomandibular space upon transverse section *(see inset)* **(B)**.

Space of the Body of the Mandible. The **space of the body of the mandible** is formed by the periosteum that is anterior to the body of the mandible, from its mandibular symphysis to the anterior borders of both the masseter and medial pterygoid muscles (Figure 11-10 and see Figure 3-52).

This potential space contains the mandible; a part of the inferior alveolar nerve, artery, and vein; and the dental and alveolar branches of these blood vessels, as well as the mental and incisive branches. If the space of the body of the mandible is involved in a dental (or odontogenic) infection, the source usually involves the mandibular

teeth. The space of the mandible communicates with the vestibular space of the mandible, as well as with the buccal, submental, submandibular, and sublingual spaces.

Submental Space. The **submental space** (sub-**men**-tuhl) is located in the midline between the mandibular symphysis and hyoid bone as part of the submandibular triangle (Figure 11-11 and see Figure 2-25). The floor of this space is the superficial cervical fascia covering the suprahyoid muscles (see Figure 4-25). The roof is the mylohyoid muscle, covered by the investing fascia. Forming the lateral borders of this space are the diverging anterior bellies of the digastric muscles.

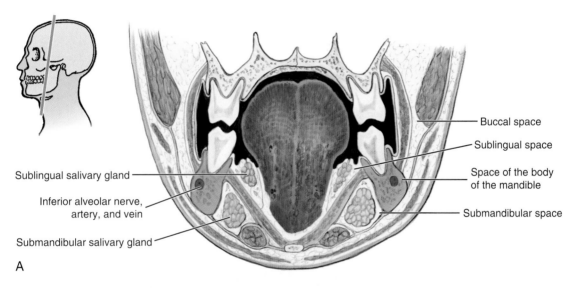

FIGURE 11-9 The skull and mandible from lateral views highlighting the submasseteric space.

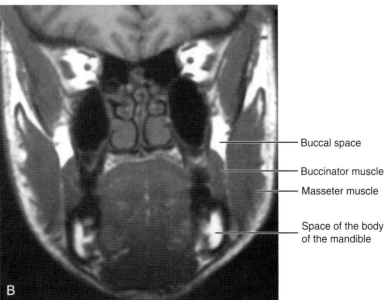

FIGURE 11-10 Frontal section of the head and neck *(see inset)* highlighting the space of the body of the mandible **(A),** with magnetic resonance imaging **(B)**. *(From Reynolds PA, Abrahams PH: McMinn's interactive clinical anatomy: head and neck, ed 2, London, 2001, Elsevier.)*

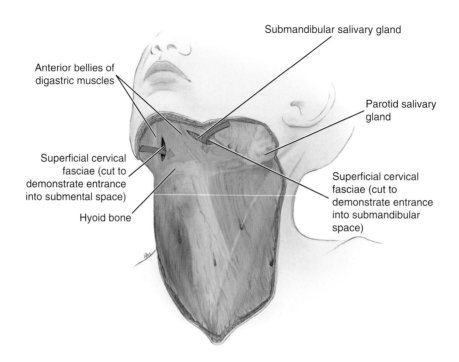

FIGURE 11-11 Anterolateral view of the neck with the skin removed, leaving the superficial cervical fasciae in place with the platysma muscle omitted. Location of both the submental space at the midline and the two lateral submandibular spaces is indicated.

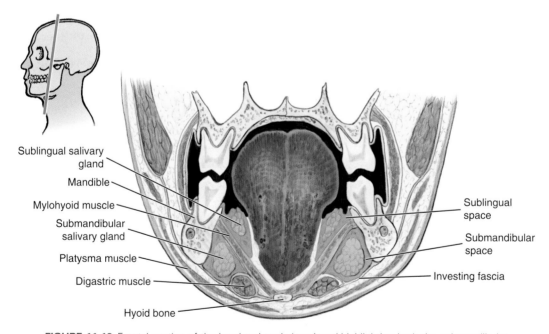

FIGURE 11-12 Frontal section of the head and neck *(see inset)* highlighting both the submandibular space and sublingual space.

The submental space contains the submental lymph nodes and the origin of the anterior jugular vein (see Figures 6-13 and 10-10). The submental space communicates with the space of the body of the mandible and the submandibular and sublingual spaces. If the submental space is involved in a dental (or odontogenic) infection, the source is usually the mandibular anterior teeth or an anterior extension of the infection from the submandibular space (see Table 12-1). With an

infection within the space, the mental region will appear glossy and swollen, with discomfort upon swallowing or dysphagia.

Submandibular Space. The **submandibular space** (sub-man-dib-u-luhr) is located lateral and posterior to the submental space on each side of the jaws as part of the submandibular triangle (Figure 11-12; see Figures 11-11 and 2-25 as well as 4-28). The cross-sectional shape of this bilateral space is triangular, with the mylohyoid line of the mandible being its superior border. The mylohyoid muscle then forms its medial border and the hyoid bone creates its medial apex (see Figure 4-25).

The submandibular space contains the submandibular lymph nodes, most of the submandibular salivary gland, and parts of the facial artery (see Figures 7-5, 6-6, and 10-10). This space communicates with the infratemporal, submental, and sublingual spaces as well as the parapharyngeal space of the neck (discussed later).

If the submandibular space is involved in a dental (or odontogenic) infection, the source usually involves the mandibular posterior teeth. With this type of infection, there can be possible loss of the firmness of the inferior border of the mandible upon palpation due to concurrent visible unilateral swelling of the submandibular region (see Table 12-1). This space also becomes involved if there is a spread of dental (or odontogenic) infection, possibly across the midline to the contralateral submandibular space, which may result in the serious complication of Ludwig angina with its bilateral submandibular space involvement (see Figure 12-12).

Sublingual Space. The **sublingual space** (sub-**ling**-gwuhl) is located deep to the oral mucosa, with the oral mucosa its roof (see Figures 11-12 and 4-28). The floor of this space is the mylohyoid muscle; thus this muscle creates the division between the submandibular and sublingual spaces with the sublingual space superior to the more inferior submandibular space (see Figure 4-28). The tongue

and its intrinsic muscles form the medial border of the sublingual space, and the mandible forms its lateral wall.

The sublingual space contains the sublingual salivary gland and ducts, the duct of the deep lobe of the submandibular salivary gland, a part of the lingual nerve and artery, and the twelfth cranial or hypoglossal nerve (see Figures 7-7 and 8-20). The space communicates with the submental and submandibular spaces as well as the space of the body of the mandible.

If the sublingual space is involved in in a dental (or odontogenic) infection, the source is usually a mandibular first molar or premolar, which may result in a swelling only of the floor of the mouth with an elevated tongue and discomfort upon swelling. However, nothing is initially visible or extraorally palpable during examination, unlike similar involvement of the submandibular space (see Table 12-1).

CERVICAL SPACES

The cervical spaces within the neck can communicate with the spaces of the face and jaws, as well as with each other. Most importantly, these spaces connect the spaces of the face and jaws with those of the thorax (chest), allowing dental (or odontogenic) infection to spread to vital organs such as the heart and lungs as well as the brain (see Chapter 12). The cervical spaces include: the previsceral, parapharyngeal, retropharyngeal, and perivertebral spaces (Figures 11-13 and 11-14; Table 11-3).

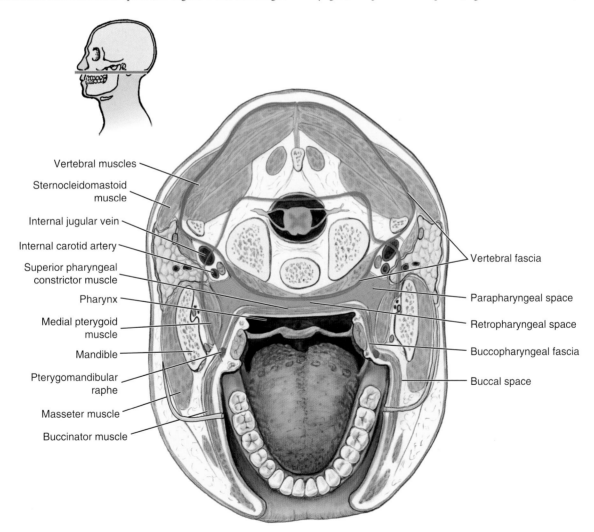

FIGURE 11-13 Transverse section of the oral cavity and neck *(see inset)* highlighting both the parapharyngeal space and retropharyngeal space.

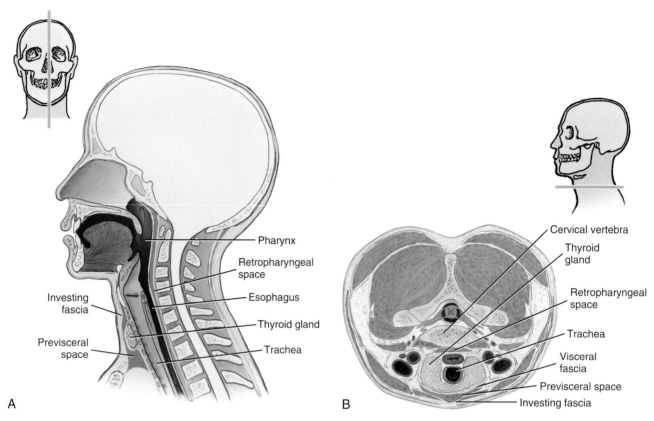

FIGURE 11-14 The head and neck highlighting both the retropharyngeal space and previsceral space upon midsagittal section (*see inset*) **(A)**, with the neck upon transverse section (*see inset*) **(B)**.

TABLE 11-3	Major Cervical Fascial Spaces		
SPACE	**LOCATION**	**CONTENTS**	**COMMUNICATION PATTERN**
Previsceral (visceral)	Between visceral and investing fasciae	Pharynx, larynx, trachea, and esophagus	Parapharyngeal spaces
Parapharyngeal (lateral pharyngeal)	Lateral to visceral fascia around pharynx	Anterior compartment: deep cervical lymph nodes	Retropharyngeal space
Retropharyngeal (retrovisceral)	Between vertebral and visceral fasciae	Retropharyngeal lymph nodes in early childhood	Parapharyngeal
Perivertebral	Posterior to retropharyngeal space	Cervical vertebrae and associated structures	

Previsceral Space. The **previsceral space** (pre-**vis**-er-al) or *visceral space* is located between the visceral and investing fasciae, anterior to the trachea. The previsceral space encases the visceral compartment of the neck, which contains the pharynx, larynx, trachea, and esophagus. The previsceral space communicates with the parapharyngeal spaces.

Parapharyngeal Space. The **parapharyngeal space** (pare-uh-fuh-**rin**-je-uhl) or *lateral pharyngeal space* is a bilateral fascial space lateral to the pharynx and medial to the medial pterygoid muscle, parallel to the carotid sheath. The space is shaped like an inverted pyramid, with the skull base superiorly and inferiorly the greater cornu of the hyoid bone at its apex. The parapharyngeal space in its posterior compartment is also adjacent to the carotid sheath, which contains the internal and common carotid arteries and the internal jugular

vein, as well as the tenth cranial or vagus nerve as discussed earlier (see Figure 6-1). The space is also adjacent to the posterior cranial nerves, the ninth or glossopharyngeal, eleventh or accessory, and twelfth or hypoglossal cranial nerves as they exit the cranial cavity.

Anteriorly, the parapharyngeal space extends to the pterygomandibular raphe, where it is continuous with the infratemporal and buccal spaces. The parapharyngeal space's anterior compartment contains the deep cervical lymph nodes. The posterior compartment extends around the pharynx, where it is continuous with another cervical fascial space, the retropharyngeal space. According to recent studies, the parapharyngeal space communicates only with the retropharyngeal space. Dental (or odontogenic) infections can become serious when they reach the parapharyngeal space because of its connection to the retropharyngeal space.

Retropharyngeal Space. The **retropharyngeal space** (ret-roh-fuh-**rin**-je-uhl) or *retrovisceral space* is a fascial space located immediately posterior to the pharynx, between the vertebral and visceral fasciae. The retropharyngeal space extends from the base of the skull, where it is posterior to the superior pharyngeal constrictor muscle and inferior to the thorax (chest). The space is divided into two lateral compartments by a fibrous raphe and contains the retropharyngeal lymph nodes in early childhood. The retropharyngeal space communicates with the parapharyngeal spaces since it is continuous with it.

Because of the rapidity with which dental (or odontogenic) infections can travel inferiorly along the retropharyngeal space to the thorax (chest), the retropharyngeal space is also known as the "danger space" of the neck by healthcare professionals when infections occur within it (see Chapter 12). Nasal and pharyngeal infections can also be involved with this space. With any dental (or odontogenic) infection within the retropharyngeal space, there can be stiffness of the neck, difficulty swallowing or dysphagia, difficult or labored breath from dyspnea, and bulging of the posterior pharyngeal wall. Complications can include airway obstruction, aspiration pneumonia, and acute inflammation of the midchest.

Perivertebral Space. Posterior to the retropharyngeal space is the **perivertebral space** (pare-ee-**ver**-tuh-bruhl) that contains the cervical vertebrae and associated structures. It is a cylinder-shaped space surrounded by the deep cervical fasciae and extends from the skull base to the lower spine. This space can be broken down to the prevertebral space anteriorly and the paravertebral space posteriorly.

CERVICAL COMPARTMENTS

When discussing the locations of the cervical fasciae, the neck can also be divided into four major cervical compartments (Figure 11-15 and Table 11-4). It is felt that the division into compartments is more appropriate than being described as "space" in the neck by many anatomists. Compartments may be bordered by bone and/or muscle, as well as fascia, and individual compartments may intercommunicate. The defining of these cervical compartments is also useful when

TABLE 11-4	**Cervical Compartments With Contents and Borders**	
CERVICAL COMPARTMENT	**CONTENTS**	**BORDER**
Vertebral compartment	Spinal cord, cervical vertebrae, associated vertebral muscles	Vertebral fascia
Visceral compartment	Thyroid, thymus, and parathyroid glands as well as the hyoid bone, larynx, trachea, esophagus, and pharynx	Visceral fascia
Vascular compartments	Internal carotid and common carotid arteries, as well as the internal jugular veins	Carotid sheaths

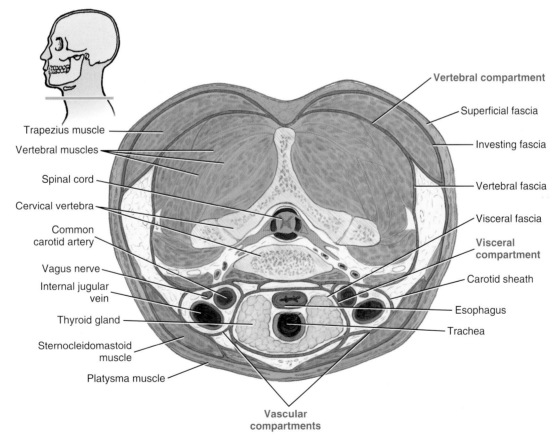

FIGURE 11-15 The neck upon transverse section (*see inset*) noting the three compartments (*dashed lines*) and their relationship to their bordering fasciae including the vertebral compartment within the vertebral fascia, visceral compartment within the visceral fascia, and the vascular compartments each within the carotid sheaths.

discussing the anatomic borders of cancer and subsequent cancer treatment. This includes cancer of the thyroid gland and its involvement with the regional cervical lymph nodes.

The single **vertebral compartment** (or posterior compartment) contains the spinal cord, cervical vertebrae, and associated vertebral muscles that support and move the head and neck. The vertebral compartment is bordered by the vertebral fascia in the neck (see Figures 11-1 to 11-3).

The single **visceral compartment** (or anterior compartment) contains the thyroid, thymus, and parathyroid glands as well as the hyoid bone, larynx, trachea, esophagus, and pharynx. This compartment is a continuation of the gastrointestinal and respiratory systems. This compartment is more moveable in comparison to the other compartments since it changes its overall shape during swallowing or speech. The visceral compartment is bordered by the visceral fascia in the neck (see Figures 11-1 to 11-3).

Finally, the two bilateral **vascular compartments** (or lateral compartments), located lateral and posterior to the pharynx, consist of two carotid sheaths bordered by each vascular compartment in the neck (see Figures 11-1 to 11-3). Thus each vascular compartment contains major blood vessels. These major blood vessels include: the internal carotid and common carotid arteries as well as the internal jugular veins.

REVIEW QUESTIONS

1. Which of the following statements CORRECTLY describes the deep fasciae?
   A. Dense and inelastic tissue forming sheaths around deep structures
   B. Fatty and elastic fibrous tissue found just deep to the skin
   C. Potential spaces containing loose connective tissue
   D. Fatty and elastic fibrous tissue forming spaces under the skin
   E. Dense and inelastic deep structures of the vascular system

2. Which of the following structures are located within the carotid sheath?
   A. Internal and common carotid arteries and tenth cranial nerve
   B. External and common carotid arteries and fifth cranial nerve
   C. External jugular vein and tenth cranial nerve
   D. Internal jugular vein and fifth cranial nerve

3. In which of the following spaces is the pterygoid plexus of veins located?
   A. Parotid space
   B. Temporal space
   C. Infratemporal space
   D. Buccal space
   E. Parapharyngeal space

4. The masticator space includes the submasseteric space and which other space?
   A. Submental space
   B. Submandibular space
   C. Sublingual space
   D. Pterygomandibular space
   E. Retropharyngeal space

5. Which of the following types of tissue surrounds the space of the body of the mandible?
   A. Fatty tissue
   B. Loose connective tissue
   C. Periosteum
   D. Elastic tissue

6. The submandibular space communicates MOST directly with which of the following spaces?
   A. Temporal space
   B. Parotid space
   C. Buccal space
   D. Sublingual space
   E. Canine space

7. The parapharyngeal space is located between the superior pharyngeal constrictor muscle and
   A. lateral pterygoid muscle.
   B. medial pterygoid muscle.
   C. mylohyoid muscle.
   D. masseter muscle.
   E. buccinator muscle.

8. Which space is located in the midline between the mandibular symphysis and the hyoid bone?
   A. Retropharyngeal space
   B. Sublingual space
   C. Submandibular space
   D. Submental space
   E. Submasseteric space

9. Which of the following nerves is located within the pterygomandibular space?
   A. Infraorbital nerve
   B. Posterior superior alveolar nerve
   C. Inferior alveolar nerve
   D. Anterior superior alveolar nerve

10. Which of the following areas MOST directly communicates with the retropharyngeal space?
    A. Masticator space
    B. Submandibular space
    C. Previsceral space
    D. Parapharyngeal space

11. Which of the following muscles forms the roof of the pterygomandibular space?
    A. Lateral pterygoid muscle
    B. Medial pterygoid muscle
    C. Temporalis muscle
    D. Sternocleidomastoid muscle

12. Which of the following blood vessels is located within the sublingual space?
    A. Facial artery
    B. Anterior jugular vein
    C. Lingual artery
    D. Inferior alveolar vein

13. Which of the following spaces is considered by healthcare professionals to be the "danger space" of the neck?
    A. Parapharyngeal space
    B. Body of the mandible
    C. Submandibular space
    D. Retropharyngeal space

14. Which of the following fascial structures is also considered part of the deep fasciae of the face?
    A. Masseteric-parotid fascia
    B. Investing fascia
    C. Visceral fascia
    D. Carotid sheath

15. Which of the following structures is located within the superficial fasciae of the head and neck?
    A. Temporalis muscle
    B. Muscles of facial expression
    C. Parotid salivary gland
    D. Thyroid gland

16. What forms the superior border of the submandibular space?
    A. Mylohyoid line
    B. Hyoid bone
    C. Angle of the mandible
    D. Trachea and larynx
17. Which of the following spaces is parallel to the carotid sheath?
    A. Temporal space
    B. Canine space
    C. Parapharyngeal space
    D. Parotid space
18. Which of the following spaces is located deep to the muscles of facial expression that elevate the upper lip?
    A. Parotid space
    B. Submandibular space
    C. Masticator space
    D. Canine space
19. Which of the following spaces is NOT part of the masticator space?
    A. Infratemporal space
    B. Temporal space
    C. Submasseteric space
    D. Parotid space
20. Which of the following fasciae listed runs deep and parallel to the carotid sheath?
    A. Temporal fascia
    B. Visceral fascia
    C. Pterygoid fascia
    D. Investing fascia

Identification Exercises

Identify the structures on the following diagrams by filling in each blank with the correct anatomic term. You can check your answers by looking back at the figure indicated in parentheses for each identification diagram.

1. (Figure 11-1, *A*)

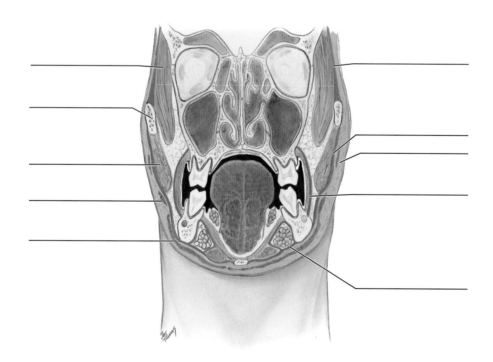

2. (Figure 11-1, *B*)

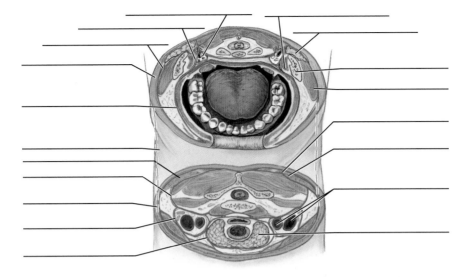

3. (Figure 11-2)

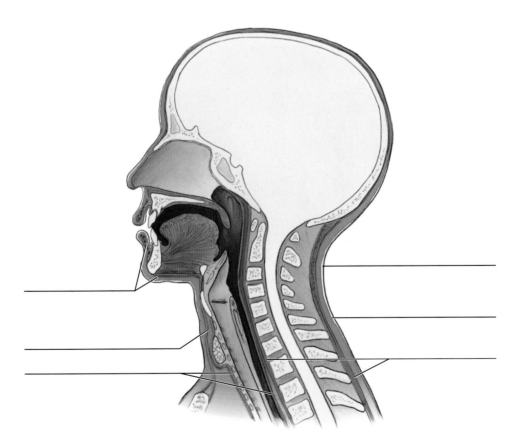

4. (Figure 11-3)

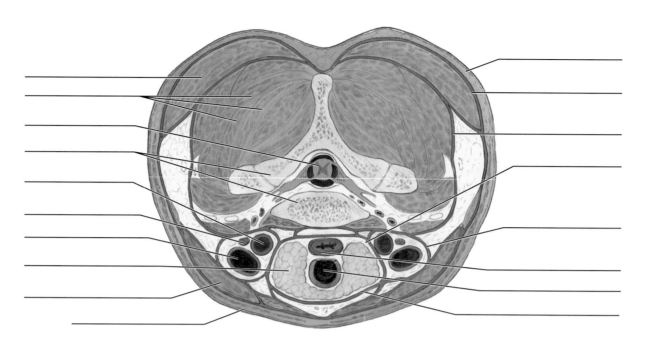

5. (Figure 11-4)

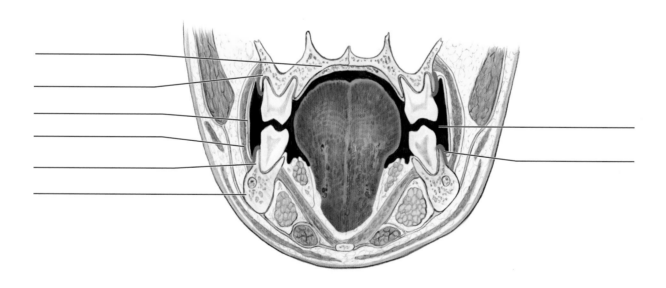

6. (Figure 11-5)

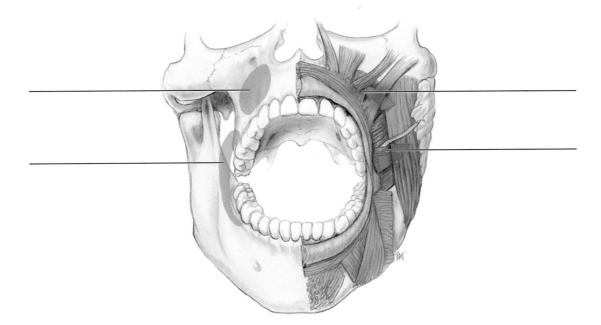

7. (Figure 11-6)

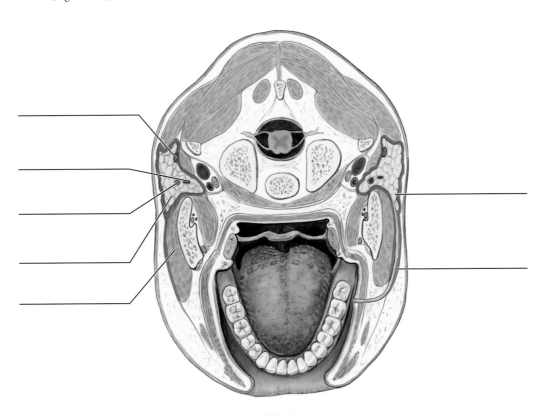

8. (Figure 11-7)

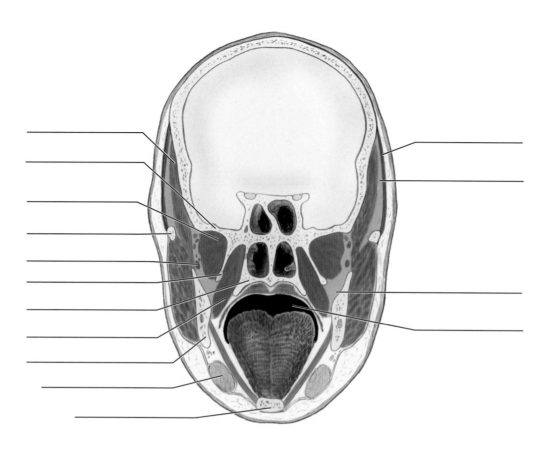

9. (Figure 11-8, *A*)

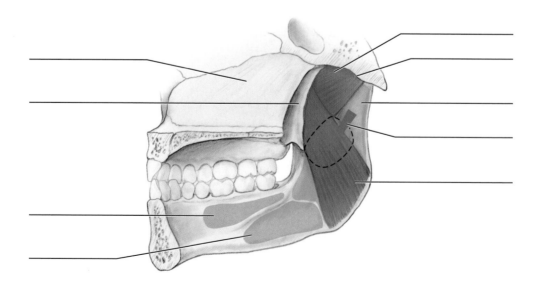

10. (Figure 11-8, *B*)

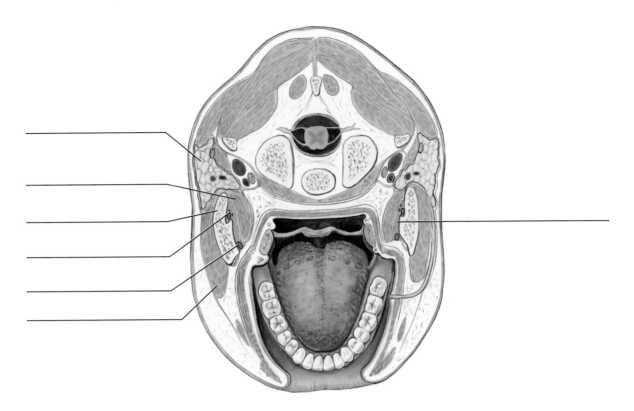

11. (Figure 11-9)

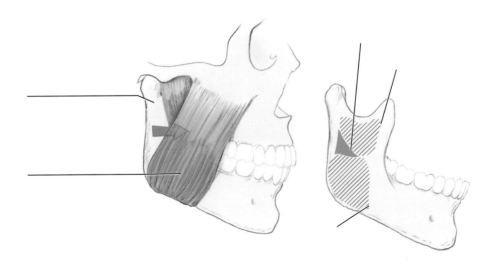

12. (Figure 11-10, *A*)

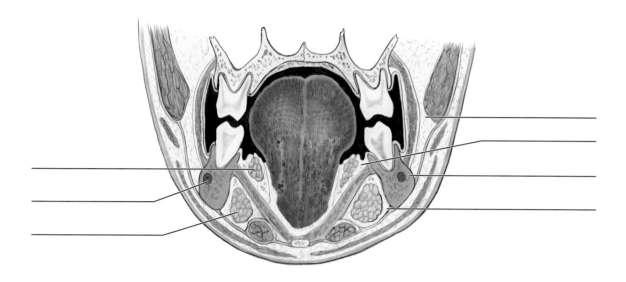

13. (Figure 11-11)

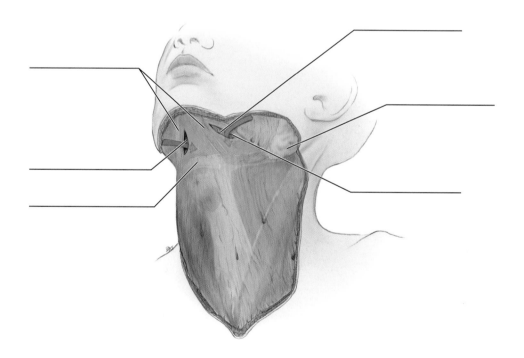

14. (Figure 11-12)

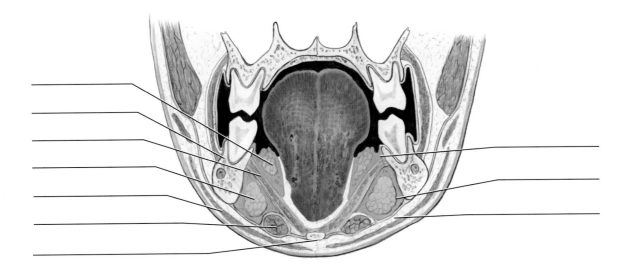

15. (Figure 11-13)

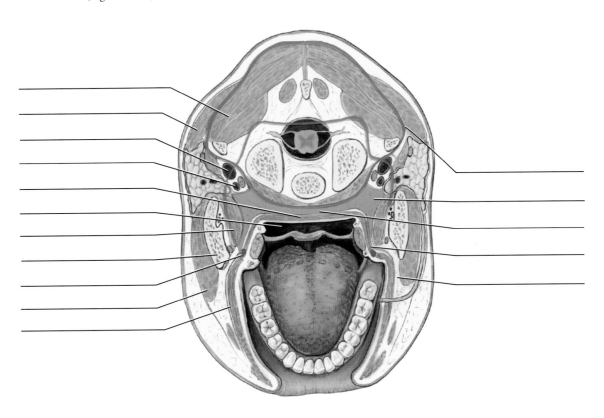

16. (Figure 11-14, *A*)

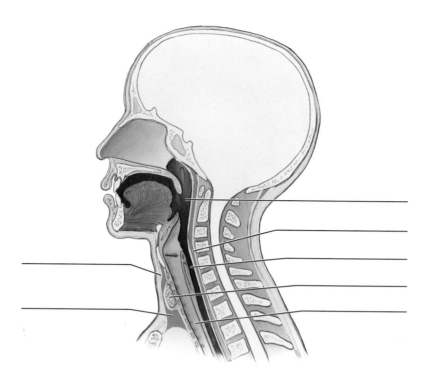

17. (Figure 11-14, *B*)

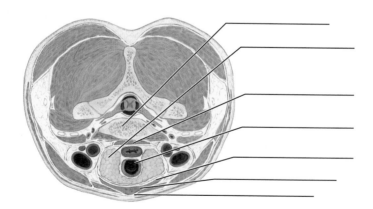

CHAPTER 12

Spread of Infection

●●● LEARNING OBJECTIVES

1. Define and pronounce the **key terms** and **anatomic terms** in this chapter.
2. Discuss the spread of odontogenic infection to the sinuses and by the vascular system, lymphatic system, and spaces in the head and neck region.
3. Trace the routes of odontogenic infection in the head and neck region on a diagram, skull, and patient.
4. Discuss the complications that can occur with the spread of odontogenic infection in the head and neck region.
5. Discuss the prevention of the spread of odontogenic infection during patient dental care.
6. Correctly complete the review questions and activities for this chapter.
7. Integrate an understanding of the anatomic considerations for the spread of odontogenic infection into clinical dental practice.

KEY TERMS

Abducens nerve paralysis (ab-**doo**-senz) (puh-**ral**-i-sis) Loss of function of sixth cranial nerve.

Abscess (**ab**-ses) Infection with suppuration resulting from pathogens in contained space.

Cavernous sinus thrombosis (**kav**-er-nus) (throm-**bo**-sis) Infection of cavernous sinus.

Cellulitis (sel-u-**ly**-tis) Diffuse inflammation of soft tissue.

Fistula/Fistulae (**fis**-tu-luh, **fis**-tu-lee) Passageway(s) in skin, mucosa, or bone allowing drainage of abscess at surface.

Infection Invasion by pathogens with multiplication of them.

Ludwig angina (**lood**-vig an-**ji**-nuh) Serious infection of submandibular space.

Maxillary sinusitis (sy-nuh-**si**-tis) Infection of maxillary sinus.

Meningitis (muh-in-**jite**-is) Inflammation of meninges of brain or spinal cord.

Odontogenic infection (o-don-toh-**jen**-ik) Infection involving teeth or associated tissue.

Opportunistic infection (op-uhr-too-**nis**-tik) Resident microbiota creating infection because body's defenses are compromised.

Osteomyelitis of the jaw (OMJ) (os-tee-o-my-uh-**ly**-tus) Inflammation of bone marrow.

Pathogens (**path**-o-jens) Microbiota that are not residents and can cause an infection.

Pustule (**pus**-tule) Small elevated and circumscribed suppuration-containing lesion of skin or oral mucosa.

Resident microbiota (my-kro-**bi**-o-tuh) Indigenous regional microorganisms usually not causing infections.

Stoma (**stoh**-muh) Opening such as fistula.

Suppuration (sup-u-**ray**-shuhn) Pus containing pathogenic bacteria, white blood cells, tissue fluid, debris.

INFECTION PROCESS OVERVIEW

The healthy body usually lives in balance with a number of **resident microbiota** that are indigenous in nature. A microbiota is a regional collection or community of microbes. The population of resident microbiota within the oral cavity is similar to most of the rest of the body in that it consists of a few eucaryotic fungi and protists, but bacteria are the most numerous and obvious microbial components. However, nonresident microorganisms called **pathogens** can invade and initiate an **infection**. Infection is a process by which there is an invasion by and multiplication of these pathogens. Pathogens can involve bacteria, viruses, fungi, and protozoa. These pathogens contain virulence factors that help further the infection process (discussed further). A dental professional should understand the infection process that allows microorganisms to create disease states.

ODONTOGENIC INFECTION

Dental infection or **odontogenic infection** (also known as *dentoalveolar infections* by the medical community) involving the teeth or associated tissue is caused by oral pathogens that are usually of more than one species or are *polymicrobial* as well as mixed in nature. In these types of infections, the presence of one microorganism species generates a niche for other pathogenic microorganism species to colonize. These infections can be of dental origin with an odontogenic infection or can arise from a nonodontogenic or secondary source. Infections of dental origin usually originate from progressive dental caries or extensive periodontal disease, or even with implant placement as with periimplantitis.

While the majority of intraoral infections are caused by the overgrowth of resident aerobic *Streptococcus viridans*, it is estimated that approximately 60% of these infections also contain anaerobic rods, such as *Peptostreptococcus*, *Fusobacterium*, and *Prevotella* species. The microbial specificity in odontogenic infections has been more clearly delineated with technologic advances in sampling and anaerobic culturing; laboratories now routinely culture for anaerobic microorganisms in oxygen-free gas environments, which increases the yield of anaerobic bacteria in culture.

These polymicrobial resident microorganisms inhabit the surfaces of the teeth and oral mucosa but always in smaller numbers until an infection occurs. They are also found as resident microbiota within the gingival sulci and saliva as part of the formation of dental biofilm (plaque). Thus most odontogenic infections result initially from the increased formation of dental biofilm (plaque) from the surrounding area. Pathogens can also be introduced deeper into the oral mucosa by the trauma caused by dental procedures such as the contamination of oral surgery sites (e.g., during tooth extraction or implant placement) and the contamination associated with needle tracts made during incorrect administration of a local anesthetic (see Chapters 9 and 11).

Each strain of pathogens has defined virulence factors and can contribute to the pathogenicity of the microorganisms. Virulence factors can include those produced by the pathogen such as bacterial toxins (including endotoxins and exotoxins), cell surface proteins that mediate attachment, platelet binding factors, cell surface carbohydrates and proteins that protect the pathogen, and hydrolytic enzymes. These are in addition to the innate anatomic features of the pathogen such as capsules, spores, and flagella that can contribute to its pathogenicity. These virulence factors, whether produced or innate, enable colonization of the pathogen as well as tissue invasion and degradation.

Specifically, more than 50% of the gram-negative anaerobic bacteria that are known pathogens for head and neck infections (see earlier discussion) are capable of producing beta-lactamases. These enzymes are responsible for resistance to a broad class of systemic beta-lactam antibiotics, including penicillin. There are several groups and classes of beta-lactamases that result in antibiotic resistance. For example, several of the class C beta-lactamases can result in cephalosporin resistance and some of the class A beta-lactamases confer resistance to oxyimino-cephalosporins, cephamycins, and carbapenems. Beta-lactamase provides antibiotic resistance by breaking the antibiotics' structure. These antibiotics all have a common element in their molecular structure, a four-atom ring known as a beta-lactam. Through hydrolysis, the lactamase enzyme breaks the beta-lactam ring open, deactivating the molecule's antibacterial properties.

Thus, the beta-lactamases are responsible for the initial tissue damage caused by head and neck infections, as well as treatment failures with odontogenic infections. These enzymes may not only survive penicillin therapy as discussed but also may shield penicillin-susceptible co-pathogens from the activity of penicillin by releasing the enzyme freely into their environment. Careful use of antimicrobials in the future may reduce and control the emergence of penicillin-resistant organisms. The only current defense is the combined use of

a beta-lactamase inhibitor with a known systemic antibiotic that the pathogen is sensitive to after culturing (see later discussion).

Odontogenic infection is the most prevalent disease globally and it is the main reason for seeking dental care. However, some odontogenic infections are secondary infections from a primary infection of orofacial tissue such as the skin, tonsils, ears, or sinuses. These nonodontogenic sources of infections must be diagnosed and treated early if noted during dental care; prompt medical referral will prevent further spread and potential complications. A dental professional may want to refer to an oral or systemic pathology text for more information on this topic (see Appendix A).

ODONTOGENIC INFECTION LESIONS

Odontogenic infections can result in various types of pathologic lesions, depending on the location of the infection and thus the type of tissue involved. Pathologic lesions in the head and neck from odontogenic infections can include an abscess, cellulitis, or osteomyelitis.

ABSCESS

An **abscess** in the oral cavity forms when there is localized entrapment of pathogens from a chronic odontogenic infection in a well circumscribed but closed tissue space such as that created by the oral mucosa (Figures 12-1 to 12-5). The abscess becomes filled with suppuration and feels fluctuant with palpation. **Suppuration** or *pus* contains pathogenic bacteria, white blood cells, tissue fluid, and debris.

Periapical abscess formation can occur with progressive caries, when pathogens invade the usually sterile pulp and the infection spreads apically. This type of abscess is the most common odontogenic emergency. In combination with the right circumstances that compromise the innate body defenses, an erupting mandibular third molar can involve a pericoronal abscess or *pericoronitis*, which is a less common type of odontogenic emergency. Pathogens can also become entrapped in deepened gingival sulci or periodontal pockets in cases of severe periodontal disease and cause a periodontal abscess, which is the least common type of odontogenic emergency.

An abscess can be either acute or chronic. Abscess formation may not be detectable on radiographs during the early acute stages. However, in the later stages of infection, chronic abscess formation

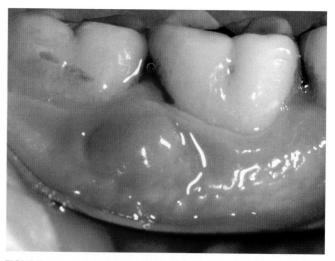

FIGURE 12-1 Intact periodontal abscess in the mandibular vestibule located between the apices of the mandibular first and second molars. *(Courtesy Margaret J. Fehrenbach, RDH, MS.)*

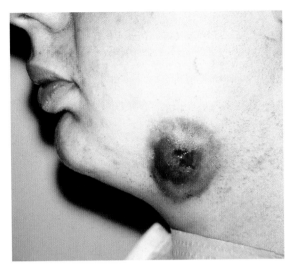

FIGURE 12-2 Chronic abscess on the buccal skin surface, with a fistula and stoma present, that involves a periapical infection of the mandibular second molar. *(Courtesy Dr. Mark Gabrielson.)*

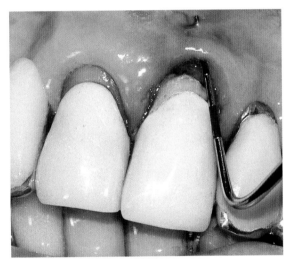

FIGURE 12-3 Periodontal abscess in the maxillary vestibule involving the maxillary central incisor, with fistula and stoma formation (see probe insertion). *(Courtesy Margaret J. Fehrenbach, RDH, MS.)*

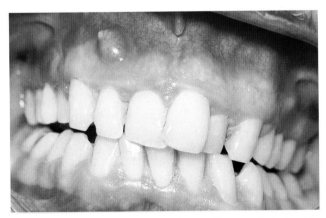

FIGURE 12-4 Periapical abscess in the maxillary vestibule involving infection of the maxillary lateral incisor, with pustule formation.

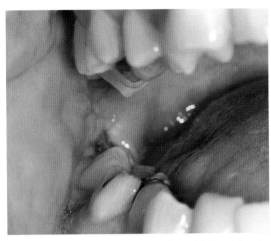

FIGURE 12-5 Pericoronal abscess or pericoronitis involving the mandibular third molar. *(Courtesy Margaret J. Fehrenbach, RDH, MS.)*

can lead to the formation of a tract(s) or fistula (plural, fistulae) in the outer skin, oral mucosa, or alveolar process. The passageways allow drainage of the infection with suppuration possibly noted on the surface (see Figures 12-2 and 12-3).

The infection process can cause the overlying tissue to undergo necrosis (or cell death), which allows this tract to form in the tissue. The opening of the fistula from the tract is called a stoma. If the alveolar process surrounds the odontogenic infection, it will break down the bone in its thinnest part (either the facial or lingual cortical plate), following the path of least resistance, and thus will then be noted as a localized radiolucency on radiographs.

The soft tissue over a fistula in the alveolar process may also have an associated extraoral or intraoral pustule. A pustule is a small elevated and circumscribed lesion of either the outer skin or oral mucosa that contains suppuration (see Figure 12-4). The position of the pustule is determined largely by the relationship between the fistula and the overlying muscle attachments. Again, the infection will follow the path of least resistance (Table 12-1). Importantly, muscle attachments to the bones, unlike the other facial soft tissue, may serve as barriers to the spread of infection.

The most common treatment for suppurating odontogenic infections is surgical drainage and the need for the definitive restoration or extraction of the infected teeth, whichever is the primary source of infection. For those involving pericoronal infections, the inflammation can usually be resolved by flushing the debris and infected material from underneath the inflamed pericoronal tissue. However, it may only resolve by extracting the associated tooth or the operculum, which is the inflamed overlying gingival tissue.

Newer studies recommended heat application in the form of moist packs and/or mouthrinses as supportive therapy in the management of these suppurating odontogenic infections. Heat produces vasodilation and increased circulation, more rapid removal of tissue breakdown products, and great influx of immune cells and antibodies. Clinical follow-up of the patient is of critical importance, especially if drainage is unproductive. In these unresolved cases, a course of systemic antibiotics may be instituted after appropriate microbial swabs are obtained and cultured to individualize the antibiotic regimen (see earlier discussion).

CELLULITIS

Cellulitis of the face and neck can also occur with odontogenic infections, resulting in an acute level of diffuse inflammation of soft tissue

TABLE 12-1	Clinical Presentations of Orofacial Abscesses*
CLINICAL PRESENTATION OF LESION	**TEETH AND ASSOCIATED PERIODONTIUM MOST COMMONLY INVOLVED**
Maxillary vestibule	Maxillary central or lateral incisor from all its surfaces and root (see Figures 12-3 and 12-4)
	Maxillary canine from all surfaces and root that is short and inferior to levator anguli oris muscle
	Maxillary premolars from buccal surfaces and roots
	Maxillary molars from buccal surfaces or buccal roots that are short and inferior to buccinator muscle
Penetration of nasal floor	Maxillary central incisor from root
Nasolabial skin region	Maxillary canine from all surfaces and root that is long and superior to levator anguli oris muscle
Palate	Maxillary lateral incisor from palatal surface and root
	Maxillary premolars from palatal surfaces and roots
	Maxillary molars from palatal surfaces and palatal roots
Perforation into maxillary sinus	Maxillary molars from buccal surfaces and buccal roots that are long
Buccal skin surface	Maxillary molars from buccal surfaces and buccal roots that are long and superior to buccinator muscle
	Mandibular first and second molars from buccal surfaces and buccal roots that are long and inferior to buccinator muscle (see Figure 12-2)
Mandibular vestibule	Mandibular incisors from all surfaces and roots that are short and superior to mentalis muscle
	Mandibular canine and premolars from all surfaces and roots that are all superior to depressor muscles
	Mandibular first and second molars from buccal surfaces and roots that are short and superior to buccinator muscle (see Figure 12-1)
Submental skin region	Mandibular incisors from roots that are long and inferior to mentalis muscle
Sublingual region	Mandibular first molar from lingual surface and roots that are all superior to mylohyoid muscle
	Mandibular second molar from lingual surface and roots that are short and superior to mylohyoid muscle
Submandibular skin region	Mandibular second molar from lingual surface and roots that are long and inferior to mylohyoid muscle
	Mandibular third molars from all surfaces and roots that are inferior to mylohyoid muscle

*Only permanent teeth are considered in this table.

spaces unlike a more localized abscess (Figure 12-6; see Chapter 11). The clinical signs and symptoms are pain, tenderness, erythema or redness, and diffuse edema of the involved soft tissue space, causing a massive and firm swelling that feels doughy to indurated (or hardened) with palpation (Table 12-2). Difficulty swallowing (or dysphagia) or restricted eye opening (or ptosis) may also happen if the cellulitis occurs within the pharynx or orbital regions, respectively.

Usually the infection forms an additional facial abscess trying to contain the infection; if not initially treated, however, it may discharge on the facial skin surface. These cases may be associated with extensive necrosis of the skin covering the abscess formation, which may eventually result in severe scarring of the surface skin with healing.

However, without any treatment, cellulitis can spread due to perforation of the surrounding facial bone, becoming more generalized and causing serious complications such as Ludwig angina (discussed later). Cellulitis is treated by administration of a course of systemic antibiotics and removal of the cause of the infection. In addition, ultrasonography (USG) is a newer and effective image modality used to diagnose as well as manage the fascial space infections.

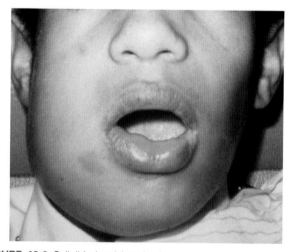

FIGURE 12-6 Cellulitis involving the buccal space resulting from an abscess of the mandibular first molar. *(Courtesy Dr. Mark Gabrielson.)*

OSTEOMYELITIS

Another type of lesion that can be related to odontogenic infection is osteomyelitis of the jaw (OMJ), an inflammation of the bone marrow. Osteomyelitis can locally involve any bone in the body or can be generalized. This inflammation develops from the invasion of the tissue of a long bone by pathogens, usually from a skin or pharyngeal infection. In osteomyelitis involving the jaw, the pathogens are most likely to derive from a periapical abscess, from an extension of cellulitis, or from contamination of an oral surgery site (Figure 12-7). It is also more common after insufficient immobilization of bony fragments resulting from oral trauma cases.

Osteomyelitis occurs more often in the mandible; it occurs only rarely in the maxillae because of the mandible's thicker cortical plates and reduced vascularization. Continuation of osteomyelitis leads to

TABLE 12-2	Clinical Presentations of Orofacial Cellulitis*	
CLINICAL PRESENTATION OF LESION	**SPACE INVOLVED**	**TEETH AND ASSOCIATED PERIODONTIUM MOST COMMONLY INVOLVED IN INFECTION**
Infraorbital, zygomatic, and buccal regions	Buccal space	Maxillary premolars and molars; mandibular molars (see Figure 12-6)
Posterior border of mandible	Parotid space	Not generally of odontogenic origin
Submental region	Submental space	Mandibular anterior teeth
Unilateral submandibular region	Submandibular space	Mandibular posterior teeth
Bilateral submandibular region	Submental, sublingual, and submandibular spaces with Ludwig angina	Spread of mandibular infection
Lateral cervical region	Parapharyngeal space	Spread of mandibular infection

*Only permanent teeth are considered in this table.

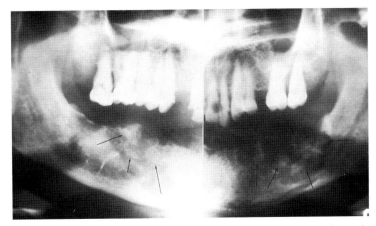

FIGURE 12-7 Panoramic radiograph of osteomyelitis with its bone resorption and associated sequestra *(arrows). (Courtesy Margaret J. Fehrenbach, RDH, MS.)*

bone resorption and formation of sequestra, which are pieces of dead bone separated from the sound bone within the area. These bony changes including the formation of sequestra can be detected by radiographic evaluation (see Figure 12-7).

Paresthesia, evidenced by burning or prickling ("pins and needles" feeling), may develop in the entire mandible if the infection involves the mandibular canal carrying the inferior alveolar nerve (see Chapters 8 and 9). Localized paresthesia of the lower lip may occur if the infection is distal to the mental foramen where the mental nerve exits. Treatment consists of drainage as discussed earlier, removal of any sequestra by surgery, and systemic antibiotic administration combined with an beta-lactamase inhibitor; in some patients the additional use of hyperbaric oxygen may be necessary. Today, osteomyelitis of the jaw is uncommon because both dental care and antibiotics are now more readily available.

MEDICALLY COMPROMISED PATIENTS

The resident microbiota found in the oral cavity usually do not create an infection. If, however, the body's innate defenses are compromised, they can create **opportunistic infections**. Medically compromised individuals include those with human immunodeficiency virus (HIV) infection, uncontrolled diabetes, anemia, and those undergoing transplant or cancer therapy (Figure 12-8). These patients also have a higher risk

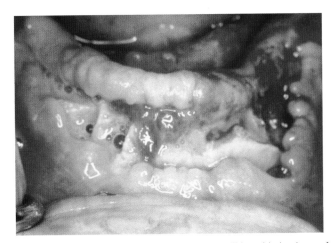

FIGURE 12-8 Osteoradionecrosis of the mandible with its loss of bone vitality and inflammation after radiation therapy for oral cancer. This therapy tends to increase the risk of secondary odontogenic infection due to the compromised health of the patient. *(Courtesy of Margaret J. Fehrenbach, RDH, MS.)*

of complications resulting from odontogenic infections because of their extensive medical histories.

SPREAD OF ODONTOGENIC INFECTION

Any odontogenic infections that start in the teeth and associated oral tissue can have significant consequences if they spread to vital structures, tissue, or organs. Usually a localized abscess establishes a fistula in the skin, oral mucosa, or the associated alveolar process, allowing natural drainage of the infection and diminishing the risk of its spread as was discussed earlier. However, fistula formation and drainage do not always occur so the risk of spreading the infection is still present.

Occasionally, odontogenic infection can spread to the paranasal sinuses or can be spread by the vascular system, lymphatic system, or spaces in the head and neck. Reviewing the communication patterns in tissue, structures, or organs is important to the understanding of the possible routes of the spread of infection with odontogenic infections.

SPREAD TO PARANASAL SINUSES

The paranasal sinuses of the skull can become infected as a result of the direct spread of infection from the teeth and associated dental tissue, resulting in secondary sinusitis (see Chapter 3). A perforation, an abnormal hole in the wall of the sinus, can also be caused by an infection, which may then further the spread of infection.

MAXILLARY SINUSITIS

Secondary sinusitis of dental origin occurs mainly in the maxillary sinuses because the roots of the maxillary posterior teeth and associated tissue are close to these sinuses (see Figure 3-46). Thus **maxillary sinusitis** can result from the spread of infection from a periapical abscess initiated by a root of a maxillary posterior tooth that perforates the sinus floor to involve the sinus mucosa. In addition, a contaminated root fragment can be displaced into the maxillary sinus during an extraction, possibly creating an infection.

However, most infections of the maxillary sinuses are not of dental origin but are caused by an upper respiratory infection, an infection in the nasal region that spreads to the sinuses, such as after the common cold. It is important to note that an infection in one sinus can travel through the nasal cavity to other sinuses and lead to serious complications for the patient such as infection of the cranial cavity and brain. Thus it is important that any sinusitis be treated aggressively by medical referral to eliminate the initial infection, especially in medically compromised patients.

The symptoms of sinusitis include headache, usually near the involved sinus, and foul-smelling nasal or pharyngeal discharge, possibly with fever and weakness. The skin over the involved sinus can be tender and hot, with erythema or redness due to the inflammation in the area when palpated and examined (see Figure 3-58). Difficulty in breathing (dyspnea) occurs, as well as pain, when the nasal passages become blocked by tissue inflammation. Early radiographic evidence of sinusitis is the thickening of the sinus walls. Subsequent radiographic evaluation shows increased radiopacity (or cloudiness) and possibly perforation, usually using bilateral comparisons of the paired sinuses; magnetic resonance imaging (MRI) may also be indicated (see Figure 3-56).

Acute sinusitis usually responds to a course of systemic antibiotics. Surgery may be necessary in cases of prolonged chronic maxillary sinusitis to enlarge the ostia of the lateral walls in the nasal cavity so that adequate drainage can diminish the effects of the infection. The approach to the maxillary sinus during surgery is through the thinner facial cortical bone of the canine fossa. Recent studies show that removal of the toxic mucus with its inflammatory products is also of prime importance in prevention of chronic sinusitis (see Chapter 3).

SPREAD BY VASCULAR SYSTEM

The vascular system of the head and neck can allow the spread of infection from the teeth and associated oral tissue because pathogens can travel in the veins into other tissue, structures, or organs after draining the infected oral site (see Chapter 6). The spread of odontogenic infection by way of the vascular system can occur because of bacteremia or an infected thrombus possibly resulting in thrombosis.

BACTEREMIA

Bacteria traveling in the vascular system can cause bacteremia, which can occur during dental treatment (see further discussion in Chapter 10). In an individual with a high risk for infective endocarditis, these bacteria may lodge in the compromised tissue and set up serious infection deep in the heart, which can result in massive and fatal heart damage. Bacteremia may also be implicated in patients at risk for deep tissue infection surrounding a newly placed prosthesis or in medically compromised patients.

CAVERNOUS SINUS THROMBOSIS

An infected intravascular clot or thrombus can dislodge from the inner blood vessel wall and travel as an infected embolus (see Figures 6-16 and 6-17). An infected embolus can travel in the veins draining the oral cavity, ending up in areas such as the dural venous sinuses within the cranial cavity. These dural venous sinuses are channels by which blood is conveyed from the cerebral veins into the veins of the head and neck, particularly the internal jugular vein. However, because of the communication of the dural sinuses with the veins of the cranial cavity and direction of blood flow, there is an increased possibility of spreading infection.

The cavernous sinus is most likely to be involved in the possible fatal spread of odontogenic infection (see Figures 6-12 and 8-6). The paired cavernous sinuses are located on each of the lateral surfaces of the body of the sphenoid bone. Each cavernous sinus communicates by anastomoses across the midline with the contralateral cavernous sinus and also with the pterygoid plexus of veins and the superior ophthalmic vein, which anastomoses with the facial vein. These major veins drain the teeth through the posterior superior and inferior alveolar veins and the lips through the superior and inferior labial veins.

It is a common misconception that the veins of the head do not contain one-way valves like other veins of the circulatory system. Most veins of the face, but not all, have valves as discussed in Chapter 8. In fact, it is not the absence of venous valves but the existence of communications between the facial vein and cavernous sinus and the direction of blood flow that are important in the spread of infection from the face. Therefore odontogenic infections that drain into these major veins may initiate an inflammatory response resulting in an increase in blood stasis and thrombus formation. The transport of the infected thrombus (or thrombi) as an embolus (or emboli) into this venous sinus thus results in **cavernous sinus thrombosis**.

Needle tract contamination can also result in the spread of infection from the infratemporal space to the pterygoid plexus of veins if a posterior superior alveolar block is incorrectly administered (see Figure 9-7). In addition, nonodontogenic infections of the area that includes the orbital region, nasal region, and paranasal sinuses may result in the spread of infection to the cavernous sinus. That is why this area is considered by medical professionals to be the "danger triangle" of the face.

The signs and symptoms of cavernous sinus thrombosis include fever, drowsiness, and rapid pulse. In addition, there is loss of function of the sixth cranial nerve or abducens because it runs through the cavernous sinus, resulting in abducens nerve paralysis. Because the muscle supplied by the nerve moves the eyeball laterally, inability to perform this movement suggests nerve damage. Additionally, the patient usually has double vision (diplopia) due to restricted movement of one eye, as well as edema of the eyelids and conjunctivae, tearing (lacrimation), and extruded eyeballs (exophthalmus), depending on the course of the infection (Figure 12-9).

With cavernous sinus thrombosis there may also be damage to the other cranial nerves such as the third cranial or oculomotor nerve and fourth cranial or trochlear nerve as well as to the ophthalmic and maxillary divisions of the fifth cranial or trigeminal nerve and changes in the tissue they innervate, since these nerves travel in the cavernous sinus wall. Finally, this infection can be fatal because it may lead to meningitis, inflammation of the meninges in the brain or spinal cord,

which requires immediate hospitalization with intravenous antibiotics and anticoagulants (see Chapter 8).

SPREAD BY LYMPHATIC SYSTEM

The lymphatic system of the head and neck can allow the spread of infection from the teeth and associated oral tissue (see Chapter 10). This occurs because the pathogens can also travel in the lymph through the lymphatic vessels that connect the series of lymph nodes from the oral cavity to other tissue, structures, or organs. Thus these pathogens can move from a primary node near the infected site to a secondary node at a distant site.

The route of odontogenic infection traveling through the lymph nodes varies according to the teeth involved. The submandibular nodes are the primary nodes for most of the teeth and associated tissue, except the maxillary third molars (with superior deep cervical nodes) and mandibular incisors (with submental nodes) (Figure 12-10 and see Table 10-1). The submandibular nodes then empty into the superior deep cervical nodes.

The superior deep cervical nodes empty into either the inferior deep cervical nodes or directly into the jugular trunk and then into the vascular system (see Figure 10-1). However, once the infection is within the vascular system, it can be spread systemically to other tissue, structures, and organs, as previously discussed, widely disseminating the infection.

LYMPHADENOPATHY

A lymph node involved in infection undergoes both hypertrophy and hyperplasia, which results in lymphadenopathy, an increase in size and a change in the consistency of the lymph node so that it becomes palpable and can even be visualized in some cases (see Figure 10-22). This change in the lymph node allows it to better fight the infection process. Evaluation of the involved nodes can determine the degree of regional involvement in the infection process, which is instrumental in the diagnosis and management of the infection.

SPREAD BY SPACES

The spaces of the head and neck can allow the spread of infection from the teeth and associated oral tissue because the pathogens can travel within the fascial spaces (or specifically, the cervical compartments), from one space near the infected site to another more distant space by means of the spread of the related inflammatory exudate (see Chapter 11). When involved in infection, the space can undergo cellulitis (see Table 12-2), which can cause a change in the usual and somewhat symmetric proportions of the face and neck (see Chapter 2).

If the maxillary teeth and associated tissue are infected, the infection can spread into the vestibular space of the maxilla, buccal space, or canine space. If the mandibular teeth and associated tissue are infected, the infection can spread into the vestibular space of the mandible, buccal space, submental space, sublingual space, submandibular space, masticator spaces, or the space of the body of the mandible, depending on the location of the tooth and extent of infection (Figures 12-10 and 12-11).

The insertion of the mylohyoid muscle along the mandible dictates which mandibular subspace is initially affected by an odontogenic infection. The apex of the mandibular first molar is superior to the mylohyoid muscle, so involvement of this tooth or teeth anterior to it will first involve the sublingual space (see Figure 11-12).

In contrast, the apices of the mandibular second and third molars are inferior to the mylohyoid muscle, and infection here will directly

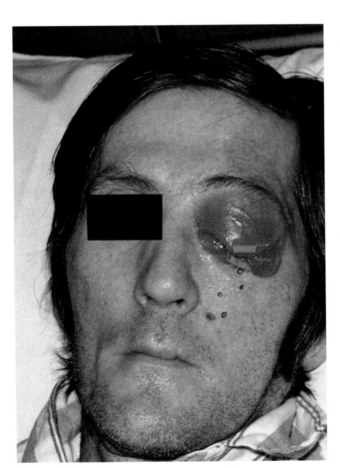

FIGURE 12-9 Cavernous sinus thrombosis, an infection of the cavernous sinus, with its edema of the eyelids and conjunctivae, tearing, and extruded eyeballs. *(From Reynolds PA, Abrahams PH: McMinn's interactive clinical anatomy: head and neck, ed 2, London, 2001, Elsevier.)*

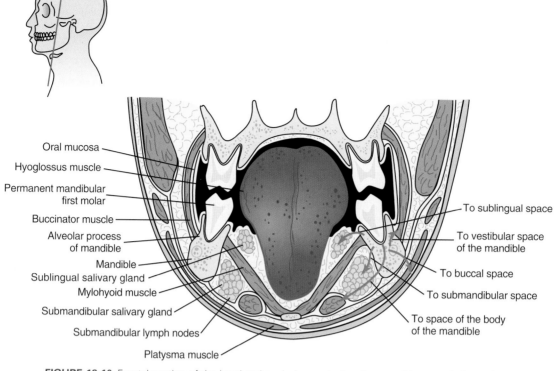

Oral mucosa
Hyoglossus muscle
Permanent mandibular first molar
Buccinator muscle
Alveolar process of mandible
Mandible
Sublingual salivary gland
Mylohyoid muscle
Submandibular salivary gland
Submandibular lymph nodes
Platysma muscle

To sublingual space
To vestibular space of the mandible
To buccal space
To submandibular space
To space of the body of the mandible

FIGURE 12-10 Frontal section of the head and neck demonstrating the possible spread of an odontogenic infection from a mandibular first molar. The infection would spread first into the sublingual space and then possibly to other spaces as noted. Note that the submandibular lymph nodes are primary nodes for most teeth and associated tissue, except for the maxillary third molars and mandibular incisors.

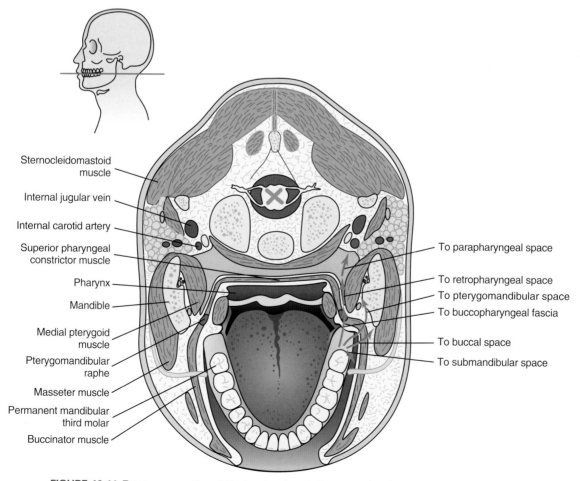

Sternocleidomastoid muscle
Internal jugular vein
Internal carotid artery
Superior pharyngeal constrictor muscle
Pharynx
Mandible
Medial pterygoid muscle
Pterygomandibular raphe
Masseter muscle
Permanent mandibular third molar
Buccinator muscle

To parapharyngeal space
To retropharyngeal space
To pterygomandibular space
To buccopharyngeal fascia
To buccal space
To submandibular space

FIGURE 12-11 Transverse section of the head and neck demonstrating the spread of an odontogenic infection from a mandibular third molar directly into the submandibular space and then possibly to other spaces as noted even to the cervical spaces that are located deep within the neck.

spread to the submandibular space. However, these spaces freely communicate around the posterior border of the mylohyoid muscle, so both subspaces may become involved if the infection continues.

From these spaces, the infection can spread into other spaces of the jaws and neck such as the parapharyngeal and retropharyngeal spaces, causing serious complications (discussed next).

LUDWIG ANGINA

One of the most serious lesions of the jaw is **Ludwig angina**, which is cellulitis of the submandibular space (Figure 12-12 and see Figure 11-12). It involves the spread of infection from an abscess from any of the mandibular teeth or associated tissue to one space initially—the submental, the sublingual, or possibly the submandibular space itself.

The infection progresses to involve the submandibular space bilaterally, with a risk of spreading to the parapharyngeal space and then onto the retropharyngeal space of the neck (see Figures 11-13 and 11-14). With this lesion, there is initially massive bilateral submandibular regional swelling, which can extend down the anterior cervical triangles to the clavicles, possibly spreading to the upper thorax (chest). Swallowing, speaking, and breathing may be difficult, with high fever and drooling evident. Respiratory obstruction develops rapidly as continued swelling elevates the tongue, displacing it backward, blocking the pharyngeal airway. Contrast-enhanced computed tomography scan has become the imaging modality of choice in the evaluation of the patient with a deep tissue cervical infection.

As the retropharyngeal space, which is considered the "danger space" of the neck by healthcare professionals, becomes involved with edema of the larynx there can be complete respiratory obstruction, resulting in asphyxiation and death. Thus Ludwig angina is an acute medical emergency requiring immediate hospitalization and may necessitate an emergency cricothyrotomy. During this emergency airway puncture, an incision is made through the skin of the neck and cricothyroid membrane underneath, which is the larger part of the laryngeal membrane, to quickly create a much-needed patent airway.

With the advent of earlier care of abscessed teeth and more routine antibiotic treatment with early signs that indicate a severe infectious state, Ludwig angina has become an uncommon dental emergency in healthy patients. However, symptoms may be masked in partially treated cases, and risk is exponentially increased in medically compromised patients (see earlier discussion). Also, with the rising popularity of oral piercings, there has been an increase in the serious infection of oral sites that can also include Ludwig angina if not treated promptly (Figure 12-13).

PREVENTION OF SPREAD OF INFECTION

To prevent the occurrence of infection due to dental treatment, a thorough medical history with periodic updates will allow the dental professional to perform effective treatment of all patients, including those who are medically compromised, to avoid serious complications due to active dental disease. A medical consultation is indicated when there is uncertainty as to the risk of opportunistic infection. Usually just rescheduling the patient for elective dental treatment after consultation for and resolution of infection may prove beneficial. In addition, before major medical surgical procedures such as heart surgery, risky teeth and any signs of infection must be addressed.

There must also be strict adherence to standard infection control measures during any type of dental treatment so as to prevent the spread of infection; for example, the removal of heavy dental biofilm (dental plaque) accumulations before restorative treatment or periodontal therapy. Particular care must be taken to avoid contaminating oral surgery sites of tooth extraction, implant placement, or periodontal therapy.

Using an antiseptic oral rinse before the treatment protocol, a rubber dam, or an antimicrobial-laced external water supply when ultrasonic instrumentation or irrigation are used may help prevent the spread of infection. Also important is not administering a local anesthetic through an area of odontogenic infection so as to avoid transferring the pathogens deeper into the tissue by needle tract contamination. After dental treatment an antiseptic oral rinse, as well as a course of systemic antibiotics, might be prescribed if the risk of infection exists.

Most importantly, early diagnosis and treatment of head and neck infections must occur in all patients. To do this, all head and neck regions should be assessed so as to obtain the presence of infection, especially in high-risk patients. For examination of the oral cavity,

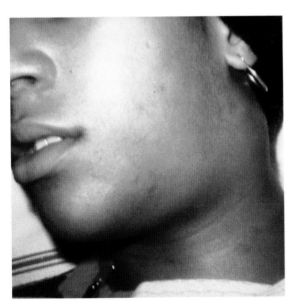

FIGURE 12-12 Ludwig angina with its massive bilateral swelling showing involvement of both the submandibular and submental spaces in this case resulting from an abscess of the mandibular third molar. *(Courtesy Dr. Mark Gabrielson.)*

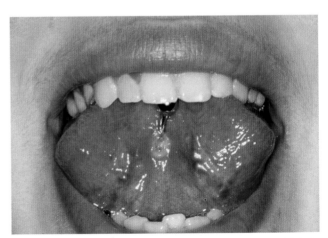

FIGURE 12-13 Localized infection with suppuration on the ventral surface of the tongue due to a tongue piercing. *(Courtesy Margaret J. Fehrenbach, RDH, MS.)*

pressure from palpation may uncover lingering tenderness that may lead the clinician to seek further clues for a differential diagnosis. Skin regions may display redness or erythema or swelling that again may be related to the spread of infection.

However, the inflammatory process of the medial aspect of the mandible may be hidden from a thorough inspection by overlying soft tissue, an area studies show is prone to serious infections from the pericoronal tissue around the mandibular third molar (discussed earlier). Additionally, the inferior border of the mandible must be palpated to exclude the extension of infection to critical areas of the neck (discussed earlier). Imaging of suspected regions using the latest technology is key to effective diagnosis for any head and neck infections.

Oral infections can have significant medical ramifications, including death. As the healthcare professional most familiar with a patient's oral health, the dental professional must be knowledgeable about the appearances, causes, and symptoms of the lesions of all types of oral infections as well as expert in the means of their prevention. In addition, the dental professional must keep up with recent guidelines for standard precautions for infection control such as those reported by the Centers for Disease Control and Prevention.

REVIEW QUESTIONS

1. Which of the following complications is MOST likely to occur with untreated Ludwig angina?
   A. Abducens nerve paralysis
   B. Meningitis
   C. Respiratory obstruction
   D. Sinus perforation
   E. Lacrimation and hematoma

2. Which of the following cranial nerves is MOST likely to be involved with a case of cavernous sinus thrombosis?
   A. Oculomotor and trochlear nerves
   B. Vagus and glossopharyngeal nerves
   C. Hypoglossal and accessory nerves
   D. Optic and olfactory nerves

3. Which of the following definitions listed below is CORRECT concerning an oral abscess?
   A. Inflammation of bone
   B. Inflammation of meninges
   C. Infection confined in oral mucosal space
   D. Diffuse inflammation of soft tissue

4. Which of the following statements is CORRECT concerning cavernous sinus thrombosis?
   A. Most major veins of the face do NOT have valves
   B. Only dental infections can spread to the maxillary sinus
   C. Orbital tissue is NOT affected
   D. Needle tract contamination may be involved

5. If an infection involves the lingual surface of the mandibular third molar, where is the swelling MOST likely to be initially observed?
   A. In the mandibular vestibule
   B. Beneath the tongue
   C. In the submandibular region
   D. In both the buccal and submental regions

6. Which of the following types of infection processes presents as a diffuse inflammation of soft tissue spaces?
   A. Meningitis
   B. Cellulitis
   C. Osteomyelitis
   D. Sinusitis

7. Which of the following is a possible virulence factor noted with gram-negative anaerobic bacteria?
   A. Ability to be killed by penicillin
   B. Production of protective cellular envelopes
   C. Ability to survive in an oxygen-heavy environment
   D. Production of beta-lactamase enzyme

8. Which of the following statements CORECTLY describes the resident microbiota of the oral cavity?
   A. Is completely dissimilar to the rest of the body
   B. Mainly consists of pathogens
   C. Mainly consists of bacteria
   D. Involves a systemic noncommunity of microbes

9. Which of the following lymph nodes are primary nodes for MOST of the teeth, except the mandibular incisors and maxillary third molars, and thus can be involved in the spread of dental infections to nearby orofacial structures?
   A. Submental nodes
   B. Submandibular nodes
   C. Superior deep cervical nodes
   D. Inferior deep cervical nodes

10. Which of the following can ONLY present as pathogens traveling in the vascular system?
    A. Thrombus
    B. Embolus
    C. Sequestra
    D. Bacteremia

11. Which of the following processes can occur to lymph nodes when involved in an infection?
    A. Paresthesia
    B. Hypertrophy
    C. Xerostomia
    D. Metastasis

12. Which of the following is NOT a sign or symptom for abducens nerve paralysis?
    A. Double vision
    B. Exophthalmus
    C. Single vision
    D. Lacrimation

13. What part of the face listed below is considered by medical professionals to be part of the "danger triangle" of the face?
    A. Temporal region
    B. Mental region
    C. Nasal region
    D. Oral region

14. When a dental patient is FIRST diagnosed with an inflammation of the meninges, what form of care is needed?
    A. Wait and see if the infection progresses to the upper thorax
    B. Drainage of the localized infection and daily systemic antibiotics
    C. Immediate hospitalization with intravenous antibiotics and anticoagulants
    D. NO treatment is possible due to the poor level of prognosis for the patient

15. What type of treatment is usually necessary in cases of prolonged chronic maxillary sinusitis?
    A. Enlargement of ostia of the lateral walls of the nasal cavity
    B. Removal of the infected nasal septum to allow for drainage
    C. Leaving the mucus to drain naturally by both the nares and pharynx
    D. Immediate hospitalization with intravenous antibiotics and saline

16. Which of the following usually CANNOT be considered part of the indigenous microorganisms within a healthy body?
    A. Dental biofilm (plaque)
    B. Resident microbiota
    C. Pathogens
    D. Resident microbiota and pathogens

17. The MOST important treatment for suppurating odontogenic infections is
    A. systemic antibiotics.
    B. surgical drainage.
    C. cold packs applied hourly.
    D. hyperbaric oxygen.

18. Which of the following situations has recently added to more cases of Ludwig angina being noted?
    A. Careful use of systemic antibiotics
    B. Early diagnosis of oral infections
    C. Popularity of oral piercings
    D. Routine culturing for anaerobic microorganisms

19. Which of the following are the USUAL symptoms noted with a maxillary sinusitis?
    A. Headache at the back of the skull
    B. Skin cold to the touch
    C. Foul-smelling nasal or pharyngeal discharge
    D. Increased energy levels

20. Which of the following cases demonstrates the MOST common cause of infections of the maxillary sinus?
    A. Spread of infection from a mandibular periapical abscess
    B. Contamination from extracted maxillary anterior tooth root fragment displaced into sinus
    C. Trauma to the nasal region that results in traveling blood clots
    D. Spread of upper respiratory infection within the nasal region to the sinus

APPENDIX A

Bibliography

Aarthi Nisha V, et al: The role of colour Doppler ultrasonography in the diagnosis of fascial space infections: a cross sectional study. *J Clin Diagn Res.* 2013;7(5):962–967.

Alves N, et al: Morphological study of the lingula in adult human mandibles of Brazilian individuals and clinical implications. *BioMed Res Int.* 2015;87:37-51.

Babbush CA, Fehrenbach MJ, Emmons M, Nunez DW, editors: *Mosby's dental dictionary*, ed 3, St Louis, 2014, Elsevier.

Bahl R, et al: Odontogenic infections: Microbiology and management. *Contemp Clin Dent.* 2014;5(3):307-311.

Burns Y, et al: Anesthetic efficacy of the palatal-anterior superior alveolar injection. *J Am Dent Assoc.* 2004;135(9):1269-1276.

Cawson RA: *Essentials of oral pathology and oral medicine*, ed 8, London, 2008, Churchill Livingstone/Elsevier.

Chong V: Cervical lymphadenopathy: What radiologists need to know. *Cancer Imaging.* 2004;4(2):116-120.

Corbett IP, et al: A comparison of the anterior middle superior alveolar nerve block and infraorbital nerve block for anesthesia of maxillary anterior teeth. *J Am Dent Assoc.* 2010;141(12):1442-1448.

Dorland's medical dictionary, ed 32, Philadelphia, 2012, Elsevier.

Drake RL, et al: *Gray's anatomy for students*, ed 2, London, 2010, Elsevier.

Eisenmenger LB, Wiggins RH: Imaging of head and neck lymph nodes. *Radiol Clin North Am.* 2015;53(1):115-132.

Fabian FM: Observation of the position of the lingula in relation to the mandibular foramen and the mylohyoid groove. *Ital J Anat Embryol.* 2006;111(3):151-158.

Federative Committee on Anatomical Terminology: *Terminologia anatomica: International anatomical terminology*, Stuttgart, Germany, 1998, Thieme.

Fehrenbach MJ: Gow-Gates mandibular nerve block: an alternative in local anesthetic use. *Access (ADHA)*, November 2002.

Fehrenbach MJ, et al: *Mosby's dental dictionary*, ed 3, St Louis, 2014, Elsevier.

Fehrenbach MJ: The incisive block: Underutilized but ultimately useful. *California Dental Hygiene Journal*, Summer 2011.

Fehrenbach MJ: Anatomic considerations for the administration of local anesthesia, maxillary nerve anesthesia, mandibular nerve anesthesia. In Logothetis DD, editor: *Local anesthesia for the dental hygienist*, ed 2, St Louis, 2017, Elsevier.

Fehrenbach MJ: Extraoral and intraoral patient assessment. In Darby ML, Walsh MM, editors: *Dental hygiene theory and practice*, ed 4, Philadelphia, 2015, Elsevier.

Fehrenbach MJ: Inflammation and repair: Immunity. In Ibsen AC, Phelan JA, editors: *Oral pathology for the dental hygienist*, ed 6, St Louis, 2014, Elsevier.

Fehrenbach MJ, editor: *Dental anatomy coloring book*, ed 2, St Louis, 2007, Elsevier.

Fehrenbach MJ, Herring SW: Spread of dental infection, *Journal of Practical Hygiene*, September/October 1997.

Fehrenbach MJ, Popowics T: *Illustrated dental embryology, histology, and anatomy*, ed 4, St Louis, 2016, Elsevier.

Goda A, et al: Analysis of the factors affecting the formation of the microbiome associated with chronic osteomyelitis of the jaw. *Clin Microbiol Infect.* 2014;20(5):O309-O317.

Guidera AK, et al: Head and neck fascia and compartments: no space for spaces. *Head Neck.* 2014;36(7):1058-68.

Gv S, et al: Facial pain followed by unilateral facial nerve palsy: a case report with literature review. *J Clin Diagn Res.* 2014;8(8):ZD34-ZD35.

Haas DA: Alternative mandibular nerve block techniques: a review of the Gow-Gates and Akinosi-Vazirani closed-mouth mandibular nerve block techniques. *J Am Dent Assoc.* 2011;142(Suppl 3):8S-12S.

Hargreaves KM, Berman LH: *Cohen's pathways of the pulp*, ed 10, Elsevier, 2010.

Hetson G, et al: Statistical evaluation of the position of the mandibular foramen. *Oral Surg Oral Med Oral Pathol.* 1988;65(1):32-34.

Jacobs S: *Human anatomy: A clinically oriented approach*, London, 2007, Churchill Livingstone.

Johnson TM, et al: Teaching alternatives to the standard inferior alveolar nerve block in dental education: outcomes in clinical practice. *J Dent Educ.* 2007;71(9):1145-1152.

Katsumi Y, et al. Variation in arterial supply to the floor of the mouth and assessment of relative hemorrhage risk in implant surgery. *Clin Oral Implants Res.* 2013;24(4):434-40.

Kumar V, et al: *Robbins & Cotran pathologic basis of disease*, ed 9, St Louis, 2015, Elsevier.

Lanter BB, Sauer K, Davies DG: Bacteria present in carotid arterial plaques are found as biofilm deposits which may contribute to enhanced risk of plaque rupture. *MBio.* 2014;10;5(3):e01206-14.

Logan BM, Reynolds PA, Hutchings RT: *Color atlas of head and neck anatomy*, ed 4, London, 2010, Elsevier.

Logothetis DD, Fehrenbach MJ: Local anesthesia options during dental hygiene care. *RDH Magazine*, June 2014.

López-Píriz R, et al: Management of odontogenic infection of pulpal and periodontal origin. *Med Oral Patol Oral Cir Bucal.* 2007;1;12(2):E154-9.

Madan GA, et al: Failure of inferior alveolar nerve block: Exploring the alternatives. *J Am Dent Assoc.* 2002;133(7):843-846.

Malamed SF: *Handbook of local anesthesia*, ed 6, St Louis, 2013, Elsevier.

Marsh PD, Devine DA: How is the development of dental biofilms influenced by the host? *J Clin Periodontol.* 2011;38(Suppl 11):28-35.

Meesa IR, Srinivasan A: Imaging of the oral cavity. *Radiol Clin North Am.* 2015;53(1):99-114.

Monnazzi MS: Anatomic study of the mandibular foramen, lingula and antilingula in dry mandibles, and its statistical relationship between the true lingula and the antilingula. *Int J Oral Maxillofac Surg.* 2012;41(1):74-78.

Montagner F, et al: Beta-lactamic resistance profiles in *Porphyromonas, Prevotella,* and *Parvimonas* species isolated from acute endodontic infections. *J Endod.* 2014;40(3):339-344.

Moore KL, Persaud TVN, Torchia MG: *The developing human: Clinically oriented embryology*, ed 10, Philadelphia, 2015, Elsevier.

Nelson SJ: *Wheeler's dental anatomy, physiology, and occlusions*, ed 10, Philadelphia, 2015, Elsevier.

Neville B, et al: *Oral and maxillofacial pathology*, ed 4, St Louis, 2016, Elsevier.

Newman MG, Takei HH, Klokkevold PR: *Clinical periodontology*, ed 12, Philadelphia, 2015, Elsevier.

Nicholson ML: A study of the position of the mandibular foramen in the adult human mandible. *Anat Rec.* 1985;212(1):110-112.

Norton NS: *Netter's head and neck anatomy for dentistry*, ed 2, Philadelphia, 2012, Elsevier.

Okeson JP: *Management of temporomandibular disorders and occlusion*, ed 7, St Louis, 2013, Elsevier.

Patankar A, et al: Evaluation of microbial flora in orofacial space infections of odontogenic origin. *Natl J Maxillofac Surg.* 2014;5(2):161–165.

Parisi E, Glick M: Cervical lymphadenopathy in the dental patient: a review of clinical approach. *Quintessence Int.* 2005;36(6):423-36.

Pogrel MA: Permanent nerve damage from inferior alveolar nerve blocks: a current update. *J Calif Dent Assoc.* 2012;40(10):795-797.

Rams TE, Degener JE, van Winkelhoff AJ: Prevalence of β-lactamase-producing bacteria in human periodontitis. *J Periodontal Res.* 2013;48(4):493-499.

Regezi, JA, Sciubba JJ, Jordan RCK. *Oral pathology: Clinical correlations*, ed 6, St. Louis, 2012, Elsevier.

Reshma VJ, et al: Characterization of cervicofacial lymph nodes - a clinical and ultrasonographic study. *J Clin Diagn Res.* 2014;8(8):ZC25-ZC28.

Rodella LF, et al: A review of the mandibular and maxillary nerve supplies and their clinical relevance. *Arch Oral Biol.* 2012;57(4):323-334.

Sarikov R, Juodzbalys G: Inferior alveolar nerve injury after mandibular third molar extraction: a literature review. *J Oral Maxillofac Res.* 2014;29;5(4):e1.

Standring S: *Gray's anatomy: the anatomical basis of clinical practice*, ed 40, London, 2008, Churchill Livingstone.

Thangavelu K, et al: Significance of localization of mandibular foramen in an inferior alveolar nerve block. *J Nat Sci Biol Med.* 2012;3(2):156-160.

Troeltzsch M, et al: A review of pathogenesis, diagnosis, treatment options, and differential diagnosis of odontogenic infections: A rather mundane pathology? *Quintessence Int.* 2015;46(4):351-361.

Velasco I, Soto R: Anterior and middle superior alveolar nerve block for anesthesia of maxillary teeth using conventional syringe. *Dent Res J.* 2012;9(5):535–540.

Wiggins RH, Srinivasan A: Head and neck imaging: Preface. *Radiol Clin North Am.* 2015;53(1):xi.

Zhang J, Stringer MD: Ophthalmic and facial veins are not valveless. *Clin. Experiment. Ophthalmol.* 2010; 38(5):502–10.

Appendix B

Extraoral and Intraoral Examinations Procedure

Before proceeding with the actual examination, it is important for the dental professional to review the patient record including the dental and medical histories, examine radiographs or other laboratory records, and explain the assessment procedure. Establishing an examination sequence and following it systematically during examination reduces the possibility of overlooking any areas during the examination. Visually dividing the head and neck into specific regions and then palpating each region bilaterally in order from superior to inferior regions is key to the system recommended.

Initially the patient is generally observed during reception and while seated to note any physical characteristics and abnormalities that may require special dental care modifications or medical as well as dental consultation.

Ask the patient to remove neck-related clothing, glasses, dentures, or appliances before examinations. Inquire about the history of any lesions if presented during general evaluation and later whether any discomfort occurs during the examination if the patient appears distressed.

Following the observation of atypical or abnormal findings, the dental professional needs to describe and document them accurately in the patient record. Precise descriptive terms enable the dental professional to communicate with other dental and healthcare professionals to help with the formation of an accurate differential diagnosis. An accurate diagnosis will then enable a clinically effective treatment plan. See related textbooks in oral pathology for further discussion as listed in Appendix A.

Finally, educating patients through instruction in self-examination techniques to identify any atypical to abnormal findings on their own allows them to assume some responsibility for the care and control of their personal oral and associated systemic health. This emphasis on continuing dental care can easily be done during the professional examination process, stressing the need for early detection and for the patient to contact dental professionals as soon as possible. Discussion of the elimination of high-risk behaviors and options to change lifestyles that predispose to orofacial cancer or other orofacial disease should also be part of the overall process, especially in those patients with related past history.

REGIONS	STEPS
Extraoral Examination	
Overall evaluation of the face, head, and neck, including the skin	• With patient sitting upright and relaxed, visually observe symmetry and coloration of the face and neck while allowing the patient to look at hand mirror throughout so as to understand the steps for self-examination.

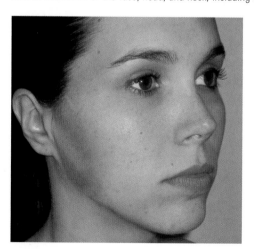

FIGURE 2-9

REGIONS	STEPS
Frontal region, including forehead and frontal sinuses 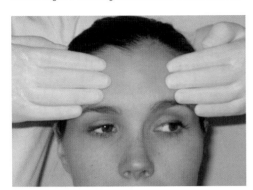 **FIGURE 2-2, *B***	• Visually inspect and bilaterally palpate the forehead including the frontal sinuses.
Parietal and occipital regions including scalp, hair, and occipital nodes 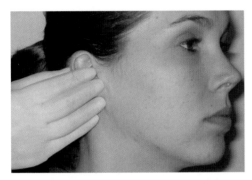 **FIGURE 2-5** 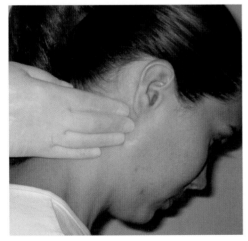 **FIGURE 10-4**	• Visually inspect the entire scalp by moving the hair, especially around the hairline, starting from one ear and proceeding to the other ear. • Then bilaterally palpate the occipital nodes on each side of the base of the head while the patient leans the head forward.

Continued

REGIONS	STEPS
Temporal and auricular regions, including scalp, ears, and auricular nodes	• Visually inspect and manually palpate the external ear, as well as the scalp, face, and auricular nodes around each ear.

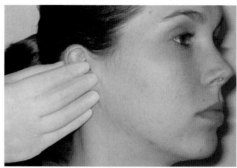
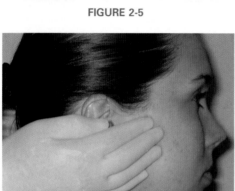

FIGURE 2-5

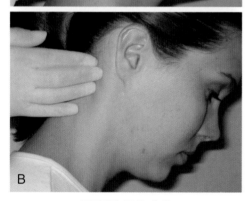

FIGURE 10-5, _A, B_

Orbital regions, including the eyes	• Visually inspect the eyes with their movements and responses to light and action.

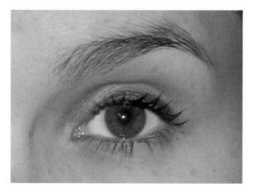

FIGURE 2-6, _B_

REGIONS	STEPS
Nasal region, including the nose	• Visually inspect and bilaterally palpate the external nose, starting at the root of the nose and proceeding to its apex.

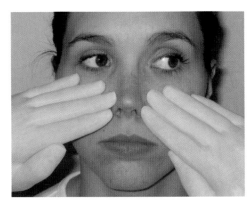

FIGURE 2-8

REGIONS	STEPS
Infraorbital and zygomatic regions, including the muscles of facial expressions, facial nodes, maxillae, maxillary sinuses, and temporomandibular joints (TMJs)	• Visually inspect inferior to the orbits, especially noting the use of the muscles of facial expression. • Visually inspect and bilaterally palpate each side of the face, moving from the infraorbital region to the labial commissure and then to the surface of the mandible. • Visually inspect and bilaterally palpate the maxillary sinuses.

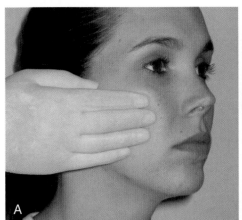 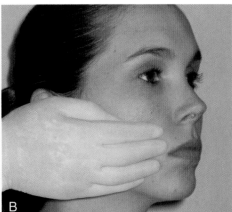

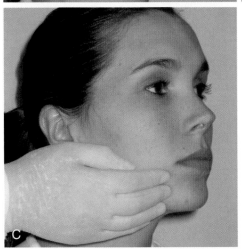

FIGURE 10-6, *A-C*

Continued

REGIONS	STEPS

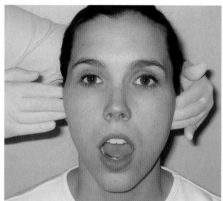

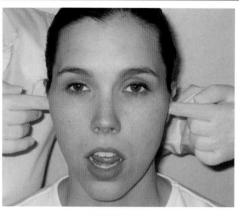

| | • Then ask the patient to open and close the mouth several times. Then ask patient to move the opened lower jaw left, then right, and then forward. Ask if there is any pain or tenderness experienced and note any sounds made by either joint.
• To further access the TMJs, gently place a finger into the outer part of each external acoustic meatus during these movements. |

FIGURE 5-7   **FIGURE 5-8**

Buccal regions, including the masseter muscles, parotid salivary glands, and mandible

• Visually inspect and bilaterally palpate the masseter and parotid gland by starting in anterior to each ear, moving to the zygomatic arch, and then inferior to the angle of the mandible.
• Then place the fingers of each hand over each masseter and ask the patient to clench the teeth together several times.

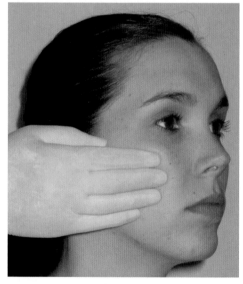

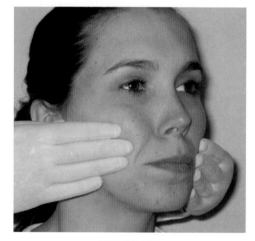

FIGURE 7-3   **FIGURE 4-20**

Mental region, including the chin

• Visually inspect and bilaterally palpate the chin.

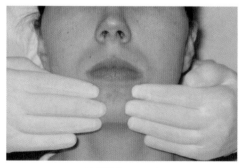

FIGURE 2-22, *B*

REGIONS	STEPS
Submandibular and submental triangles, including submandibular and sublingual salivary glands and associated nodes	• Have the patient lower the chin and manually palpate directly the submandibular and sublingual glands as well as the associated nodes underneath the chin and on the inferior border of the mandible. • Then push the tissue in the area over the bony inferior border of the mandible on each side, where it is grasped and rolled.

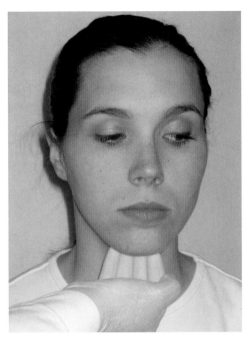

FIGURE 10-12

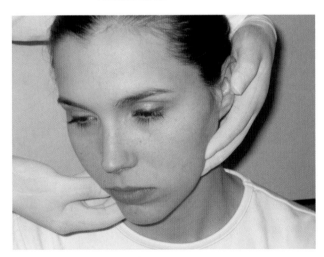

FIGURE 10-13

Continued

REGIONS	STEPS
Anterior and posterior cervical triangles, including sternocleidomastoid muscles (SCMs) and associated cervical nodes	• Have the patient look straight ahead and manually palpate on each side of the neck the superficial cervical nodes starting inferior to the ear and continuing the whole length of the SCMs surface to the clavicles. • Then have the patient tilt the head to the one side and then to the other to allow palpation of the superior deep cervical nodes on the underside of the anterior and posterior aspects of the SCMs as before. • Then have the patient raise the shoulders up and forward to palpate over each trapezius muscle surface the inferior deep cervical, accessory, and supraclavicular nodes.

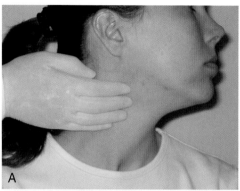

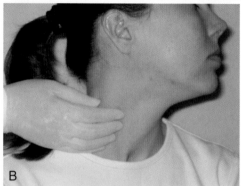

FIGURE 10-14, *A, B*

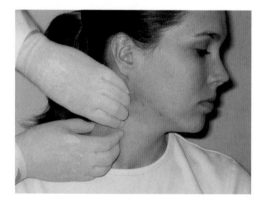

FIGURE 10-17

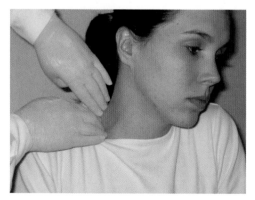

FIGURE 10-18

REGIONS	STEPS
Anterior midline cervical region, including hyoid bone, thyroid gland, thyroid cartilage, and larynx 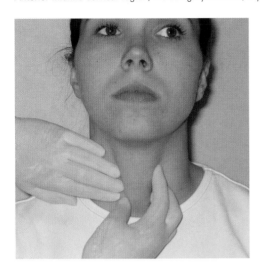 **FIGURE 7-12**	• Locate the thyroid cartilage and pass the fingers up and down the thyroid gland, examining for abnormal masses and overall size. • Then place one hand on each side of the trachea and gently displace the thyroid tissue to the contralateral side of the neck for each side, while the other hand manually palpates the displaced glandular tissue. • Then compare the two lobes of the gland for size and texture using visual inspection as well as manual or bimanual palpation. • Ask the patient to swallow to check for gland mobility by visually inspecting it while it moves superiorly and then back inferiorly, possibly with a glass of water for the patient to swallow. • Finally, bidigitally palpate both the hyoid and larynx and deliberately move each one gently.

Intraoral Examination

Oral cavity, including lips, labial commissures, buccal mucosa and labial mucosa, parotid salivary glands and ducts, alveolar processes, and attached gingiva 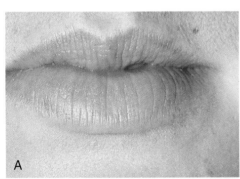 A 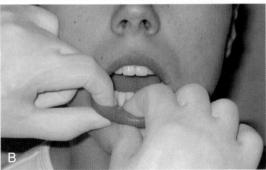 B **FIGURE 2-10, *A, B***	• Look at the lips overall. • Have the patient smile and then open the mouth slightly and bidigitally palpate, as well as visually inspect, the lower and upper lip in a systematic manner from one commissure to the other. • Then gently pull the lower and upper lip away from the teeth to observe the labial mucosa and then bidigitally palpate the inner lips.

Continued

REGIONS	**STEPS**
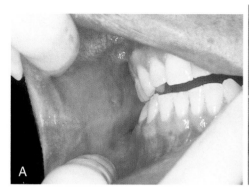 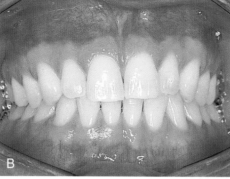 FIGURE 2-12 FIGURE 2-13	• Then gently pull the buccal mucosa slightly away from the teeth to bidigitally palpate the inner cheek on each side, using circular compression. • Dry the area with gauze and observe the salivary flow from each parotid duct near the parotid papillae. • Retract both the buccal mucosa and labial mucosa to visually inspect the vestibular area and gingival tissue, including the maxillary tuberosity and retromolar pad on each side. • Then bidigitally palpate these inner areas using circular compression.
Palate and pharynx, including the hard and soft palates, faucial pillars, palatine tonsils, uvula, and visible parts of oropharynx and nasopharynx 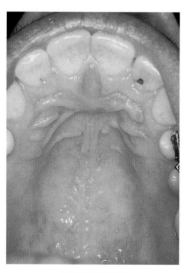 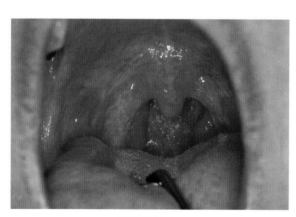 FIGURE 2-15 FIGURE 4-31	• Have the patient tilt the head back slightly and extend the tongue to view the palatal and pharyngeal regions while using the mouth mirror to intensify the light source. • Gently place the mouth mirror with mirror side down on the middle of the dorsal surface of the tongue and ask the patient to say "ah." As this is done, again visually observe the soft palate with uvula as well as the visible parts of the pharynx. • Compress the hard palate with the first or second finger of one hand, avoiding circular compression as well as avoiding palpation on the soft palate so as to prevent initiating the gag reflex.

REGIONS	STEPS
Tongue, including all surfaces from tip to base, as well as swallowing pattern	<ul><li>Have the patient slightly extend the tongue and wrap gauze around the anterior third of the tongue in order to obtain a firm grasp to visually inspect and then digitally palpate the dorsal surface.</li><li>Then turn the tongue slightly on its side to visually inspect its base and lateral borders and bidigitally palpate the lateral borders.</li><li>Have the patient lift the tongue to visually inspect and digitally palpate the ventral surface.</li><li>Ask the patient to swallow and observe the swallowing pattern while holding the lips apart, possibly with a glass of water for the patient to swallow.</li></ul>

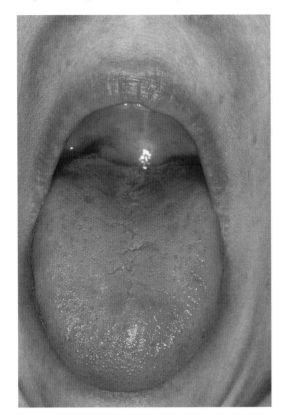

FIGURE 2-17, *B*

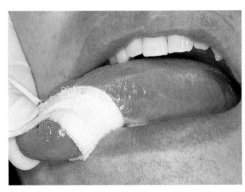

FIGURE 2-16

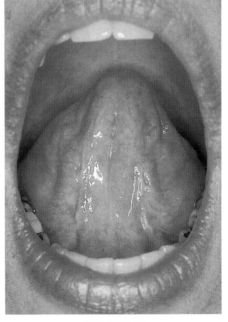

FIGURE 2-18

Continued

REGIONS	STEPS
Floor of the mouth, including the submandibular and sublingual salivary glands and ducts 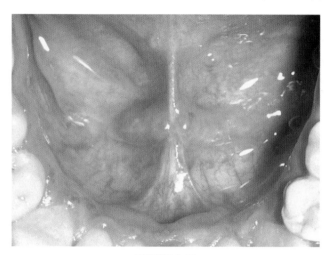 FIGURE 2-19 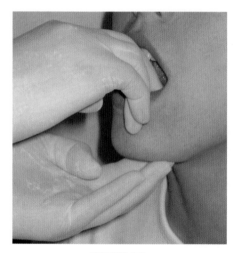 FIGURE 7-8	• While the patient lifts the tongue to the palate and using the mouth mirror to intensify the light source, visually inspect the mucosa of the floor of the mouth and check the lingual frenum. • Dry each sublingual caruncle with gauze and observe the salivary flow from the ducts. • Then bimanually palpate the sublingual region by placing an index finger intraorally behind each mandibular canine, and the index finger of the opposite hand extraorally under the chin, compressing the tissue between the fingers.

Glossary of Key Terms and Anatomic Structures

A

Abducens nerve (ab-**doo**-suhnz) Sixth cranial nerve (VI) serving as eye muscle.

Abducens nerve paralysis (puh-**ral**-i-sis) Loss of function of sixth cranial nerve.

Abscess (**ab**-ses) Infection with suppuration resulting from pathogens in contained space.

Accessory lymph nodes Deep cervical nodes located along accessory nerve.

Accessory nerve Eleventh cranial nerve (XI) serving trapezius and sternocleidomastoid muscles as well as palatal and pharyngeal muscles.

Accessory middle meningeal artery (muh-**nin**-je-uhl) Artery off first part of maxillary artery that supplies meninges.

Action Movement by a muscle when fibers contract.

Action potential (po-**ten**-shuhl) Rapid depolarization of cell membrane resulting in nerve impulse along membrane.

Adenoids (**ad**-uh-noids) Another term for pharyngeal tonsils.

Afferent nerve (**af**-uhr-uhnt) Sensory nerve carrying information from periphery to brain or spinal cord.

Afferent nervous system Sensory nerve system carrying information from receptors to brain or spinal cord.

Afferent vessels Lymphatic vessel with lymph flowing into lymph node.

Ala, alae (**ah**-luh, ah-**lee**) Winglike cartilaginous structure(s) that laterally borders the naris (nares).

Alveolar mucosa (al-**vee**-uh-luhr mu-**ko**-suh) Mucosa lining vestibules of oral cavity.

Alveolar process of the mandible (**man**-di-buhl) Part of mandible containing roots of mandibular teeth.

Alveolar process of the maxilla (mak-**sil**-uh) Part of maxilla containing roots of maxillary teeth.

Alveolus, alveoli (**al**-vee-uh-luhs, **al**-vee-uh-ly) Tooth socket in alveolar process surrounding tooth root.

Anastomosis, anastomoses (uh-nuhs-tuh-**moh**-sis, uh-nuhs-tuh-**moh**-sees) Communication of blood vessel(s) with other vessel(s).

Anatomic nomenclature (an-uh-**tom**-ik **no**-muhn-klay-chuhr) System of names of anatomic structures.

Anatomic position Erect position, arms at sides, palms and toes directed forward, with eyes looking forward.

Anesthesia (an-es-**thee**-zhuh) Loss of feeling or sensation resulting from drugs or gases.

Angle of the mandible (**man**-di-buhl) Bend of the mandible at intersection of posterior and inferior borders of mandibular ramus.

Angular artery (**ang**-u-lar) Artery branching at termination of facial artery supplying side of nose.

Anterior Front of area.

Anterior arch Arch of atlas or first cervical vertebra.

Anterior auricular lymph nodes (aw-**rik**-u-luhr) Superficial nodes located anterior to ear.

Anterior cervical triangle Anterior region of neck.

Anterior ethmoidal nerve (eth-**moy**-duhl) Nerve from nasal cavity and paranasal sinuses forming nasociliary nerve.

Anterior faucial pillar (**faw**-shuhl **pil**-uhr) Vertical fold anterior to each palatine tonsil created by palatoglossal muscle.

Anterior jugular lymph nodes (**jug**-u-luhr) Superficial cervical nodes located along anterior jugular vein.

Anterior jugular vein Vein that begins inferior to chin draining into external jugular vein.

Anterior middle superior alveolar (ASMA) block (al-**vee**-uh-luhr) Injection that anesthetizes anterior and middle superior alveolar nerves as well as nasopalatine and greater palatine nerves that results in numbness of maxillary teeth and associated facial and lingual periodontium and gingiva, except for structures innervated by posterior superior alveolar nerve.

Anterior superior alveolar artery Arterial branch from infraorbital artery giving rise to branches for maxillary anteriors.

Anterior superior alveolar (ASA) block Injection that anesthetizes anterior superior alveolar nerve that results in numbness of maxillary anteriors and associated labial periodontium and gingiva.

Anterior superior alveolar (ASA) nerve Nerve serving maxillary anteriors and associated labial periodontium and gingiva that later joins infraorbital nerve.

Anterior suprahyoid muscle group (**soo**-pruh-**hi**-oid) Suprahyoid muscles located anterior to hyoid that include anterior belly of digastric, mylohyoid, and geniohyoid muscles.

Anterior tympanic artery Artery off first part of maxillary artery that supplies inner surface of tympanic membrane.

Antitragus (an-te-**tray**-guhs) Flap of tissue opposite tragus of ear.

Aorta (ay-**or**-tuh) Major artery giving rise to common carotid and subclavian arteries on left side and brachiocephalic artery on right side.

Aperture (**ap**-uhr-chuhr) Narrow opening in a bone.

Apex, apices (**ay**-peks, **ay**-pih-sees) Pointed end(s) of conical structure.

Apex of the nose Tip of nose.

Apex of the tongue Tip of tongue.

Arch Prominent bridgelike bony structure.

Arterial plaque Substance lining arteries consisting mainly of cholesterol.

Arteriole (ahr-**tare**-ee-ole) Smaller artery branching off artery and connecting with capillary.

Artery Blood vessel carrying blood away from the heart.

Articular eminence (ahr-**tik**-u-luhr **em**-i-nuhns) Structure on temporal bone articulating with mandible at temporomandibular joint.

Articular fossa (**fos**-uh) Fossa on temporal bone articulating with mandible at temporomandibular joint.

Articulating surface of the condyle (ahr-**tik**-u-late-ing) (**kon**-dyl) Part of head of mandibular condyle articulating with temporal bone at temporomandibular joint.

Articulation (ahr-tik-u-**lay**-shuhn) Area where bones are joined to each other.

Ascending palatine artery (**pal**-uh-tine) Artery branching from facial artery supplying palatine muscles and tonsils.

Ascending pharyngeal artery (fuh-**rin**-je-uhl) Medial artery branching from external carotid artery supplying pharyngeal walls, soft palate, and brain tissue.

Atherosclerosis (ath-uhr-o-skluh-**roh**-sis) Narrowing and blocking of the arteries by fatty arterial plaque.

Atlas (**at**-luhs) First cervical vertebra that articulates with the occipital bone.

Attached gingiva (jin-**ji**-vuh) Gingiva tightly adhering to bone over roots of teeth.

Auricle (**aw**-ri-kuhl) Oval flap of external ear.

Auricular region (aw-**rik**-u-luhr) Region of head with external ear as prominent feature.

Auriculotemporal nerve (aw-**rik**-u-lo-**tem**-puh-ruhl) Nerve that serves ear and scalp and parotid and joins posterior trunk of mandibular division of trigeminal nerve.

Autonomic nervous system (ANS) (aw-toh-**nom**-ik) Subdivision of efferent division of peripheral nervous system that operates without conscious control and is subdivided into sympathetic and parasympathetic.

Axis (**ak**-sis) Second cervical vertebra articulating with first and third cervical vertebrae.

B

Bacteremia (bak-tuhr-**ee**-me-uh) Bacteria traveling within vascular system.

Base of the tongue Posterior third or root of tongue.

Basilar part of the occipital bone (**bay**-si-luhr) (ok-**sip**-i-tuhl) Plate anterior to the foramen magnum.

Bell palsy (**pawl**-ze) Unilateral facial paralysis involving facial nerve.

Body of the hyoid bone (**hi**-oid) Anterior midline part of hyoid.

Body of the mandible (**man**-di-buhl) Base or horizontal part of mandible.

Body of the maxilla (**max**-sil-uh) Horizontal part of each maxilla containing maxillary sinus.

Body of the sphenoid bone (**sfe**-noid) Middle part of bone containing sphenoidal sinuses.

Body of the tongue Anterior two thirds of tongue.

Bones Mineralized structures protecting internal soft tissue and serving as biomechanic basis for movement.

Brachiocephalic artery (bray-kee-o-suh-**fal**-ik) Artery branching directly off aorta on right side of body giving rise to right common carotid and subclavian arteries.

Brachiocephalic vein Vein formed from merger of internal jugular and subclavian veins with right and left brachiocephalic veins forming superior vena cava.

Brain Division of central nervous system subdivided into cerebrum, cerebellum, and brainstem.

Brainstem Division of brain that includes medulla, pons, midbrain.

Bridge of the nose Bony structure inferior to nasion in nasal region.

Buccal (**buk**-uhl) Structure closest to inner cheek.

Buccal artery Artery branching from maxillary artery supplying buccinator muscle and cheek.

Buccal block Injection that anesthetizes the buccal nerve that results in numbness of the associated buccal periodontium and gingiva of mandibular molars.

Buccal fat pad Dense pad of tissue in cheek covered by buccal mucosa.

Buccal lymph nodes Superficial facial nodes located at mouth angle and superficial to buccinator muscle.

Buccal mucosa (mu-**ko**-suh) Mucosa that lines inner cheek.

Buccal nerve Nerve serving skin of cheek and buccal mucosa as well as the associated buccal periodontium and gingiva of mandibular molars and joining muscular nerve branches forming anterior trunk of mandibular division of trigeminal nerve.

Buccal region Region of head composed of soft tissue of cheek.

Buccal space Fascial space between buccinator and masseter muscles.

Buccinator muscle (**buk**-sin-nay-tuhr) Muscle of facial expression forming part of cheek.

Buccopharyngeal fascia (buk-ko-fuh-**rin**-je-uhl **fash**-e-uh) Deep cervical fasciae enclosing entire upper part of alimentary canal.

C

Canal Longer narrow, tubelike opening in a bone.

Canines (**kay**-nines) Anteriors that are third teeth from midline in each quadrant.

Canine eminence (**em**-i-nuhns) Facial ridge of bone over maxillary canine.

Canine fossa (**fos**-uh) Fossa superior to the roots of maxillary canines.

Canine space Fascial space located lateral to maxillary canine apex.

Capillary (**kap**-i-lare-ee) Smaller blood vessel branching off an arteriole to supply blood directly to tissue.

Carotid canal (kuh-**rot**-id) Canal in temporal bone carrying internal carotid artery among other vessels.

Carotid pulse Reliable pulse palpated from common carotid artery.

Carotid sheath Deep cervical fasciae forming a tube running down the side of neck.

Carotid sinus Swelling in artery just before common carotid artery bifurcates into internal and external carotid arteries.

Carotid triangle Smaller triangular region of neck superior to omohyoid muscle and part of anterior cervical triangle.

Cavernous sinus (**kav**-er-nuhs) Venous sinus located on side of sphenoid that communicates with pterygoid plexus of veins and superior ophthalmic vein.

Cavernous sinus thrombosis (throm-**boh**-sis) Infection of cavernous sinus.

Cellulitis (sel-u-**ly**-tis) Diffuse inflammation of soft tissue.

Central nervous system (CNS) Division of nervous system consisting of spinal cord and brain.

Cerebellum (suhr-uh-**bel**-uhm) Second largest division of brain that coordinates muscles, maintains muscle tone and posture, and coordinates balance.

Cerebrum (suh-**ree**-bruhm) Largest division of brain that coordinates sensory data and motor functions, as well as governs many aspects of intelligence and reasoning, learning, and memory.

Cervical lymph node levels Division of nodes in neck by region using Roman numerals.

Cervical muscles Muscles of the neck including sternocleidomastoid and trapezius muscles.

Cervical vertebra, vertebrae (**ver**-tuh-bruh, **ver**-tuh-bree) Vertebrae in vertebral column between skull and thoracic vertebrae.

Chorda tympani nerve (**kor**-duh **tim**-pan-ee) Branch of facial nerve serving submandibular and sublingual glands and tongue.

Ciliary nerves (**sil**-ee-a-re) Nerves to or from eyeball, with some converging with branches from nose forming nasociliary nerve.

Circumvallate lingual papillae (sur-kuhm-**val**-ate ling-gwuhl puh-**pil**-ee) Larger mushroom-shaped lingual papillae anterior to sulcus terminalis.

Common carotid artery (kuh-**rot**-id) Artery travelling in carotid sheath in neck branching into internal and external carotid arteries.

Condyle (**kon**-dyl) Oval bony prominence typically found at articulations.

Condyloid process (**kon**-duh-loid) Large and posterior projection off mandible.

Conjunctiva (kuhn-**junk**-ti-vuh) Membrane lining inside of eyelids at front of eyeball.

Contralateral (kon-truh-**lat**-uhr-uhl)) Structure on opposite side.

Cornu (**kor**-noo) Small, hornlike prominence of a bone.

Coronal suture (**kor**-o-nuhl) Suture between frontal and parietal bones.

Coronoid notch (**kor**-uh-noid) Notch in anterior border of mandibular ramus.

Coronoid process Anterior superior projection of mandibular ramus.

Corrugator supercilii muscle (kor-uh-**gay**-tuhr soo-per-**sil**-ee-eye) Muscle of facial expression in eye region used when frowning.

Cranial bones (**kray**-nee-uhl) Skull bones forming cranium including occipital, frontal, parietal, temporal, sphenoid, ethmoid.

Cranial nerves Part of peripheral nervous system connected to brain carrying information to and from it.

Cranium (**kray**-nee-uhm) Structure formed by cranial bones including occipital, frontal, parietal, temporal, sphenoid, ethmoid.

Crest Roughened border or ridge on bone surface.

Cribriform plate (**krib**-ri-form) Horizontal plate of ethmoid perforated with numerous foramina for olfactory nerves.

Crista galli (**kris**-tuh **gal**-ee) Vertical midline continuation of perpendicular plate of ethmoid into cranial cavity.

Crossover-innervation Overlap of terminal nerve fibers from contralateral side of dental arch.

D

Deep Structure located inwards and away from surface.

Deep auricular artery (aw-**rik**-u-luhr) Artery off first part of maxillary artery that supplies auricular region and outer surface of tympanic membrane.

Deep cervical lymph nodes Nodes located along internal jugular vein dividing into superior and inferior based on point where omohyoid muscle crosses.

Deep lingual artery (**ling**-gwuhl) Artery supplies from ventral surface to apex of tongue.

Deep lingual vein Vein supplies from ventral surface to apex of tongue.

Deep parotid lymph nodes (puh-**rot**-id) Nodes located deep to parotid gland.

Deep temporal arteries (**tem**-puh-ruhl) Artery branching from maxillary artery supplying temporalis muscle.

Deep temporal nerves Nerves for temporalis muscle.

Dens (denz) Odontoid process of second cervical vertebra.

Dental plexus (**plek**-suhs) Network of vessels or nerves within both maxillary and mandibular dental arches.

Depression of the mandible (de-**presh**-uhn) (**man**-di-buhl) Lowering of lower jaw.

Depressor anguli oris muscle (de-**pres**-uhr **an**-gu-ly **or**-is) Muscle of facial expression in mouth region depressing angle of mouth.

Depressor labii inferioris muscle (**lay**-be-eye in-**fere**-ee-o-ris) Muscle of facial expression in the mouth region depressing lower lip.

Descending palatine artery (**pal**-uh-tine) Branch of maxillary artery terminating in greater palatine artery and lesser palatine artery.

Diencephalon (dy-uhn-**sef**-uh-lon) Division of brain consisting of thalamus and hypothalamus.

Digastric fossa (di-**gas**-trik **fos**-uh) Anterior belly of digastric muscle insertion site.

Digastric muscle Suprahyoid muscle with anterior and posterior belly.

Distal (**dis**-tuhl) Area farther away from median plane.

Dry eye syndrome (DES) Lacrimal glands producing less lacrimal fluid.

Dorsal (**dor**-suhl) Back of an area.

Dorsal lingual arteries (**ling**-gwuhl) Arteries supplying posterior dorsal surface of tongue.

Dorsal lingual veins Veins supplying dorsal surface of tongue.

Dorsal surface of the tongue Top surface of tongue.

Dorsum sellae (**dor**-suhm **sell**-ee) Part on superior surface of the sphenoid bone.

Duct Passageway to carry secretion from exocrine gland to set location.

E

Efferent nerve (**ef**-uhr-uhnt) Motor nerve carrying information away from brain or spinal cord to periphery.

Efferent nervous system Motor nerve system carrying information from brain or spinal cord to muscles or glands.

Efferent vessel Lymphatic vessel with lymph flowing out of lymph node from node's hilus.

Elevation of the mandible (el-uh-**vay**-shuhn) (**man**-di-buhl) Raising of lower jaw.

Embolus, emboli (**em**-bo-lus, **em**-bo-ly) Foreign materials such as thrombus (or thrombi) traveling in blood to block vessel.

Eminence (**em**-i-nuhns) Tubercle or rounded elevation on bony surface.

Endocrine gland (**en**-doh-krin)) Ductless gland with secretion being poured directly into vascular system.

Epicondyle (ep-i-**kon**-dyl) Small prominence located superior to or upon a condyle.

Epicranial aponeurosis (ep-ee-**kray**-nee-uhl ap-o-noo-**roh**-sis) Scalpal tendon from epicranial muscle.

Epicranial muscle Muscle of facial expression in scalp with frontal and occipital bellies.

Epiglottis (ep-i-**glot**-is) Flap of cartilage folding back to cover entrance to larynx during swallowing.

Ethmoid bone (**eth**-moid) Single midline cranial bone of skull.

Ethmoidal sinuses (eth-**moy**-duhl) Paired paranasal sinuses located in ethmoid.

Ethmoidal spine Prominent spine on sphenoid bone.

Exocrine gland (**ek**-soh-krin) Gland with associated duct serving as passageway for secretion to be emptied directly into site of use.

External Outer side of the wall of hollow structure.

External acoustic meatus (uh-**koos**-tik me-**ay**-tuhs) Canal leading to tympanic cavity.

External carotid artery (kuh-**rot**-id) Artery arising from common carotid artery supplying extracranial tissue of head and neck.

External jugular lymph nodes (**jug**-u-luhr) Superficial cervical nodes located along external jugular vein.

External jugular vein Vein forming from posterior division of retromandibular vein.

External nasal nerve (**nay**-zuhl) Nerve from nasal surface converging with other branches forming nasociliary nerve.

External nose Surface anatomic feature of the nose.

External oblique line (o-**bleek**) Crest on lateral side of the mandible where the mandibular ramus joins the body.

External occipital protuberance (ok-**sip**-i-tuhl pro-**too**-buhr-uhns) Midline prominence on posterior surface of occipital bone.

Extrinsic tongue muscles (eks-**trin**-sik) Tongue muscles with different origins outside the tongue.

Eyelids Movable upper and lower tissue covering and protecting each eyeball.

F

Facial Structure closest to facial surface.

Facial artery Anterior artery branching from external carotid artery with complicated path giving rise to ascending palatine, submental, inferior and superior labial, angular arteries.

Facial bones Skull bones creating the face including lacrimal bones, nasal bones, vomer, inferior nasal conchae, zygomatic bones, maxillae, mandible.

Facial lymph nodes Superficial nodes located along facial vein that include malar, nasolabial, buccal, mandibular.

Facial nerve Seventh cranial nerve (VII) serving the muscles of facial expression, posterior suprahyoid muscles, lacrimal gland, sublingual and submandibular glands, tongue part, and part of skin through its greater petrosal, chorda tympani, posterior auricular nerves and muscular branches.

Facial paralysis (puh-**ral**-i-sis) Loss of the action of facial muscles.

Facial vein Vein draining into internal jugular vein after draining facial areas.

Fascia, fasciae (**fas**-she-uh, **fas**-she-ee) Layer(s) of fibrous connective tissue underlying the skin and surrounding muscles, bones, vessels, nerves, organs, other structures.

Fascial spaces (**fas**-she-uhl) Potential spaces between layers of fascia.

Fauces (**faw**-seez) Junction between oral region and oropharynx.

Filiform lingual papillae (**fil**-i-form **ling**-gwuhl puh-**pil**-ee) Papillae giving the tongue its velvety texture.

Fissure (**fish**-uhr) Narrow and cleftlike opening in a bone.

Fistula/Fistulae) (**fis**-tu-luh, **fis**-tu-lee) Passageway(s) in the skin, mucosa, or bone allowing drainage of abscess at surface.

Foliate lingual papillae (**fo**-lee-uht **ling**-gwuhl puh-**pil**-ee) Ridges of papillae on lateral tongue surface.

Foramen/Foramina) (fo-**ray**-muhn, fo-**ram**-i-nuh) Short window-like opening(s) in a bone.

Foramen cecum (**see**-kuhm) Depression on dorsal surface of tongue where sulcus terminalis points backward toward pharynx.

Foramen lacerum (**las**-er-uhm) Foramen among sphenoid, occipital, and temporal bones filled with cartilage.

Foramen magnum (**mag**-nuhm) Foramen in occipital carrying spinal cord, vertebral arteries, eleventh cranial nerve.

Foramen ovale (o-**vuh**-lee) Foramen in sphenoid carrying mandibular division of trigeminal or fifth cranial nerve.

Foramen rotundum (roh-**tun**-dum) Foramen in sphenoid carrying trigeminal or fifth cranial nerve.

Foramen spinosum (**spine**-o-sum) Foramen in sphenoid carrying middle meningeal artery.

Fossa, fossae (**fos**-uh, **fos**-ee) Deeper depression(s) on a bony surface.

Frontal bone Single cranial bone forming forehead and part of orbits.

Frontal eminence (**em**-i-nuhns) Prominence of forehead.

Frontalis muscle (frun-**tal**-is) Frontal belly of epicranial muscle.

Frontal nerve Nerve from merger of the supraorbital and supratrochlear nerves that continues into the ophthalmic nerve when joined by the lacrimal and nasociliary nerves.

Frontal plane Plane related to an imaginary line dividing the body at any level into anterior and posterior parts.

Frontal process of the maxilla (mak-**sil**-uh) Process forming part of orbital rim.

Frontal process of the zygomatic bone (zy-go-**mat**-ik) Process forming part of orbital wall.

Frontal region Region of the head that includes forehead and supraorbital area.

Frontal section Section through any frontal plane.

Frontal sinuses Paired paranasal sinuses located internally in frontal bone.

Frontonasal duct (frun-toh-**nay**-zuhl) Drainage canal of each frontal sinus to nasal cavity.

Fungiform lingual papillae (**fun**-ji-form **ling**-gwuhl puh-**pil**-ee) Smaller papillae with mushroom-shaped appearance.

G

Ganglion, ganglia (**gang**-gle-on, **gang**-gle-uh) Accumulation(s) of neuron cell bodies outside central nervous system.

Genial tubercles (juh-**ni**-uhl) Midline bony projections or mental spines on medial aspect of mandible.

Genioglossus muscle (ji-nee-o-**gloss**-us) Extrinsic tongue muscle arising from genial tubercles.

Geniohyoid muscle (ji-nee-o-**hi**-oid) Anterior suprahyoid muscle deep to mylohyoid muscle.

Gingiva, gingivae (jin-**ji**-vuh, jin-**ji**-vee) Mucosa(e) surrounding maxillary and mandibular teeth.

Glabella (gluh-**bell**-uh) Smooth elevated area on frontal bone between supraorbital ridges.

Gland Structure producing chemical secretion necessary for body functioning.

Glandular tissue In the head and neck area includes lacrimal, salivary, thyroid, parathyroid, and thymus.

Glossopharyngeal nerve (**gloss**-o-fuh-**rin**-je-uhl) Ninth cranial nerve (IX) serving parotid, pharyngeal muscle, tongue.

Goiter (**goi**-tuhr) Enlarged thyroid gland due to disease process.

Golden Proportions Guidelines for considering vertical dimensions of face to create pleasing proportion.

Gow-Gates mandibular block (man-**dib**-u-luhr) Injection that anesthetizes entire mandibular nerve that results in numbness of mandibular teeth and associated facial and lingual periodontium and gingiva.

Greater cornu (**kor**-nu) Pair of projections from sides of the body of hyoid.

Greater palatine artery (**pal**-uh-tine) Artery branching from maxillary artery travelling to palate.

Greater palatine (GP) block Injection that anesthetizes greater palatine nerve that results in numbness of associated palatal periodontium and gingiva of maxillary posteriors.

Greater palatine foramen (fo-**ray**-muhn) Foramen in palatine bone carrying greater palatine nerve and blood vessels.

Greater palatine (GP) nerve Nerve serving posterior hard palate and associated palatal periodontium and gingiva of the maxillary posteriors that joins maxillary nerve.

Greater petrosal nerve (puh-**tro**-suhl) Branch of facial nerve serving lacrimal gland, nasal cavity, and minor salivary glands of the hard and soft palates.

Greater wing Posterolateral process of body of sphenoid.

H

Hamulus, hamuli (**ham**-u-lis, **ham**-u-ly) Process of medial pterygoid plate of sphenoid.

Hard palate (**pal**-uht) Anterior part of palate formed by palatine processes of maxillae and posterior part by horizontal plates of palatine bones.

Head Rounded structure projecting from a bony surface by a neck.

Helix (**he**-liks) Superior and posterior free margin of auricle.

Hematoma (he-muh-**toh**-muh) Bruise resulting when blood vessel is injured and small amount of blood escapes into surrounding tissue and then clots.

Hemorrhage (**hem**-uh-ruhj) Large amounts of blood escaping into surrounding tissue without clotting when blood vessel is seriously injured.

Hilus (**hi**-luhs) Depression on side of lymph node where lymph flows out by way of efferent lymphatic vessel.

Horizontal plane Plane related to an imaginary line dividing the body at any level into superior and inferior parts.

Horizontal plates of the palatine bones (**pal**-uh-tine) Plates forming posterior part of hard palate.

Hyoglossus muscle (hi-o-**gloss**-us) Extrinsic tongue muscle originating from hyoid.

Hyoid bone (**hi**-oid) Bone suspended in the neck allowing attachment of many muscles.

Hyoid muscles Muscles that attach to hyoid classified by whether superior or inferior to it.

Hypoglossal canal (hi-poh-**gloss**-uhl) Canal in occipital carrying twelfth cranial nerve.

Hypoglossal nerve Twelfth cranial nerve (XII) serving muscles of tongue.

Hypophyseal fossa (hi-**pof**-uh-ze-uhl **fos**-uh) Deepest part of sella turcica containing pituitary gland.

Hyposalivation (hi-poh-sal-i-**vay**-shuhn) Reduced saliva production by salivary glands.

Hypothalamus (**hi**-poh-**thal**-uh-muhs) Part of diencephalus regulating homeostasis.

I

Incisive artery (in-**sy**-siv) Artery branching from inferior alveolar artery supplying mandibular anteriors.

Incisive block Injection that anesthetizes incisive and mental nerves that results in numbness of mandibular anteriors and premolars as well as associated facial periodontium and gingiva.

Incisive foramen (fo-**ray**-muhn) Foramen between palatal process of maxillae that carries branches of both nasopalatine nerves and blood vessels and is marked by incisive papilla.

Incisive nerve Nerve formed from dental and interdental branches of mandibular anteriors and merging with mental nerve forming inferior alveolar nerve and that serves mandibular anteriors and premolars as well as associated facial periodontium and gingiva.

Incisive papilla (puh-**pil**-uh) Bulge of tissue on anterior hard palate over incisive foramen.

Incisors (in-**sy**-zuhrs) Anteriors first and second from midline consisting of both centrals and laterals, respectively.

Incisura (in-si-**su**-ruh) Indentation or notch at edge of a bone.

Infection Invasion by pathogens with multiplication of them.

Inferior Area facing away from the head and toward the feet.

Inferior alveolar artery (al-**vee**-uh-luhr) Artery branching from maxillary artery supplying mandibular posteriors that branches into mental and incisive arteries.

Inferior alveolar (IA) block Injection that anesthetizes inferior alveolar nerve and its nerve branches as well as lingual nerve that results in numbness of mandibular teeth and associated lingual periodontium and gingiva as well as associated facial periodontium and gingiva of mandibular anteriors and premolar.

Inferior alveolar (IA) nerve Nerve formed from merger of incisive and mental nerves serving tissue of the chin, lower lip, and labial mucosa as well as mandibular teeth and associated periodontium and gingiva of mandibular anteriors and premolars that later joins posterior trunk of mandibular division of trigeminal nerve.

Inferior alveolar vein Vein draining mandibular teeth as well as chin.

Inferior articular processes (ahr-**tik**-u-luhr) Processes of first and second cervical vertebrae allowing articulation with inferior vertebrae.

Inferior labial artery (**lay**-be-uhl) Artery branching from facial artery supplying lower lip area.

Inferior labial vein Vein draining lower lip area and then draining into facial vein.

Inferior nasal concha, conchae (**kong**-kah, **kong**-kee) Paired facial bones projecting inwardly from maxillae forming walls of nasal cavity.

Inferior nuchal line (**noo**-kuhl) Inferior ridge on posterior surface of occipital bone.

Inferior orbital fissure (**or**-bi-tuhl) Fissure between greater wing of sphenoid and each maxilla carrying infraorbital and zygomatic nerves as well as infraorbital artery and inferior ophthalmic vein.

Inferior temporal line (**tem**-puh-ruhl) Inferior ridge on lateral skull surface.

Inferior thyroid artery (**thy**-roid) Branch off thyrocervical trunk of subclavian artery to supply thyroid gland.

Infrahyoid muscles (in-fruh-**hi**-oid) Hyoid muscles inferior to hyoid.

Infraorbital artery (in-fruh-**or**-bi-tuhl) Artery branching from the maxillary artery giving rise to anterior superior alveolar artery and branches to orbit.

Infraorbital (IO) block Injection that anesthetizes both anterior superior alveolar and middle superior alveolar nerves as well as the nearby infraorbital nerve that results in numbness of maxillary anteriors and premolars and associated facial periodontium and gingiva.

Infraorbital canal Canal off infraorbital sulcus terminating on surface of each maxilla as infraorbital foramen.

Infraorbital foramen (fo-**ray**-muhn) Foramen of each maxilla inferior to infraorbital rim that transmits infraorbital nerve and blood vessels.

Infraorbital (IO) nerve Nerve forming maxillary nerve and formed from branches of upper lip, cheek, lower eyelid, side of nose that joins with anterior and middle superior alveolar nerves.

Infraorbital region Region of head located inferior to orbital region and lateral to nasal region.

Infraorbital rim Inferior margin of orbit.

Infraorbital sulcus (**sul**-kuhs) Groove in floor of orbital surface.

Infratemporal crest (in-fruh-**tem**-puh-ruhl) Crest dividing each greater wing of sphenoid into temporal and infratemporal surfaces.

Infratemporal fossa (**fos**-uh) Fossa inferior to temporal fossa and infratemporal crest on greater wing of the sphenoid.

Infratemporal space Space that occupies infratemporal fossa.

Infratrochlear nerve (**in**-fruh-**trok**-lere) Nerve from medial eyelid and side of nose converging with other branches forming the nasociliary nerve.

Innervation (in-uhr-**vay**-shuhn) Supply of nerves to tissue or organs.

Insertion End of the muscle attached to more movable structure.

Interdental gingiva (in-tuhr-**den**-tuhl) Attached gingiva between teeth.

Intermaxillary suture (in-tuhr-**mak**-sil-lare-ee) Suture between two maxilla forming maxillae.

Intermediate tendon of the digastric muscle (di-**gas**-trik) Tendon between two muscle bellies of digastric muscle.

Internal Inner side of the wall of hollow structure.

Internal acoustic meatus (uh-**koos**-tik me-**ay**-tuhs) Bony meatus in temporal bone carrying seventh and eighth cranial nerves.

Internal carotid artery (kuh-**rot**-id) Artery off common carotid artery giving rise to ophthalmic artery and supplying intracranial structures.

Internal jugular vein (**jug**-u-luhr) Vein travelling in carotid sheath from jugular foramen that drains head and neck.

Internal nasal nerves (**nay**-zuhl) Nerves from nasal cavity converging with other branches to form nasociliary nerve.

Intertragic notch (in-tuhr-**tray**-jic) Small groove between tragus and antitragus on surface of ear.

Intrinsic tongue muscles (in-**trin**-sik) Muscles located inside tongue.

Investing fascia (**fash**-e-uh) Most external layer of deep cervical fasciae.

Ipsilateral (ip-see-**lat**-uhr-uhl) Structure on same side.

Iris (**eye**-ris) Central colored area of eyeball.

J

Joint Junction or union between two or more bones.

Joint disc Fibrous disc located between temporal bone and mandibular condyle.

Joint capsule Fibrous capsule enclosing temporomandibular joint.

Jugular foramen (**jug**-u-luhr fo-**ray**-muhn) Foramen between occipital and temporal bones carrying internal jugular vein and ninth, tenth, and eleventh cranial nerves.

Jugular notch of the occipital bone (ok-**sip**-i-tuhl) Occipital or medial part of jugular foramen.

Jugular notch of the temporal bone (**tem**-puh-ruhl) Temporal or lateral part of jugular foramen.

Jugular trunk Lymphatic vessel draining one side of head and neck emptying into that side's lymphatic duct.

Jugulodigastric lymph node (**jug**-u-lo-di-**gas**-trik) Superior deep cervical node located inferior to posterior belly of digastric muscle.

Jugulo-omohyoid lymph node (**jug**-u-lo-o-moh-**hi**-oid) Inferior deep cervical node located at crossing of omohyoid muscle and internal jugular vein.

L

Labial (**lay**-be-uhl) Structure closest to lips.

Labial commissure (**kom**-uh-shur) Corner of mouth where upper and lower lips meet.

Labial frenum/frena (**free**-nuhm, **free**-nuh) Fold of tissue or frenulum located at midline between labial mucosa and alveolar mucosa of maxillae or mandible.

Labial mucosa (mu-**ko**-suh) Lining of inner parts of lips.

Labiomental groove (lay-be-o-**men**-tuhl) Groove separating lower lip from chin.

Lacrimal bone (**lak**-ri-muhl) Paired facial bone forming medial wall of orbit.

Lacrimal ducts Ducts in orbital part of gland draining lacrimal fluid or tears.

Lacrimal fluid Tears or watery fluid excreted by lacrimal gland.

Lacrimal fossa (**fos**-uh) Fossa of frontal bone containing lacrimal gland.

Lacrimal gland Glands in lacrimal fossa of frontal bone producing lacrimal fluid or tears.

Lacrimal nerve Nerve serving lateral part of eyelid and other eye tissue and joining frontal and nasociliary nerves forming ophthalmic nerve.

Lacrimal punctum (plural, **puncta**) (**punk**-tum, **punk**-tah) Small holes found at the medial canthus of both upper and lower eyelids.

Lambdoidal suture (lam-**doid**-uhl) Suture between occipital and both parietal bones.

Laryngopharynx (luh-ring-go-**fare**-inks) Inferior part of pharynx close to laryngeal opening.

Larynx (**lare**-inks) Upper part of lower airway.

Lateral Area farther away from median plane.

Lateral canthus, canthi (**kan**-thus, **kan**-thy) Outer corner(s) of eye.

Lateral deviation of the mandible (de-vee-**ay**-shuhn) (**man**-di-buhl) Shifting of lower jaw to one side.

Lateral masses of the atlas (**at**-luhs) Lateral parts of first cervical vertebra articulating superiorly with occipital and inferiorly with axis.

Lateral masses of the ethmoid bone (**eth**-moid) Lateral parts of ethmoid that contain ethmoidal sinuses.

Lateral pterygoid muscle (**ter**-i-goid) Muscle of mastication lying in infratemporal fossa.

Lateral pterygoid nerve Muscular branch from anterior trunk of mandibular division of trigeminal nerve serving lateral pterygoid muscle.

Lateral pterygoid plate Part of pterygoid process.

Lateral surface of the tongue Side of tongue.

Lesser cornu (**kor**-nu) Pair of projections off hyoid.

Lesser palatine artery (**pal**-uh-tine) Artery branching from maxillary artery traveling to soft palate.

Lesser palatine foramen (fo-**ray**-munh) Foramen in palatine bone transmitting lesser palatine nerve and blood vessels.

Lesser palatine nerve Nerve serving soft palate and palatine tonsils tissue along with posterior nasal cavity that then joins maxillary nerve.

Lesser petrosal nerve (puh-**tro**-suhl) Parasympathetic fibers from ninth cranial nerve exiting skull through foramen ovale of sphenoid.

Lesser wing Anterior process of the body of sphenoid.

Levator anguli oris muscle (le-**vay**-tuhr **an**-gu-ly **or**-is) Muscle of facial expression in mouth region elevating angle of the mouth.

Levator labii superioris alaeque nasi muscle (**lay**-be-eye **soo**-per-ee-**or**-is **a**-luh-kwee **nay**-zi) Muscle of facial expression in the mouth region elevating upper lip and ala of nose.

Levator labii superioris muscle Muscle of facial expression in the mouth region elevating upper lip.

Levator veli palatini muscle (**vee**-ly pal-uh-**ti**-ni) Muscle of soft palate rising to close off nasopharynx.

Ligament (**lig**-uh-muhnt) Band of fibrous tissue connecting bones.

Line Small straight ridge of a bone.

Lingual (**ling**-gwuhl) Structure closest to tongue.

Lingual artery Anterior artery branching from external carotid artery supplying structures superior to hyoid.

Lingual foramen Tiny foramen on medial surface of mandible at midline.

Lingual frenum (**free**-nuhm) Midline fold of tissue between ventral surface of tongue and floor of mouth.

Lingual nerve Nerve that serves the tongue, floor of the mouth, and associated lingual periodontium and gingiva of mandibular teeth that joins posterior trunk of mandibular division of trigeminal nerve.

Lingual papillae (puh-**pil**-ee) Small elevated structures covering dorsal surface of the body of tongue.

Lingual tonsil (**ton**-sil) Indistinct lymphoid tissue located on dorsal surface at tongue's base.

Lingual veins Veins that include deep lingual, dorsal lingual, sublingual veins.

Lingula (**ling**-gu-luh) Bony spine overhanging mandibular foramen.

Lobule (**lob**-yule) Inferior fleshy protuberance from helix of auricle.

Ludwig angina (**lood**-vig an-**ji**-nuh) Serious infection of submandibular space.

Lymph (limf) Tissue fluid draining from surrounding region and into lymphatic vessels.

Lymphadenitis (lim·fad·uh·**ny**·tis) Inflammation of lymph node.

Lymphadenopathy (lim-fad-uh-**nop**-uh-thee) Process with increase in size and change in lymphoid tissue consistency.

Lymphatic ducts (lim-**fat**-ik) Larger lymphatic vessels draining smaller vessels and then emptying into venous component of vascular system.

Lymphatic system Part of immune system consisting of vessels, nodes, ducts, tonsils.

Lymphatic vessels System of channels draining tissue fluid from surrounding regions.

Lymph nodes Organized bean-shaped lymphoid tissue filtering lymph by way of lymphocytes.

M

Major salivary glands (**sal**-i-vare-ee) Large paired glands with associated named ducts that include parotid, submandibular, and sublingual.

Malar lymph nodes (**may**-luhr) Superficial facial nodes in infraorbital region.

Mandible (**man**-di-buhl) Single facial bone articulating bilaterally with temporal bones at temporomandibular joint.

Mandibular canal (man-**dib**-u-luhr) Canal in mandible where inferior alveolar nerve and blood vessels travel.

Mandibular condyle (**kon**-dyl) Projection of bone from mandibular ramus that participates in temporomandibular joint.

Mandibular foramen (fo-**ray**-munh) Foramen of mandible carrying inferior alveolar nerve and blood vessels.

Mandibular incisive canal (in-**sy**-siv) Continuation of mandibular canal with incisive nerve.

Mandibular lymph nodes Superficial facial nodes over surface of mandible.

Mandibular nerve Third division of trigeminal nerve formed by merger of posterior and anterior trunks joining with ophthalmic and maxillary nerves forming trigeminal ganglion of trigeminal nerve.

Mandibular notch Notch located on mandible between condyle and coronoid process.

Mandibular ramus, rami (**ray**-muhs, **ray**-my) Plate(s) of mandible extending superiorly from body of mandible.

Mandibular symphysis (**sim**-fi-sis) Midline ridge showing fusion of mandibular processes.

Mandibular teeth Teeth within mandible.

Marginal gingiva (**mar**-ji-nuhl jin-**ji**-vuh) Nonattached gingiva at gingival margin of each tooth.

Masseter muscle (mass-**see**-tuhr) Most obvious and strongest muscle of mastication.

Masseteric artery (mass-i-**tare**-ik) Artery branching from maxillary artery supplying masseter muscle.

Masseteric nerve Muscular nerve branching from anterior trunk of mandibular division of trigeminal nerve serving masseter muscle and temporomandibular joint.

Masseteric-parotid fascia (mass-i-**tare**-ik-puh-**rot**-id **fash**-e-uh) Deep fascia located inferior to zygomatic arch and over masseter muscle.

Masticator space (mass-ti-**kay**-tuhr) Fascial space including entire area of mandible and muscles of mastication.

Mastoid air cells (**mass**-toid) Air spaces in mastoid process of temporal bone communicating with middle ear cavity.

Mastoid notch Notch on mastoid process of temporal bone.

Mastoid process Area on petrous part of temporal bone with air cells where cervical muscles attach.

Maxilla, maxillae (mak-**sil**-uh, mak-**sil**-ee) Complete (maxillae) or partial upper jaw (maxilla).

Maxillary artery (**mak**-sil-lare-ee) Terminal artery branching from external carotid artery.

Maxillary nerve Second division of sensory root of trigeminal nerve formed by convergence of many nerves including infraorbital nerve and serving many maxillary structures.

Maxillary process of the zygomatic bone (zy-go-**mat**-ik) Process forming part of infraorbital rim and orbital wall.

Maxillary sinuses Paranasal sinuses in each body of maxilla.

Maxillary sinusitis (sy-nuhs-**i**-tis) Infection of maxillary sinus.

Maxillary teeth Teeth within maxillae.

Maxillary tuberosity (too-buh-**ros**-i-tee) Elevation on posterior aspect of each maxilla.

Maxillary vein Vein that collects from pterygoid plexus and merges with superficial temporal vein forming retromandibular vein.

Meatus (me-**ay**-tuhs) Opening or canal in a bone.

Medial (**me**-dee-uhl) Area closer to median plane, considered mesial within dentition.

Medial canthus, canthi (**kan**-thus, **kan**-thy) Inner angle(s) of eye.

Medial pterygoid muscle (**ter**-i-goid) Muscle of mastication inserting on medial surface of mandible.

Medial pterygoid nerve Nerve for medial pterygoid, tensor tympani, and tensor veli palatini muscles.

Medial pterygoid plate Part of pterygoid process.

Median (**me**-dee-uhn) Structure at median plane.

Median lingual sulcus (**ling**-gwuhl **sul**-kuhs) Midline depression on dorsal surface of tongue corresponding to deeper median septum.

Median palatine raphe (**pal**-uh-tine **ray**-fee) Midline tendinous band on palate superficial to median palatine suture.

Median palatine suture Midline suture between palatine processes of maxillae and horizontal plates of palatine bones.

Median pharyngeal raphe (fuh-**rin**-je-uhl **ray**-fee) Midline tendinous band on posterior wall of the pharynx.

Median plane Plane related to imaginary line dividing the body into right and left halves.

Median septum (**sep**-tuhm) Midline tendinous structure dividing tongue corresponding to median lingual sulcus on dorsal surface of tongue.

Medulla (muh-**dul**-uh) Division of brainstem involved with regulation of heartbeat, breathing, vasoconstriction, reflex centers.

Meninges (**muh**-nin-jez) System of membranes protecting the central nervous system.

Meningitis (muh-in-**jite**-is) Inflammation of meninges of brain or spinal cord.

Mental artery (**men**-tuhl) Artery branching from inferior alveolar artery exiting mental foramen and supplying the chin.

Mental block Injection that anesthetizes mental nerve that results in numbness of associated facial periodontium and gingiva of mandibular anteriors and premolars.

Mental foramen (fo-**ray**-munh) Foramen inferior to apices of mandibular premolars transmitting mental nerve and blood vessels.

Mental nerve Nerve joining incisive nerve to form inferior alveolar nerve serving chin and lower lip and labial mucosa of mandibular anteriors as well as associated facial periodontium and gingiva of mandibular anteriors and premolars.

Mental protuberance (pro-**too**-buhr-uhns) Mandibular bony prominence of chin.

Mental region Region of head where chin is major feature.

Mentalis muscle (ment-**ta**-lis) Muscle of facial expression in mouth region helping raise chin.

Metastasis (muh-**tas**-tuh-sis) Spread of cancer from primary site to secondary site.

Midbrain Division of brainstem that includes relay stations for hearing, vision, motor pathways.

Middle meningeal artery (muh-**nin**-je-uhl) Artery branching from maxillary artery supplying meninges of brain by way of foramen spinosum.

Middle meningeal vein Vein draining blood from the meninges of brain into pterygoid plexus of veins.

Middle nasal concha, conchae (**nay**-zuhl) (**kong**-kah, **kong**-kee) Lateral part of ethmoid in nasal cavity.

Middle superior alveolar (MSA) block (al-**vee**-uh-luhr) Injection that anesthetizes middle superior alveolar nerve if present that results in numbness of maxillary premolars and mesiobuccal root of maxillary first molar as well as associated buccal periodontium and gingiva.

Middle superior alveolar (MSA) nerve Nerve that when present may innervate maxillary premolars and associated buccal periodontium and gingiva as well as mesiobuccal root of maxillary first molar that later joins infraorbital nerve.

Middle temporal artery (**tem**-puh-ruhl) Artery branching from superficial temporal artery supplying temporalis muscle.

Midsagittal section (mid-**saj**-i-tuhl) Section of body through median plane.

Minor salivary glands (**sal**-i-vare-ee) Small glands scattered in tissue of buccal, labial, and lingual mucosa, soft and hard palates, and floor of the mouth, as well as associated with circumvallate lingual papillae.

Molars (**moh**-luhrs) Most distal of posteriors including firsts, seconds, thirds.

Motor root of the trigeminal nerve (try-**jem**-i-nuhl) Root of trigeminal nerve.

Mucobuccal fold (mu-ko-**buk**-uhl) Fold in the vestibule where labial or buccal mucosa meets alveolar mucosa.

Mucocutaneous junction (**mu**-ko-ku-tay-nee-uhs) Lips outlined from surrounding skin.

Mucogingival junction (mu-ko-**jin**-ji-vuhl) Border between alveolar mucosa and attached gingiva.

Mucosa (mu-**ko**-suh) Mucous membrane such as that lining oral cavity.

Mumps Contagious viral infection usually involving enlargement of both parotid salivary glands.

Muscle Body tissue that shortens under neural control, causing soft tissue and bony structures to move.

Muscle of the uvula (**u**-vu-luh) Muscle of soft palate within uvula.

Muscles of facial expression Paired muscles that give the face expression located in superficial fasciae of facial tissue.

Muscles of mastication (mass-ti-**kay**-shuhn) Pairs of muscles attached to and moving mandible including temporalis, masseter, medial and lateral pterygoid muscles.

Muscles of the pharynx (**fare**-inks) Muscles that include stylopharyngeus, pharyngeal constrictor, soft palate muscles.

Muscles of the soft palate (**pal**-uht) Muscles that include palatoglossal, palatopharyngeus, levator veli palatini, tensor veli palatini, muscle of the uvula.

Muscles of the tongue Muscles of tongue that include intrinsic or extrinsic.

Muscular system Includes skeletal muscle tissue as well as other types of muscle tissue.

Muscular triangle Smaller triangular region of the neck inferior to omohyoid muscle and part of anterior cervical triangle.

Mylohyoid artery (my-lo-**hi**-oid) Artery branching from inferior alveolar artery supplying floor of the mouth and mylohyoid muscle.

Mylohyoid groove Groove on mandible where mylohyoid nerve and blood vessels travel.

Mylohyoid line Line on medial aspect of mandible.

Mylohyoid muscle Anterior suprahyoid muscle forming floor of mouth.

Mylohyoid nerve Nerve branching from inferior alveolar nerve serving mylohyoid muscle and anterior belly of digastric muscle.

Mylohyoid raphe (**ray**-fee) Midline connection between right and left mylohyoid muscles.

N

Naris, nares (**nay**-ris, **nay**-reez) Nostril(s) of nose.

Nasal bones (**nay**-zuhl) Paired facial bones forming bridge of nose.

Nasal cavity Cavity of nose within nasal region.

Nasal meatus (me-**ay**-tuhs) Groove beneath each nasal concha containing openings for communication with paranasal sinuses or nasolacrimal duct.

Nasal region Region of head where external nose is main feature.

Nasal septal cartilage (**sep**-tuhl) Inferior part of nasal septum.

Nasal septum (**sep**-tuhm) Vertical partition of nasal cavity.

Nasion (**nay**-ze-on) Midline junction between nasal and frontal bones.

Nasociliary nerve (nay-zo-**sil**-ee-a-re) Nerve joining frontal and lacrimal nerves and forming ophthalmic nerve.

Nasolabial lymph nodes (nay-zo-**lay**-be-uhl) Superficial facial nodes along nasolabial sulcus.

Nasolabial sulcus (**sul**-kuhs) Groove running upward between labial commissure and ala of nose.

Nasolacrimal duct (nay-zo-**lak**-ri-muhl) Duct formed at junction of lacrimal bone and maxilla draining lacrimal fluid or tears.

Nasolacrimal sac Lacrimal fluid within sac after passing over eyeball.

Nasopalatine branch (nay-zo-**pal**-uh-tine) Branch off sphenopalatine artery.

Nasopalatine (NP) block Injection that anesthetizes both nasopalatine nerves that results in numbness of associated palatal periodontium and gingiva for maxillary anteriors bilaterally.

Nasopalatine groove Groove on lateral surface of vomer that lodges nasopalatine nerve and branches of sphenopalatine blood vessels.

Nasopalatine (NP) nerve Nerve serving anterior hard palate and associated palatal periodontium and gingiva of maxillary anteriors bilaterally that then joins maxillary nerve.

Nasopharynx (nay-zo-**fare**-inks) Part of pharynx superior to level of soft palate.

Nerve Bundle of neural processes outside central nervous system and part of peripheral nervous system.

Nerve block Injection that anesthetizes larger area than supraperiosteal injection because local anesthetic agent is deposited near larger nerve trunks.

Nervous system Extensive, intricate network of neural structures that activates, coordinates, and controls all functions.

Neuron (**noor**-on) Cellular component of nervous system composed of cell body and neural processes.

Neurotransmitter (noor-o-**trans**-mit-uhr) Chemical agent of neuron that discharges with arrival of action potential, diffuses across synapse, and binds to receptors on other cell's membrane.

Notch Indentation at edge of bone.

O

Occipital artery (ok-**sip**-i- tuhl) Posterior artery branching from external carotid artery supplying suprahyoid and sternocleidomastoid muscles and posterior scalp tissue.

Occipital bone Single cranial bone in most posterior part of skull.

Occipital condyles (**kon**-dyls) Projections of occipital articulating with lateral masses of first cervical vertebra.

Occipitalis muscle (ok-sip-i-**ta**-lis) Occipital belly of epicranial muscle.

Occipital lymph nodes Superficial nodes located on posterior base of head.

Occipital region Region of head overlying occipital bone and covered by scalp.

Occipital triangle Smaller triangular region of neck superior to omohyoid muscle and part of posterior cervical triangle.

Oculomotor nerve (ok-u-lo-**moh**-tuhr) Third cranial nerve (III) serving certain eye muscles.

Odontogenic infections (o-don-toh-**jen**-ik) Dental infections involving teeth or associated tissue.

Olfactory nerve (ol-**fak**-tuh-ree) First cranial nerve (I) transmits smell from nose to brain.

Omohyoid muscle (o-moh-**hi**-oid) Infrahyoid muscle with superior and inferior bellies.

Ophthalmic artery (of-**thal**-mik) Artery branching from internal carotid artery supplying the eye, orbit, lacrimal gland.

Ophthalmic nerve First division of sensory root of trigeminal nerve arising from frontal, lacrimal, nasociliary nerves.

Ophthalmic veins Veins draining tissue of orbit.

Opportunistic infections (op-uhr-too-**nis**-tik) Resident microbiota creating infection because body's defenses are compromised.

Optic canal (**op**-tik) Canal in orbital apex between roots of the lesser wing of the sphenoid bone.

Optic nerve Second cranial nerve (II) transmitting sight from the eye to the brain.

Oral cavity Inside of the mouth.

Oral region Region of head containing lips, oral cavity, palate, tongue, floor of the mouth, parts of pharynx.

Orbicularis oculi muscle (or-bik-u-**lare**-is **ok**-yule-eye) Muscle of facial expression encircling eye.

Orbicularis oris muscle (**or**-is) Muscle of facial expression encircling mouth.

Orbit (**or**-bit) Eye cavity containing eyeball.

Orbital apex (**or**-bi-tuhl) Deepest part of orbit composed of parts of sphenoid and palatine bones.

Orbital plate of the ethmoid bone (**eth**-moid) Plate forming most of medial orbital wall.

Orbital region Region of head with eyeball and supporting structures.

Orbital walls Walls of orbit composed of parts of frontal, ethmoid, lacrimal, maxilla, zygomatic, sphenoid.

Origin End of muscle attached to least movable structure.

Oropharynx (or-o-**fare**-inks) Part of pharynx between soft palate and opening of larynx.

Osteomyelitis of the jaw (OMJ) (os-tee-o-my-uh-**ly**-tus) Inflammation of bone marrow.

Ostium, ostia (**os**-tee-uhm, **os**-tee-uh) Smaller opening(s) in a bone.

Otic ganglion (**ot**-ik **gang**-gle-on) Ganglion associated with lesser petrosal nerve and branches of mandibular nerve.

P

Palatal (**pal**-uh-tuhl) Structure closest to palate.

Palate (**pal**-uht) Roof of mouth.

Palatine bones (**pal**-uh-tine) Paired bones of the skull consisting of vertical and horizontal plates.

Palatine process of the maxilla (mak-**sil**-uh) Paired processes articulating with each other and forming anterior part of hard palate.

Palatine rugae (**roo**-gee) Irregular ridges of tissue surrounding incisive papilla on hard palate.

Palatine tonsils (**ton**-sils) Tonsils between anterior and posterior faucial pillars.

Palatoglossal muscle (pal-uh-toh-**gloss**-el) Muscle of soft palate forming anterior faucial pillar.

Palatopharyngeus muscle (pal-uh-toh-fuh-**rin**-je-us) Muscle of soft palate forming posterior faucial pillar.

Paranasal sinuses (pare-uh-**nay**-zuhl) Paired air-filled cavities in bone including frontal, sphenoidal, ethmoidal, maxillary.

Parapharyngeal space (pare-uh-fuh-**rin**-je-uhl) Fascial space located lateral to pharynx.

Parasympathetic nervous system (pare-uh-sim-puh-**thet**-ik) Division of autonomic nervous system involved in "rest or digest."

Parathyroid glands (pare-uh-**thy**-roid) Small endocrine glands located close to or within thyroid.

Parathyroid hormone Hormone produced and secreted by parathyroid glands directly into the blood to regulate calcium and phosphorus levels.

Paresthesia (pare-es-**thee**-zhuh) Abnormal sensation of burning or prickling from an area.

Parietal bone Paired cranial bone of the skull articulating with same bone as well with other skull bones.

Parietal region Region of head that overlies parietal bones covered by scalp.

Parotid duct (puh-**rot**-id) Duct associated with parotid that opens into oral cavity at parotid papilla.

Parotid papilla (puh-**pil**-uh) Small elevation of tissue that marks opening of parotid located opposite maxillary second molar on inner cheek.

Parotid salivary gland (**sal**-i-vare-ee) Major salivary gland over mandibular ramus and divided into superficial and deep lobes.

Parotid space Fascial space created within investing fascial layer of the deep cervical fasciae as it envelops the parotid gland.

Pathogens (**path**-o-juhns) Microbiota that are not resident microbiota and can cause infection.

Perforation (pur-fuh-**ray**-shuhn) Abnormal hole in a hollow organ such as in the wall of a sinus.

Peripheral nervous system (PNS) (puh-**rif**-uhr-uhl) Division of nervous system consisting of afferent and efferent nervous systems.

Perpendicular plate (per-pen-**dik**-u-luhr) Midline vertical plate of ethmoid.

Petrotympanic fissure (pet-roh-tim-**pan**-ik) Fissure between tympanic and petrosal parts of temporal bone through which chorda tympani nerve emerges.

Petrous part of the temporal bone (**pet**-ruhs) (**tem**-puh-ruhl) Inferior part of bone containing mastoid process and air cells.

Pharyngeal branch (fuh-**rin**-je-uhl) Branch of ascending pharyngeal artery.

Pharyngeal constrictor muscles (kuhn-**strik**-tor) Three paired muscles forming lateral and posterior walls of pharynx.

Pharyngeal tonsil Tonsil on posterior wall of nasopharynx.

Pharyngeal tubercle Midline projection of the basilar part of the occipital bone.

Pharynx (**fare**-inks) Part of both respiratory and digestive tracts divided into nasopharynx, oropharynx, and laryngopharynx.

Philtrum (**fil**-truhm) Vertical groove on skin in midline superior to upper lip.

Piriform aperture (**pir**-i-form) Anterior opening of the nasal cavity.

Plate Flat structure of a bone.

Platysma muscle (pluh-**tiz**-muh) Muscle of facial expression that runs from the neck to the mouth.

Plica fimbriata, plicae fimbriatae (**pli**-kuh fim-bree-**ay**-tuh, **pli**-kee fim-bree-**ay**-tee) Fold(s) with fringelike projections on ventral surface of tongue.

Pons (ponz) Division of brainstem that connects medulla with cerebellum.

Posterior Back of area.

Posterior arch Arch on first cervical vertebra.

Posterior auricular artery (aw-**rik**-u-luhr) Posterior artery branching from external carotid artery supplying the ear.

Posterior auricular lymph nodes Superficial nodes located posterior to ear.

Posterior auricular nerve Branch of facial nerve serving occipital belly of epicranial muscle, stylohyoid muscle, posterior belly of digastric muscle.

Posterior cervical triangle Lateral region of neck.

Posterior digastric nerve (di-**gas**-trik) Nerve supplying posterior belly of digastric muscle.

Posterior ethmoidal nerve (eth-**moy**-duhl) Nerve from nasal cavity and paranasal sinuses forming nasociliary nerve.

Posterior faucial pillar (**faw**-shuhl **pil**-uhr) Vertical fold posterior to each palatine tonsil created by palatopharyngeus muscle.

Posterior nasal apertures (**nay**-zuhl) Posterior openings of nasal cavity or choanae.

Posterior superior alveolar artery (al-**vee**-uh-luhr) Artery branching from maxillary artery supplying maxillary posteriors and maxillary sinus.

Posterior superior alveolar (PSA) block Injection that in most cases anesthetizes posterior superior alveolar nerve that results in numbness of maxillary molars and associated buccal periodontium and gingiva.

Posterior superior alveolar foramina (fo-**ram**-i-nuh) Foramina on infratemporal surface of maxilla carrying posterior superior alveolar nerve and blood vessels.

Posterior superior alveolar (PSA) nerve Nerve directly joining maxillary nerve after serving maxillary molars and associated buccal peridontium and gingiva.

Posterior superior alveolar vein Vein formed from merger of dental and alveolar branches serving maxillary teeth.

Posterior suprahyoid muscle group (**soo**-pruh-**hi**-oid) Suprahyoid muscles posterior to hyoid including posterior belly of digastric and stylohyoid muscles.

Postglenoid process (post-**gle**-noid) Process of temporal bone.

Premolars (pre-**moh**-luhrs) Posteriors that are fourth and fifth from midline in permanent dentition including firsts and seconds, respectively.

Perivertebral space (pare-ee-**ver**-tuh-bruhl) Cervical space contains cervical vertebrae and posterior to retropharyngeal space.

Previsceral space (pre-**vis**-er-uhl) Fascial space located between visceral and investing fasciae.

Primary node Lymph node draining lymph from particular region.

Primary sinusitis (sy-nuhs-**i**-tis) Inflammation of sinus.

Process General term for any prominence on bony surface.

Protrusion of the mandible (pro-**troo**-zhuhn) (**man**-di-buhl) Bringing of lower jaw forward.

Proximal (**prok**-si-muhl) Area closer to median plane.

Pterygoid arteries (**ter**-i-goid) Artery branching from maxillary artery supplying pterygoid muscles.

Pterygoid canal Small canal at the superior border of each posterior nasal aperture.

Pterygoid fascia (**fash**-e-uh) Deep fascia located on medial surface of medial pterygoid muscle.

Pterygoid fossa (**fos**-uh) Fossa between medial and lateral pterygoid plates of the sphenoid.

Pterygoid fovea (**fo**-vee-uh) Depression on anterior surface of mandibular condyle.

Pterygoid plexus of veins (**plek**-suhs) Collection of veins around pterygoid muscles and maxillary arteries draining deep face and alveolar veins into maxillary vein.

Pterygoid process Part of sphenoid forming lateral borders of posterior nasal apertures.

Pterygomandibular fold (**ter**-i-go-man-**dib**-u-luhr) Fold of tissue in oral cavity superficial to pterygomandibular raphe.

Pterygomandibular raphe (**ray**-fee) Tendinous band extending from hamulus to posterior end of mylohyoid line.

Pterygomandibular space Fascial space that is part of infratemporal space.

Pterygopalatine fossa (**ter**-i-go-**pal**-uh-tine **fos**-uh) Fossa deep to infratemporal fossa and between pterygoid process and maxillary tuberosity.

Pterygopalatine ganglion (**gang**-gle-on) Ganglion associated with greater petrosal nerve and branches of maxillary nerve.

Pupil (**pu**-pil) Black area in center of iris that responds to changing light conditions.

Pustule (**pus**-tule) Small elevated and circumscribed, suppuration-containing lesion of skin or oral mucosa.

Pyramidal process of the palatine bone (pi-**ram**-i-duhl) (**pal**-uh-tine) Projects posteriorly and lateralward from junction of horizontal and vertical plates.

R

Regions of the head Regions that include frontal, parietal, occipital, temporal, auricular, orbital, nasal, infraorbital, zygomatic, buccal, oral, mental regions.

Regions of the neck Regions that include anterior and posterior cervical triangles.

Resident microbiota (my-kro-**bi**-o-tuh) Indigenous regional microorganisms usually not causing infections.

Resting potential (po-**ten**-shuhl) Charge difference between fluid outside and inside cell resulting in differences in distribution of ions.

Retraction of the mandible (re-**trak**-shuhn) (**man**-di-buhl) Bringing of lower jaw backward.

Retromandibular vein (ret-roh-man-**dib**-u-luhr) Vein formed by merger of superficial temporal and maxillary veins dividing into anterior and posterior divisions inferior to parotid.

Retromolar pad (ret-roh-**moh**-luhr) Dense pad of tissue distal to the most distal tooth of mandible and covering retromolar triangle.

Retromolar triangle Part of alveolar process of mandible just posterior to most distal mandibular molar and covered by retromolar pad.

Retropharyngeal lymph nodes (ret-roh-fuh-**rin**-je-uhl) Deep nodes near deep parotid nodes at level of first cervical vertebra.

Retropharyngeal space Fascial space immediately posterior to pharynx.

Right lymphatic duct (lim-**fat**-ik) Duct formed from convergence of lymphatic system of right arm and thorax or chest and right jugular trunk draining same side of head and neck.

Risorius muscle (ri-**sore**-ee-us) Muscle of facial expression in mouth region used when smiling widely.

Root of the nose Area of nasal region between eyes.

S

Sagittal plane (**saj**-i-tuhl) Planes related to any imaginary plane parallel to median plane.

Sagittal suture Suture between paired parietal bones.

Saliva (suh-**ly**-vuh) Product produced by salivary glands.

Salivary gland (**sal**-i-vare-ee) Gland producing saliva lubricating and cleansing the oral cavity and helping in digestion.

Salivary stone Formation of stone within a salivary gland.

Scalp Layers of soft tissue overlying bones of cranium.

Sclera (**skleer**-uh) White area of eyeball.

Secondary node Lymph node draining lymph from primary node.

Secondary sinusitis (sy-nuhs-**i**-tis) Inflammation of the sinus related to another source.

Sella turcica (**sell**-uh **tur**-ki-kuh) Depression on sphenoid bone.

Sensory root of the trigeminal nerve (try-**jem**-i-nuhl) Root of trigeminal nerve having ophthalmic, maxillary, mandibular divisions.

Skeletal system Consists of bones, associated cartilage, and joints.

Skull Structure composed of both cranial bones or cranium and facial bones.

Soft palate (**pal**-uht) Posterior nonbony part of palate.

Somatic nervous system (SNS) (so-**mat**-ik) Subdivision of efferent division of peripheral nervous system including nerves controlling muscular system and external sensory receptors.

Space of the body of the mandible (**man**-di-buhl) Fascial space formed by periosteum covering body of mandible.

Sphenoid bone (**sfe**-noid) Single midline cranial bone consisting of body and processes.

Sphenoidal sinuses (**sfe**-noid-uhl) Paired sinuses in body of sphenoid.

Sphenomandibular ligament (**sfe**-no-man-**dib**-u-luhr **lig**-uh-muhnt) Ligament connecting spine of sphenoid with lingula of mandible.

Sphenopalatine artery (sfe-no-**pal**-uh-tine) Terminal artery branching from maxillary artery supplying nose including a branch through incisive foramen.

Spine Abrupt small prominence of a bone.

Spinal cord Division of central nervous system running along dorsal side of body linking brain to rest of body.

Spine of the sphenoid bone Spine located at posterior extremity of sphenoid.

Squamosal suture (**skway**-moh-suhl) Suture between temporal and parietal bones.

Squamous part of the temporal bone (**skway**-muhs) (**tem**-puh-ruhl) Part forming braincase and parts of zygomatic arch and temporomandibular joint.

Sternocleidomastoid branches (stir-no-kli-doh-**mass**-toid) Branches off occipital artery.

Sternocleidomastoid (SCM) muscle Paired cervical muscle serving as landmark of neck.

Sternohyoid muscle (ster-no-**hi**-oid) Infrahyoid muscle superficial to thyroid gland and cartilage.

Sternothyroid muscle (ster-no-**thy**-roid) Infrahyoid muscle inserting on thyroid cartilage.

Stoma (**stoh**-muh) Opening such as fistula.

Styloglossus muscle (sty-lo-**gloss**-us) Extrinsic tongue muscle originating from styloid process of temporal bone.

Stylohyoid muscle (sty-lo-**hi**-oid) Posterior suprahyoid muscle originating from styloid process of temporal bone.

Stylohyoid nerve Branch of the facial nerve supplying stylohyoid muscle.

Styloid process (**sty**-loid) Bony projection of temporal bone serving as attachment for muscles and ligaments.

Stylomandibular ligament (sty-lo-man-**dib**-u-luhr **lig**-uh-muhnt) Ligament connecting styloid process with angle of mandible.

Stylomastoid artery (sty-lo-**mass**-toid) Artery branching from posterior auricular artery supplying mastoid air cells.

Stylomastoid foramen (fo-**ray**-muhn) Foramen in temporal bone carrying facial or seventh cranial nerve.

Stylopharyngeus muscle (sty-lo-fuh-**rin**-je-us) Paired longitudinal muscle of pharynx arising from styloid process.

Subclavian artery (sub-**klay**-vee-uhn) Artery arising from aorta on left and brachiocephalic artery on right and giving rise to branches to supply both intracranial and extracranial structures, as well as arm.

Subclavian triangle Smaller triangular region of neck inferior to omohyoid muscle and part of posterior cervical triangle.

Subclavian vein Vein from the arm draining external jugular vein then joining with internal jugular vein and forming brachiocephalic vein.

Sublingual artery (sub-**ling**-gwuhl) Artery branching from lingual artery supplying sublingual gland, floor of the mouth, mylohyoid muscle.

Sublingual caruncle (**kar**-ung-uhl) Papilla near midline of floor of mouth where sublingual and submandibular ducts open into oral cavity.

Sublingual duct Duct associated with sublingual gland that opens at sublingual caruncle.

Sublingual fold Fold of tissue on each side of floor of mouth where smaller ducts of sublingual gland open into oral cavity.

Sublingual fossa (**fos**-uh) Fossa on medial surface of mandible containing sublingual gland.

Sublingual salivary gland (**sal**-i-vare-ee) Major salivary gland in sublingual fossa.

Sublingual space Fascial space inferior to oral mucosa making this tissue its roof.

Subluxation (sub-luhk-**say**-shuhn) Acute episode with both joints becoming dislocated.

Submandibular fossa (sub-man-**dib**-u-luhr **fos**-uh) Fossa on medial surface of mandible containing submandibular gland.

Submandibular ganglion (**gang**-gle-on) Ganglion superior to deep lobe of submandibular gland communicating with chorda tympani and lingual nerves.

Submandibular lymph nodes Superficial cervical nodes at inferior border of mandibular ramus.

Submandibular salivary gland (**sal**-i-vare-ee) Major salivary gland in submandibular fossa.

Submandibular space Paired fascial space lateral and posterior to submental space on each side.

Submandibular triangle Part of the anterior cervical triangle formed by mandible and anterior and posterior bellies of digastric muscle.

Submasseteric space (sub-mass-et-**tehr**-ik) Fascial space between masseter muscle and external surface of vertical mandibular ramus.

Submental artery (sub-**men**-tuhl) Artery branching from the facial artery supplying submandibular nodes, submandibular glands, and mylohyoid and digastric muscles.

Submental lymph nodes Superficial cervical nodes inferior to the chin.

Submental space Single fascial space midline between the symphysis and hyoid.

Submental triangle Single midline part of anterior cervical triangle created by right and left anterior bellies of digastric muscle and hyoid.

Submental vein Vein draining chin and then draining into facial vein.

Sulcus, sulci (**sul**-kuhs, **sul**-ky) Shallow depression or groove such as that on a bony surface or between a tooth and the inner surface of the marginal gingiva.

Sulcus terminalis (tur-**mi**-nal-is) V-shaped groove on dorsal surface of tongue.

Superficial Structure located toward surface.

Superficial parotid lymph nodes (puh-**rot**-id) Nodes just superficial to parotid gland.

Superficial temporal artery (**tem**-puh-ruhl) Terminal artery branching from external carotid artery arising in parotid gland and giving rise to transverse facial and middle temporal arteries as well as frontal and parietal branches.

Superficial temporal vein Vein draining side of scalp going on to form retromandibular vein along with maxillary vein.

Superior Area facing toward the head and away from the feet.

Superior articular processes (ahr-**tik**-u-luhr) Processes from vertebra allowing articulation with superior vertebra.

Superior labial artery (**lay**-be-uhl) Artery branching from facial artery supplying upper lip area.

Superior labial vein Vein draining upper lip area and then draining into facial vein.

Superior nasal concha, conchae (**nay**-zuhl **kong**-kay, **kong**-kee) Lateral part of ethmoid in nasal cavity.

Superior nuchal line (**noo**-kuhl) Superior ridge on posterior surface of occipital bone.

Superior orbital fissure (**or**-bi-tuhl) Fissure between greater and lesser wings of sphenoid transmitting structures from cranial cavity to orbit.

Superior temporal line (**tem**-puh-ruhl) Superior ridge on lateral skull surface.

Superior thyroid artery (**thy**-roid) Artery branching from external carotid artery supplying structures inferior to hyoid including thyroid.

Superior thyroid notch Deep notch in middle of superior border of thyroid cartilage.

Superior vena cava (**vee**-nuh **kay**-vuh) Vein formed from union of brachiocephalic veins emptying into heart.

Suppuration (sup-u-**ray**-shuhn) Pus containing pathogenic bacteria, white blood cells, tissue fluid, debris.

Supraclavicular lymph nodes (soo-pruh-**klah**-vik-u-luhr) Deep cervical nodes along clavicle.

Suprahyoid branch (soo-pruh-**hi**-oid) Branch of lingual nerve supplying suprahyoid muscles.

Suprahyoid muscles Hyoid muscles superior to hyoid divided by an anterior or posterior relationship to hyoid.

Supraorbital nerve (**soo**-pruh-**or**-bi-tuhl) Nerve from the forehead and anterior scalp merging with supratrochlear nerve forming frontal nerve.

Supraorbital notch Foramen on supraorbital ridge of frontal bone.

Supraorbital ridge Ridge over orbit on frontal bone.

Supraorbital rim Superior margin of orbit.

Supraorbital vein Vein joining supratrochlear vein forming facial vein in frontal region.

Supraperiostal injection (**soo**-pruh-**pare**-e-os-te-uhl) Injection anesthetizing small area because local anesthetic agent is deposited near terminal nerve endings.

Supratrochlear vein (**soo**-pruh-**trok**-lere) Vein joining supraorbital vein forming facial vein in frontal region.

Surface anatomy Study of structural relationships of external features to internal organs and parts.

Suture (**soo**-chuhr) Generally immovable articulation joining bones by fibrous tissue.

Sympathetic nervous system (sim-puh-**thet**-ik) Division of autonomic nervous system involved in "fight or flight."

Synapse (**sin**-aps) Junction between two neurons or between neuron and effector organ transmitting neural impulses by electrical or chemical means.

Synovial cavities (sy-**no**-vee-uhl) Upper and lower spaces created by division of joint by disc.

Synovial fluid Fluid secreted by membranes lining synovial cavities.

T

T-cell lymphocytes (**lim**-fo-sites) White blood cells maturing in thymus.

Temple Superficial side of head posterior to eyes.

Temporal bones (**tem**-puh-ruhl) Paired cranial bone forming lateral cranial walls and articulating with mandible at temporomandibular joint.

Temporal fascia (**fash**-e-uh) Deep fascia covering temporalis muscle down to zygomatic arch.

Temporal fossa (**fos**-uh) Fossa on lateral surface of skull containing temporalis muscle.

Temporalis muscle (tem-puh-**ruhl**-is) Muscle of mastication filling temporal fossa.

Temporal process of the zygomatic bone (zy-go-**mat**-ik) Process forming part of zygomatic arch.

Temporal region Region of the head where external ear is prominent feature.

Temporal space Fascial space formed by temporal fascia covering temporalis muscle.

Temporomandibular disorder (TMD) (tem-poh-roh-man-**dib**-u-luhr) Disorder involving one or both temporomandibular joints.

Temporomandibular joint (TMJ) Articulation between temporal bone and mandible allowing movement of mandible.

Temporomandibular joint ligament (**lig**-uh-muhnt) Ligament associated with temporomandibular joint.

Temporozygomatic suture (tem-puh-roh-zi-go-**mat**-ik) Suture between temporal and zygomatic bones.

Tensor veli palatini muscle (**ten**-sor **vee**-ly pal-uh-**ti**-ni) Muscle of soft palate stiffening it.

Thalamus (**thal**-uh-muhs) Part of diencephalon serving as central relay point for incoming nervous impulses.

Thoracic duct (thuh-**ras**-ik) Lymphatic duct draining lower half of body and left side of thorax or chest and draining left side of head and neck through left jugular trunk.

Thrombus, thrombi (**throm**-buhs, **throm**-by) Clot(s) forming on inner blood vessel wall.

Thymus gland (**thy**-mus) Endocrine gland inferior to thyroid and deep to sternum.

Thyrohyoid muscle (thy-roh-**hi**-oid) Infrahyoid muscle appearing as continuation of sternothyroid muscle.

Thyroid gland (**thy**-roid) Endocrine gland having two lobes and inferior to thyroid cartilage.

Thyroid ima artery Variable artery of thyroid gland from brachiocephalic trunk of the arch of aorta.

Thyroxine (thy-**rok**-sin) Hormone produced and secreted by thyroid directly into blood.

Tonsils (**ton**-sils) Masses of lymphoid tissue including palatine, lingual, pharyngeal, tubal tonsils.

Tragus (**tray**-guhs) Flap of tissue of auricle and anterior to external acoustic meatus.

Transverse facial artery (tranz-**vurs**) Artery branching from superficial temporal artery supplying parotid gland.

Transverse foramen (fo-**ray**-munh) Foramen on transverse processes of each cervical vertebra carrying vertebral artery.

Transverse palatine suture (**pal**-uh-tine) Suture between palatine processes of maxillae and horizontal plates of palatine bones.

Transverse process Lateral projections of cervical vertebrae.

Transverse section Section through any horizontal plane.

Trapezius muscle (truh-**pee**-zee-us) Cervical muscle covering lateral and posterior neck surfaces.

Trigeminal ganglion (try-**jem**-i-nuhl **gang**-gle-on) Sensory ganglion located intracranially on petrous part of temporal bone.

Trigeminal nerve Fifth cranial nerve (V) serving muscles of mastication and cranial muscles through its motor root and also serving teeth, tongue, oral cavity, and most of facial skin through its sensory root.

Trigeminal neuralgia (TN) (noo-**ral**-juh) Lesion of trigeminal nerve involving facial pain.

Trismus (**triz**-muhs) Reduced opening of the jaws.

Trochlear nerve (**trok**-lere) Fourth cranial nerve (IV) that serves eye muscle.

Tubal tonsil (**too**-buhl **ton**-sil) Tonsil located in nasopharynx near auditory tube.

Tubercle (**too**-buhr-kuhl) Eminence or small rounded elevation on bony surface.

Tubercle of the upper lip Thicker area in termination of midline of upper lip.

Tuberculum sellae (too-**bur**-ku-luhm **sell**-ee) Slight elevation on superior surface of sphenoid bone.

Tuberosity (too-buh-**ros**-i-tee) Large, often rough prominence on bony surface.

Tympanic part of the temporal bone (tim-**pan**-ik) (**tem**-puh-ruhl) Part forming most of external acoustic meatus.

U

Uvula of the palate (**u**-vu-luh) (**pal**-uht) Midline muscular structure hanging from posterior margin of soft palate.

V

Vagus nerve (**vay**-guhs) Tenth cranial nerve (X) serving muscles of soft palate, pharynx and larynx, ear skin, and many organs of thorax or chest and abdomen.

Vascular plexus (**plek**-suhs) Large network of blood vessels, usually veins.

Vascular compartments Two compartments of the neck that are surrounded by carotid sheath and include its contents.

Vascular system Consists of arterial blood supply, capillary network, venous drainage.

Vazirani-Akinosi mandibular block (vaz-i-**ron**-ee **ak**-ee-no-see man-**dib**-u-luhr) Injection that anesthetizes mandibular nerve similarly to inferior alveolar block but also includes mylohyoid nerve that results in similar numbness and can be used in a closed-mouth situation.

Vein Blood vessel traveling to the heart carrying blood.

Venous sinuses (**vee**-nuhs) Blood-filled space between two layers of tissue.

Ventral (**ven**-truhl) Front of area.

Ventral surface of the tongue Underside of tongue.

Venule (**ven**-yule) Smaller vein draining capillaries then joining larger veins.

Vermilion zone (vuhr-**mil**-yon) Outline of entire lip from surrounding skin.

Vertebral compartment (**ver**-tuh-bruhl) Compartment of the neck that is surrounded by the vertebral fascia and include its contents.

Vertebral fascia (**fash**-e-uh) Deep cervical fasciae covering spinal cord, cervical vertebrae, associated vertebral muscles.

Vertebral foramen (fo-**ray**-munh) Central foramen in the vertebrae for spinal cord and associated tissue.

Vertical dimension of the face Face divided into thirds.

Vertical muscle Paired muscle of the intrinsic tongue muscles that runs in vertical direction.

Vertical plates of the palatine bones (**pal**-uh-tine) Plates forming part of lateral walls of nasal cavity and orbital apex.

Vestibular fornix (ve-**stib**-u-luhr **for**-niks) Deepest recess of each vestibule.

Vestibular space of the mandible (**man**-di-buhl) Space of lower jaw.

Vestibular space of the maxilla (**mak**-sil-uh) Space of upper jaw.

Vestibules (**ves**-ti-bules) Upper and lower spaces between cheeks, lips, gingival tissue in oral region.

Vestibulocochlear nerve (vuhs-**tib**-u-lo-**kok**-luhr) Eighth cranial nerve (VIII) conveying signals from inner ear to brain.

Visceral compartment (**vis**-er-uhl) Compartment of the neck surrounded by the visceral fascia and include its contents.

Visceral fascia (**fash**-e-uh) Deep cervical fasciae formed into single midline tube running down neck.

Vomer (**vo**-muhr) Single facial bone forming posterior part of nasal septum.

von Ebner glands (**eb**-nuhr) Minor salivary glands associated with circumvallate lingual papilla.

X

Xerostomia (zeer-o-**stoh**-me-uh) Dry mouth.

Z

Zygomatic arch (zy-go-**mat**-ik) Arch formed by union of temporal process of zygomatic bone and zygomatic process of temporal bone.

Zygomatic bones Paired facial bones forming cheekbones.

Zygomatic nerve Nerve formed from the merger of zygomaticofacial and zygomaticotemporal nerves joining maxillary nerve.

Zygomatic process of the frontal bone (**frun**-tual) Process lateral to orbit.

Zygomatic process of the maxilla (mak-**sil**-uh) Process forming part of infraorbital rim.

Zygomatic process of the temporal bone (**tem**-puh-ruhl) Process consisting of the squamous part of the temporal bone that forms part of the zygomatic arch.

Zygomatic region Region of the head overlying cheekbone.

Zygomaticofacial nerve (zy-go-**mat**-i-ko-**fay**-shuhl) Nerve serving skin of cheek and joining with zygomaticotemporal nerve forming zygomatic nerve.

Zygomaticomaxillary suture (zy-go-**mat**-i-ko-**mak**-sil-lare-ee) Suture between maxillary process of zygomatic bone and zygomatic process of the maxilla.

Zygomaticotemporal nerve (zy-go-**mat**-i-ko-**tem**-puh-ruhl) Nerve serving skin of temporal region then joining with zygomaticofacial nerve forming zygomatic nerve.

Zygomaticus major muscle (zy-go-**mat**-i-kus) Muscle of facial expression in mouth region when smiling.

Zygomaticus minor muscle Muscle of facial expression in mouth region elevating upper lip.

Index

Page numbers followed by "*f*" indicate figures, "*t*" indicate tables, and "*b*" indicate boxes.

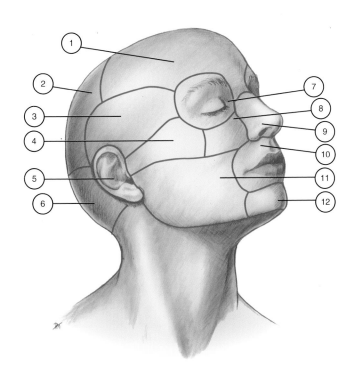

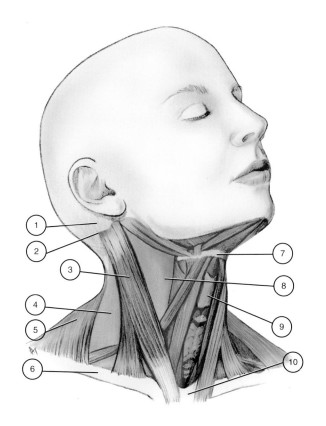

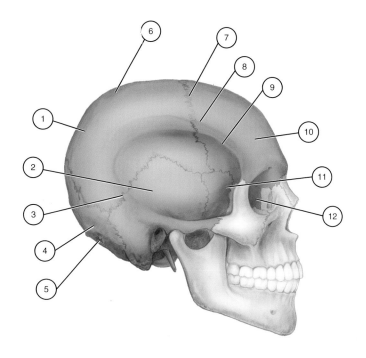

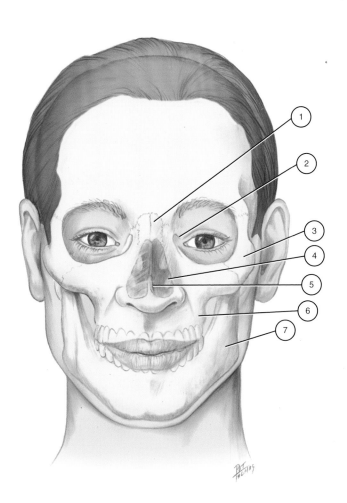

NECK REGIONS AND CERVICAL MUSCLES

1. Mastoid process of the temporal bone
2. Superior nuchal line of the occipital bone
3. Sternocleidomastoid muscle
4. Posterior cervical triangle
5. Trapezius muscle
6. Clavicle
7. Hyoid bone
8. Anterior cervical triangle
9. Thyroid cartilage
10. Sternum

HEAD REGIONS

1. Frontal region
2. Parietal region
3. Temporal region
4. Zygomatic region
5. Auricular region
6. Occipital region
7. Orbital region
8. Infraorbital region
9. Nasal region
10. Oral region
11. Buccal region
12. Mental region

FACIAL BONES—ANTERIOR VIEW

1. Nasal bone
2. Lacrimal bone
3. Zygomatic bone
4. Inferior nasal concha
5. Vomer
6. Maxilla
7. Mandible

CRANIAL BONES—LATERAL VIEW

1. Parietal bone
2. Temporal bone
3. Squamosal suture
4. Occipital bone
5. Lambdoidal suture
6. Sagittal suture
7. Coronal suture
8. Superior temporal line
9. Inferior temporal line
10. Frontal bone
11. Sphenoid bone
12. Ethmoid bone

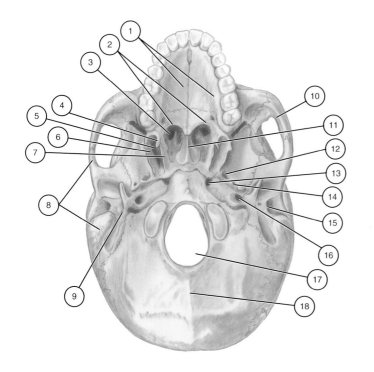

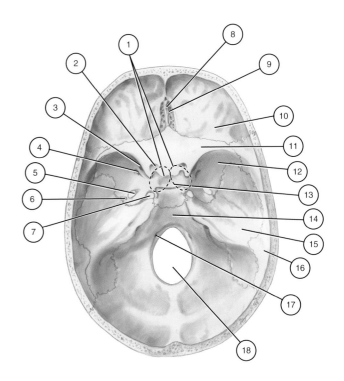

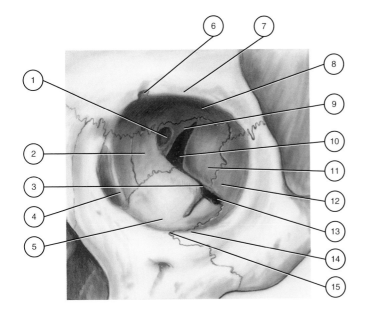

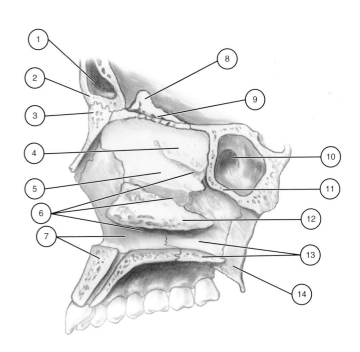

INTERNAL SKULL—SUPERIOR VIEW

1. Sphenoidal sinuses of the sphenoid bone
2. Optical canal
3. Superior orbital fissure
4. Foramen rotundum
5. Foramen ovale
6. Foramen spinosum
7. Carotid canal
8. Crista galli of the ethmoid bone
9. Cribriform plate of the ethmoid bone
10. Frontal bone
11. Lesser wing of the sphenoid bone
12. Greater wing of the sphenoid bone
13. Body of the sphenoid bone
14. Occipital bone
15. Temporal bone
16. Parietal bone
17. Hypoglossal canal
18. Foramen magnum

EXTERNAL SKULL—INFERIOR VIEW

1. Maxillae
2. Palatine bones
3. Posterior nasal aperture
4. Hamulus of the medial plate
5. Pterygoid fossa
6. Lateral plate of the sphenoid bone
7. Medial plate of the sphenoid bone
8. Temporal bone
9. Stylomastoid foramen
10. Zygomatic bone
11. Vomer
12. Foramen ovale
13. Foramen lacerum
14. External acoustic meatus
15. External acoustic meatus
16. Carotid canal
17. Foramen magnum
18. Occipital bone

NASAL CAVITY—LATERAL WALL

1. Frontal sinus
2. Frontal bone
3. Nasal bone
4. Superior nasal concha of the ethmoid bone
5. Middle nasal conchae of the ethmoid bone
6. Nasal meatuses: superior, middle, inferior
7. Maxilla
8. Crista galli of the ethmoid bone
9. Cribriform plate of the ethmoid bone
10. Sphenoidal sinus of the sphenoid bone
11. Sphenoid bone
12. Inferior nasal concha
13. Palatine bone
14. Medial pterygoid plate of the sphenoid bone

ORBIT—ANTERIOR VIEW

1. Optic canal
2. Ethmoid bone
3. Palatine bone
4. Lacrimal bone
5. Maxilla
6. Supraorbital notch
7. Supraorbital rim
8. Frontal bone
9. Lesser wing of the sphenoid bone
10. Superior orbital fissure
11. Greater wing of the sphenoid bone
12. Zygomatic bone
13. Inferior orbital fissure
14. Infraorbital rim
15. Zygomaticomaxillary suture

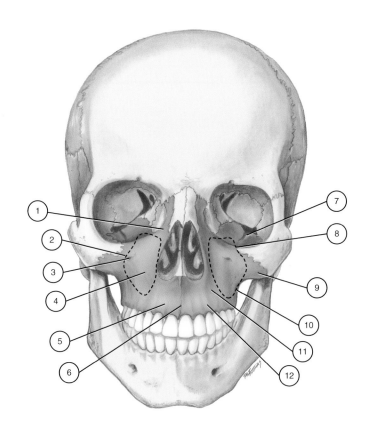

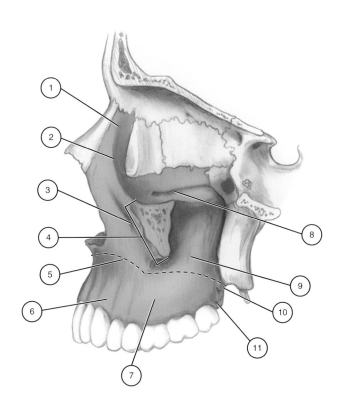

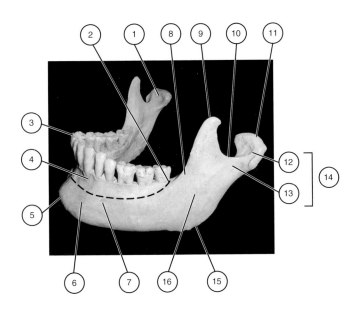

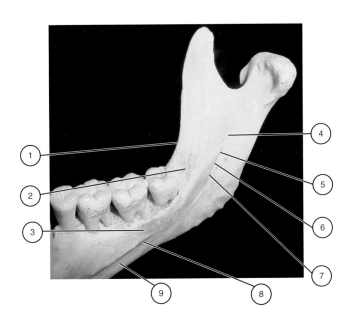

MAXILLA—LATERAL VIEW

1. Frontal process of the maxilla
2. Infraorbital rim
3. Infraorbital foramen
4. Zygomatic process of the maxilla
5. Canine fossa
6. Canine eminence
7. Alveolar process of the maxilla
8. Infraorbital sulcus
9. Body of the maxilla
10. Posterior superior alveolar foramina
11. Maxillary tuberosity

MAXILLAE—ANTERIOR VIEW

1. Frontal process of the maxilla
2. Location of the maxillary sinus
3. Infraorbital foramen
4. Body of the maxilla
5. Alveolar process of the maxilla
6. Intermaxillary suture
7. Infraorbital sulcus
8. Infraorbital rim
9. Zygomatic process of the maxilla
10. Location of maxillary sinus
11. Canine fossa
12. Canine eminence

MANDIBLE—MEDIAL VIEW

1. Coronoid notch
2. Retromolar triangle
3. Sublingual fossa
4. Mandibular ramus
5. Mandibular foramen
6. Lingula
7. Mylohyoid groove
8. Mylohyoid line
9. Submandibular fossa

MANDIBLE—LATERAL VIEW

1. Pterygoid fovea
2. External oblique line
3. Mandibular teeth
4. Alveolar process of the mandible
5. Mental protuberance
6. Body of the mandible
7. Mental foramen
8. Coronoid notch
9. Coronoid process
10. Mandibular notch
11. Articulating surface of the mandibular condyle
12. Neck of the mandibular condyle
13. Mandibular condyle
14. Condyloid process
15. Angle of the mandible
16. Mandibular ramus

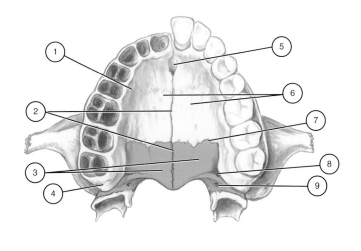

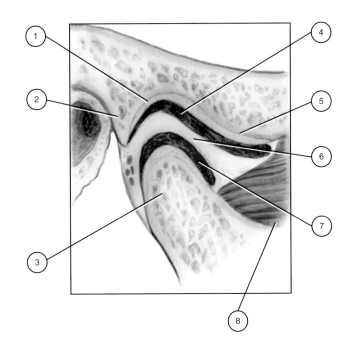

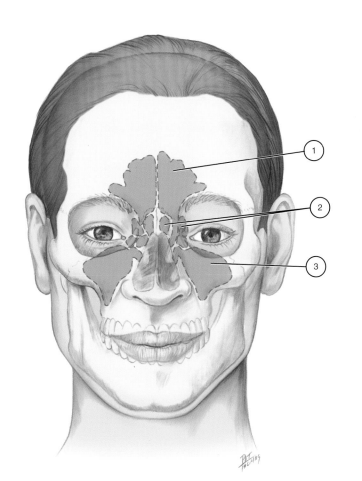

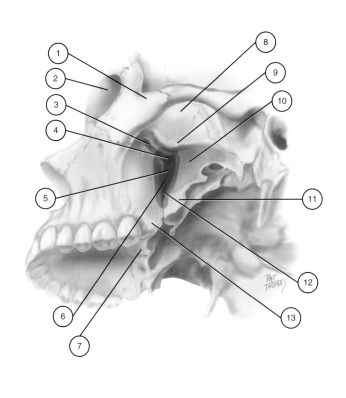

TEMPOROMANDIBULAR JOINT—SAGITTAL SECTION

1. Articular fossa
2. Postglenoid process
3. Mandibular condyle
4. Upper synovial cavity
5. Articular eminence
6. Joint disc of the temporomandibular joint
7. Lower synovial cavity
8. Lateral pterygoid muscle

HARD PALATE—INFERIOR VIEW

1. Alveolar process of the maxilla
2. Median palatine suture
3. Horizontal plates of the palatine bones
4. Maxillary tuberosity
5. Incisive foramen
6. Palatine processes of the maxillae
7. Transverse palatine suture
8. Greater palatine foramen
9. Lesser palatine foramen

SKULL FOSSAE AND BORDERS—OBLIQUE LATERAL VIEW

1. Zygomatic arch
2. Orbit
3. Inferior orbital fissure
4. Sphenopalatine foramen
5. Pterygopalatine fossa
6. Pterygomaxillary fissure
7. Palatine bone
8. Temporal fossa
9. Infratemporal crest of greater wing of sphenoid bone
10. Infratemporal fossa
11. Lateral pterygoid plate of the sphenoid bone
12. Pterygopalatine canal
13. Maxillary tuberosity

PARANASAL SINUSES

1. Frontal sinus of the frontal bone
2. Ethmoidal sinuses of the ethmoid bone
3. Maxillary sinus of the maxilla

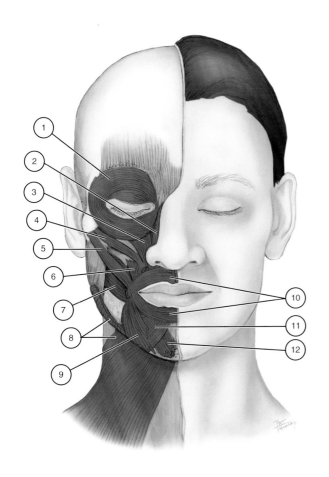
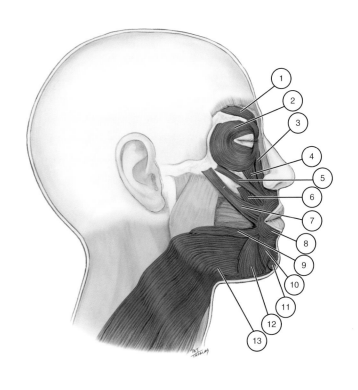
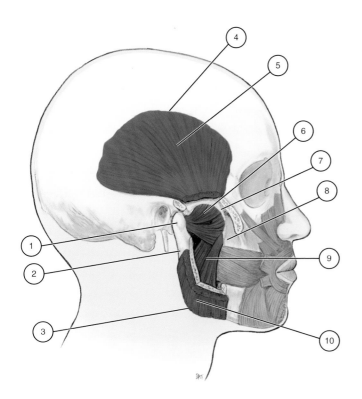
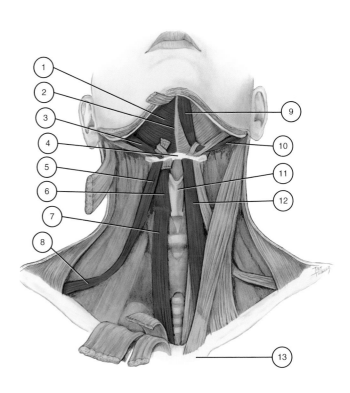

MUSCLES OF FACIAL EXPRESSION—LATERAL VIEW

1. Corrugator supercilii muscle
2. Orbicularis oculi muscle
3. Levator labii superioris alaeque nasi muscle
4. Levator labii superioris muscle
5. Zygomaticus minor muscle
6. Levator anguli oris muscle
7. Zygomaticus major muscle
8. Orbicularis oris muscle
9. Risorius muscle
10. Depressor labii inferioris muscle
11. Mentalis muscle
12. Depressor anguli oris muscle
13. Platysma muscle

MUSCLES OF FACIAL EXPRESSION—FRONTAL VIEW

1. Orbicularis oculi muscle
2. Levator labii superioris alaeque nasi muscle
3. Levator labii superioris muscle
4. Zygomaticus minor muscle
5. Zygomaticus major muscle
6. Levator anguli oris muscle
7. Buccinator muscle
8. Platysma muscle
9. Depressor anguli oris muscle
10. Orbicularis oris muscle
11. Depressor labii inferioris muscle
12. Mentalis muscle

HYOID MUSCLES—ANTERIOR VIEW

1. Mylohyoid muscle
2. Mylohyoid raphe
3. Stylohyoid muscle
4. Hyoid bone
5. Superior belly of the omohyoid muscle
6. Thyrohyoid muscle
7. Sternothyroid muscle
8. Inferior belly of the omohyoid muscle
9. Anterior belly of the digastric muscle
10. Posterior belly of the digastric muscle
11. Thyroid cartilage
12. Sternohyoid muscle
13. Sternum

MUSCLES OF MASTICATION—LATERAL VIEW

1. Mandibular condyle
2. Mandibular ramus
3. Angle of the mandible
4. Inferior temporal line
5. Temporalis muscle
6. Lateral pterygoid muscle
7. Sphenoid bone
8. Maxilla
9. Medial pterygoid muscle
10. Masseter muscle

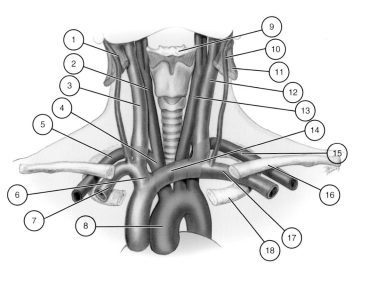

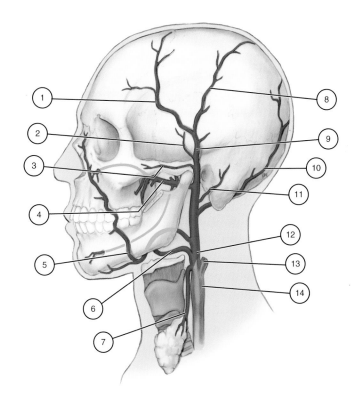

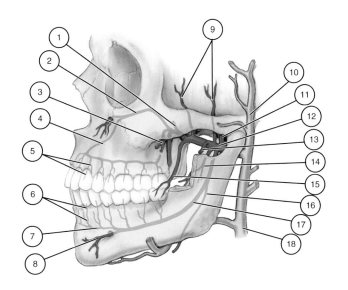

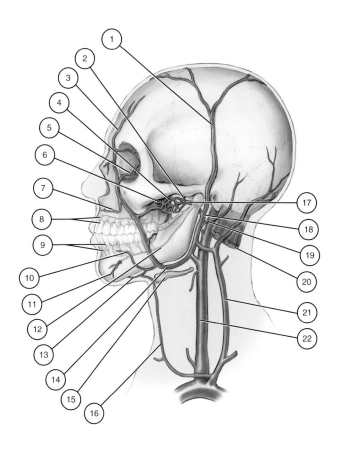

EXTERNAL CAROTID ARTERY—LATERAL VIEW

1. Frontal branch of superficial temporal artery
2. Middle temporal artery
3. Transverse facial artery
4. Maxillary artery
5. Facial artery
6. Lingual artery
7. Superior thyroid artery
8. Parietal branch of superficial temporal artery
9. Superficial temporal artery
10. Occipital artery
11. Posterior auricular artery
12. External carotid artery
13. Internal carotid artery
14. Common carotid artery

MAJOR BLOOD VESSELS OF HEAD AND NECK—ANTERIOR VIEW

1. Right external jugular vein
2. Right common carotid artery
3. Right internal jugular vein
4. Brachiocephalic artery
5. Right subclavian artery
6. Right brachiocephalic vein
7. Right subclavian vein
8. Aorta
9. Hyoid bone
10. Left external jugular vein
11. Sternocleidomastoid muscle
12. Left internal jugular vein
13. Left common carotid artery
14. Left brachiocephalic vein
15. Left subclavian artery
16. Clavicle
17. Left subclavian vein
18. First rib

VEINS OF THE HEAD—LATERAL VIEW

1. Superficial temporal vein
2. Middle meningeal vein
3. Supraorbital vein
4. Pterygoid plexus of veins
5. Ophthalmic vein
6. Posterior superior alveolar veins
7. Superior labial vein
8. Alveolar and dental branches of posterior superior alveolar vein
9. Alveolar and dental branches of inferior alveolar vein
10. Inferior labial vein
11. Mental branch of inferior alveolar vein
12. Inferior alveolar vein
13. Submental vein
14. Facial vein
15. Hyoid bone
16. Anterior jugular vein
17. Maxillary vein
18. Retromandibular vein
19. Posterior auricular vein
20. Sternocleidomastoid muscle
21. External jugular vein
22. Internal jugular vein

MAXILLARY ARTERY—LATERAL VIEW

1. Sphenopalatine artery
2. Infraorbital artery
3. Posterior superior alveolar artery
4. Anterior superior alveolar artery
5. Dental and alveolar branches of superior alveolar artery
6. Dental and alveolar branches of incisive artery
7. Incisive artery
8. Mental artery
9. Deep temporal arteries
10. Superficial temporal artery
11. Middle meningeal artery
12. Maxillary artery
13. Masseteric artery
14. Pterygoid arteries
15. Buccal artery
16. Mylohyoid artery
17. Inferior alveolar artery
18. Left external carotid artery

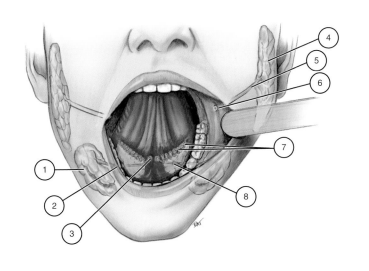

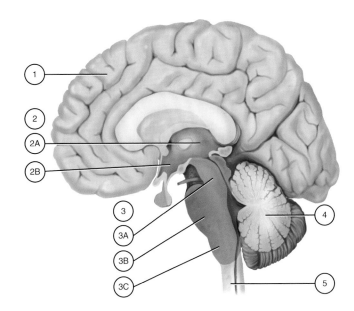

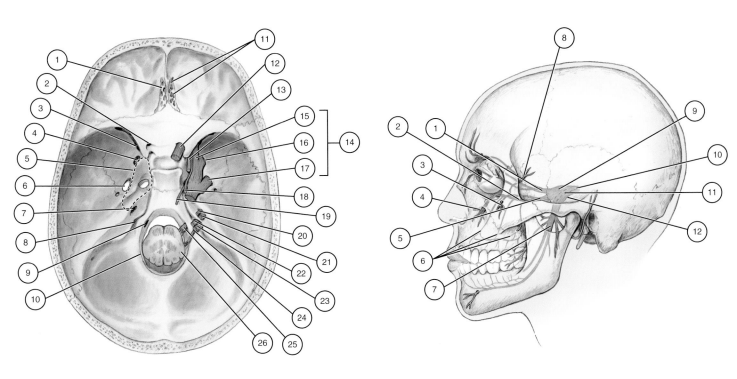

BRAIN—SAGITTAL SECTION

1. Cerebral hemisphere
2. Diencephalon
2A. Thalamus
2B. Hypothalamus
3. Brainstem
3A. Midbrain
3B. Pons
3C. Medulla
4. Cerebellum
5. Spinal cord

SALIVARY GLANDS

1. Submandibular salivary gland
2. Submandibular duct
3. Sublingual caruncle
4. Parotid salivary gland
5. Parotid duct
6. Parotid papilla
7. Sublingual ducts
8. Sublingual salivary gland

TRIGEMINAL NERVE—LATERAL VIEW

1. Ophthalmic division (V_1)
2. Zygomatic nerve
3. Zygomaticofacial nerve
4. Infraorbital nerve
5. Maxillary division (V_2)
6. Superior alveolar nerves
7. Mandibular division (V_3)
8. Zygomaticotemporal nerve
9. Trigeminal ganglion
10. Trigeminal nerve (V)
11. Motor root
12. Sensory root

CRANIAL NERVES AND INTERNAL SKULL—SUPERIOR VIEW

1. Cribriform plate of the ethmoid bone
2. Optic canal
3. Superior orbital fissure
4. Foramen rotundum
5. Location of cavernous sinus
6. Foramen ovale
7. Internal acoustic meatus
8. Jugular foramen
9. Hypoglossal canal
10. Foramen magnum
11. Olfactory nerve (I) fibers
12. Optic nerve (II)
13. Oculomotor nerve (III)
14. Trigeminal nerve (V)
15. Ophthalmic nerve (V_1)
16. Maxillary nerve (V_2)
17. Mandibular nerve (V_3)
18. Trochlear nerve (IV)
19. Abducens nerve (VI)
20. Facial nerve (VII)
21. Vestibulocochlear nerve (VIII)
22. Glossopharyngeal nerve (IX)
23. Vagus nerve (X)
24. Accessory nerve (XI)
25. Hypoglossal nerve (XII)
26. Spinal cord

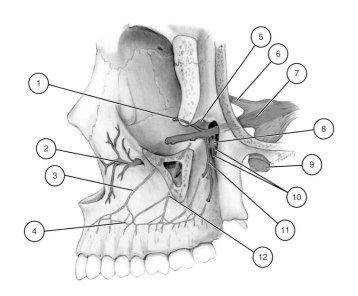

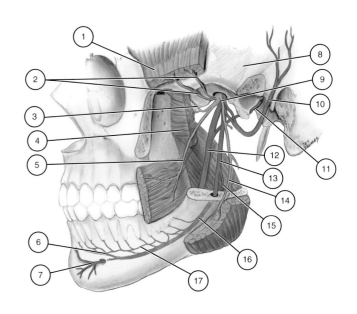

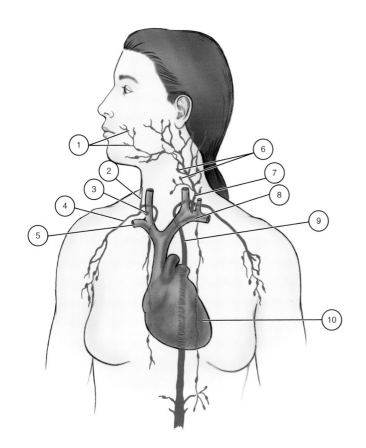

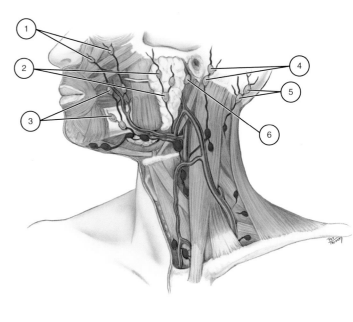

MANDIBULAR NERVE—LATERAL VIEW

1. Temporalis muscle
2. Anterior and posterior deep temporal nerves
3. Lateral pterygoid nerve
4. Lateral pterygoid muscle
5. Buccal nerve
6. Incisive nerve
7. Mental nerve
8. Location of trigeminal ganglion
9. Mandibular nerve
10. Auriculotemporal nerve
11. Chorda tympani nerve in petrotympanic fissure
12. Lingual nerve
13. Inferior alveolar nerve
14. Masseteric nerve
15. Mylohyoid nerve
16. Inferior alveolar nerve
17. Inferior dental plexus

MAXILLARY NERVE—LATERAL VIEW

1. Zygomatic nerve
2. Infraorbital nerve
3. Anterior superior alveolar nerve
4. Superior dental plexus
5. Inferior orbital fissure
6. Ophthalmic nerve
7. Maxillary nerve
8. Pterygopalatine ganglion
9. Mandibular nerve
10. Greater and lesser palatine nerves
11. Posterior superior alveolar nerve
12. Middle superior alveolar nerve

SUPERFICIAL LYMPH NODES OF THE HEAD

1. Facial lymph nodes
2. Superficial parotid lymph nodes
3. Facial lymph nodes
4. Posterior auricular lymph nodes
5. Occipital lymph nodes
6. Anterior auricular lymph nodes

LYMPHATIC SYSTEM

1. Facial lymph nodes
2. Right jugular trunk
3. Right lymphatic duct
4. Right subclavian trunk
5. Right subclavian vein
6. Cervical lymph nodes
7. Left jugular trunk
8. Left subclavian trunk
9. Thoracic duct
10. Heart

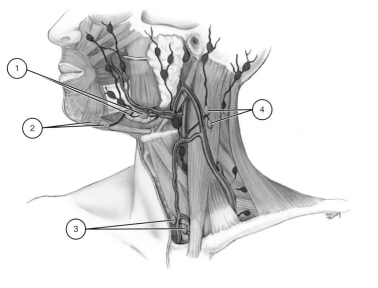

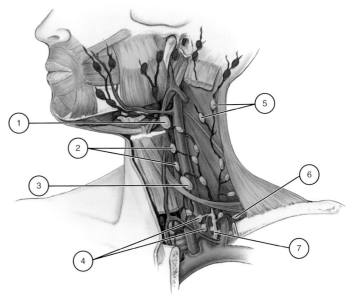

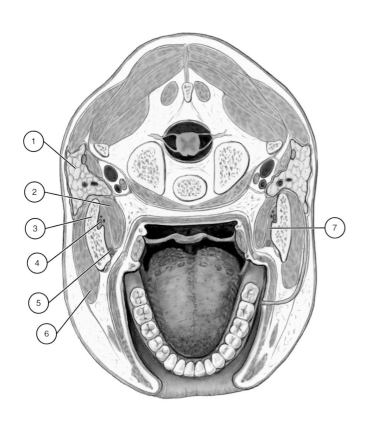

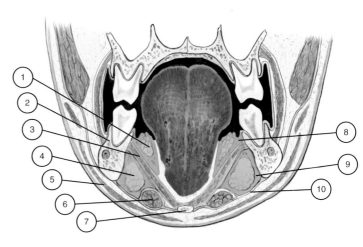

DEEP CERVICAL LYMPH NODES

1. Jugulodigastric lymph node
2. Superior deep cervical lymph nodes
3. Jugulo-omohyoid lymph node
4. Inferior deep cervical lymph nodes
5. Accessory lymph nodes
6. Supraclavicular lymph node
7. Thoracic duct

SUPERFICIAL CERVICAL LYMPH NODES

1. Submandibular lymph nodes
2. Submental lymph nodes
3. Anterior jugular lymph nodes
4. External jugular lymph nodes

SUBMANDIBULAR AND SUBLINGUAL SPACES—FRONTAL HEAD AND NECK SECTION

1. Sublingual salivary gland
2. Mandible
3. Mylohyoid muscle
4. Submandibular salivary gland
5. Platysma muscle
6. Digastric muscle
7. Hyoid bone
8. Sublingual space
9. Submandibular space
10. Investing fascia

PTERYGOMANDIBULAR SPACE—TRANSVERSE HEAD AND NECK SECTION

1. Parotid salivary gland
2. Medial pterygoid muscle
3. Mandible
4. Inferior alveolar nerve
5. Lingual nerve
6. Masseter muscle
7. Pterygomandibular space